Nurse's Chemotherapy Quick Pocket Reference

Debra S. Prescher-Hughes, RN, OCN
Director of Clinical Operations
Comprehensive Cancer Center at
Exempla Saint Joseph Hospital
Denver, CO

Cynthia J. Shyrock, RN, OCN
Manager Infusion Center
Comprehensive Cancer Center at
Exempla Saint Joseph Hospital
Denver, CO

JONES AND BARTLETT PUBLISHERS
Sudbury, Massachusetts
BOSTON   TORONTO   LONDON   SINGAPORE

World Headquarters

Jones and Bartlett
    Publishers
40 Tall Pine Drive
Sudbury, MA 01776
978-443-5000
info@jbpub.com
www.jbpub.com

Jones and Bartlett
    Publishers Canada
6339 Ormindale Way
Mississauga, Ontario
L5V 1J2
Canada

Jones and Bartlett
    Publishers International
Barb House, Barb Mews
London W6 7PA
United Kingdom

Jones and Bartlett's books and products are available through most bookstores and online booksellers. To contact Jones and Bartlett Publishers directly, call 800-832-0034, fax 978-443-8000, or visit our website www.jbpub.com.

Substantial discounts on bulk quantities of Jones and Bartlett's publications are available to corporations, professional associations, and other qualified organizations. For details and specific discount information, contact the special sales department at Jones and Bartlett via the above contact information or send an email to specialsales@jbpub.com.

The authors, editor, and publisher have made every effort to provide accurate information. However, they are not responsible for errors, omissions, or for any outcomes related to the use of the contents of this book and take no responsibility for the use of the products and procedures described. Treatments and side effects described in this book may not be applicable to all people; likewise, some people may require a dose or experience a side effect that is not described herein. Drugs and medical devices are discussed that may have limited availability controlled by the Food and Drug Administration (FDA) for use only in a research study or clinical trial. Research, clinical practice, and government regulations often change the accepted standard in this field. When consideration is being given to use of any drug in the clinical setting, the health care provider or reader is responsible for determining FDA status of the drug, reading the package insert, and reviewing prescribing information for the most up-to-date recommendations on dose, precautions, and contraindications, and determining the appropriate usage for the product. This is especially important in the case of drugs that are new or seldom used.

Production Credits

Publisher: Kevin Sullivan
Acquisitions Editor: Emily Ekle
Acquisitions Editor: Amy Sibley
Associate Editor: Patricia Donnelly
Editorial Assistant: Rachel Shuster
Production Editor: Dan Stone

Manufacturing and Inventory Control
    Supervisor: Amy Bacus
Composition: Auburn Associates, Inc.
Printing: Malloy
Cover Printing: Malloy
Cover Image: © Tiplyashin Anatoly/
    Shutterstock, Inc.

Library of Congress Cataloging-in-Publication Data
Prescher-Hughes, Debra S.
    Nurse's chemotherapy quick pocket reference / Debra Prescher-Hughes, Cynthia Shyrock.
    p. ; cm.
    Includes bibliographical references and inde
    ISBN-13: 978-0-7637-5824-0
    ISBN-10: 0-7637-5824-8
    1. Cancer—Chemotherapy—Handbooks, m   —Nursing—Handbooks, manuals, etc. 3. Antineoplastic   manuals, etc.
I. Title.
    [DNLM: 1. Neoplasms—drug therapy—Ha   stic Agents—administration & dosage—Handbooks. 3. Co   py—methods—Handbooks. QZ 39 P928n 2009]
    RC271.C5P7295 2009
    616.99'4061—dc22   2008029365

RC
271
.C5
P7295
2009

6048
Printed in the United States of America

12 11 10 09 08   10 9 8 7 6 5 4 3 2 1

CONTENTS

PREFACE

As oncology nurses we are in the midst of caring for cancer patients throughout the continuum of care. Staying abreast of the current treatments for our patients is a constant challenge. In 2007 and 2008 alone there were nine new agents approved. Since the year 2000 there have been 46. The science involved in the research and development of these drugs is remarkable. These developments also require additional educational needs for oncology nursing.

Not only do nurses need to know how to mix and administer each chemotherapy agent, but they need to know the side effects of these agents and be able to teach our patients about these side effects and how to manage them properly. *Clinical Practice Protocols in Oncology Nursing* was written as a set of protocols that could be used as an order set. *Nurse's Chemotherapy Quick Pocket Reference* condenses the information into a more readily available pocket version. We have made every attempt to be as up-to-date as possible as well as accurate and concise. Having the information available by protocol rather than each individual drug allows nurses to do a quick review of the protocol in a few paragraphs. This book is not intended to be all-inclusive of all side effects of the drugs in each protocol, but is an attempt to include the most common side effects. For all the side effect profiles we recommend that you refer to the package insert of the individual drugs.

We hope that *Nurse's Chemotherapy Quick Pocket Reference* will be an additional reference to oncology nurses and other healthcare providers who administer chemotherapy to oncology patients.

We want to thank our families and our co-workers for their patience with us as we worked on developing *Nurse's Chemotherapy Quick Pocket Reference*. Their support is greatly appreciated. We would also like to acknowledge Dan Stone at Jones and Bartlett for his attempts at keeping us on task and on time. We couldn't have done this without him.

Debra S. Prescher-Hughes
Cynthia J. Shyrock

ANAL CANCER

5-FU + Mitomycin + Radiation Therapy (Wayne State Regimen)[1,2]

Prechemo: CBC, Chem, CEA. Central line placement. 5-HT$_3$ and dexamethasone 10. Mildly to moderately emetogenic.

5-Fluorouracil 1000 mg/m^2/day: IV continuous infusion, days 1–4, and 29–32.

Mitomycin 15 mg/m^2: IV P through side arm of free-flowing IV day 1. Vesicant.

Radiation therapy: 200 cGy/day on days 1–5, 8–12, and 15–19 (total dose, 3000 cGy). Chemotherapy given concurrently with radiation therapy.

Side effects: Bone marrow depression. Nausea and vomiting mild to moderate. Mucositis and diarrhea. Local tissue irritation progressing to desquamation in radiation fields. No oil-based lotions in radiation field. Hand-foot syndrome. Photophobia, increased lacrimation, acute and chronic conjunctivitis, blepharitis, and blurred vision. Interstitial pneumonitis.

Chair time: 1 hour on days 1 and 29. Total cycle 32 days.

5-FU + Mitomycin + Radiation Therapy (EORTC Regimen)[1,3]

Prechemo: CBC, Chem, CEA. Central line placement. 5-HT$_3$ and dexamethasone. Mildly to moderately emetogenic.

Fluorouracil 750 mg/m^2/day: IV continuous infusion days 1–5 and 29–33

Mitomycin 15 mg/m^2: IV P through side arm of free flowing day 1. Vesicant.

Radiation therapy: 180 cGy/day over 5-week period. Total dose, 4500 cGy. Chemotherapy is given concurrently with radiation therapy. With partial or complete response, boost of 1500–2000 cGy is given.

Side effects: Bone marrow depression, delayed nadir. Nausea and vomiting. Mucositis and diarrhea. Local tissue irritation progressing to desquamation in radiation therapy fields. No oil-based lotions in radiation field. Hyperpigmentation, photosensitivity, and nail changes may occur. Hand-foot syndrome can be dose-limiting. Photophobia, increased lacrimation, acute and chronic conjunctivitis, blepharitis, and blurred vision. Interstitial pneumonitis.

Chair time: 1 hour on days 1 and 29. Total cycle 32 days.

5-FU + Cisplatin + Radiation Therapy (MD Anderson Regimen)[1,4]

Prechemo: CBC, Chem, Mg^{2+}, and CEA. Central line placement. $5-HT_3$ and dexamethasone. Moderately to highly emetogenic.

Chemotherapy and radiation therapy given concurrently.

Fluorouracil 250 mg/m²/day: IV continuous infusion days 1–5 of each week.

Cisplatin 4 mg/m²/day: IV continuous infusion days 1–5 of each week.

Radiation therapy: Total dose 5500 cGy over 6 weeks.

Side effects: Hypersensitivity reactions. Bone marrow depression. Nausea and vomiting, acute or delayed. Mucositis and diarrhea can be severe. Nephrotoxicity, electrolyte imbalance, alopecia. Local tissue irritation progressing to desquamation in radiation field. No oil-based lotions in radiation field. Hyperpigmentation, photosensitivity, and nail changes may occur. Hand-foot syndrome can be dose-limiting. Photophobia, increased lacrimation, acute and chronic conjunctivitis, blepharitis, and blurred vision.

Chair time: 2 hours on day 1 of each week of radiation therapy.

METASTATIC DISEASE AND/OR SALVAGE CHEMOTHERAPY

5-FU and Cisplatin[1,5]

Prechemo: CBC, Chem, Mg^{2+}, and CEA. Central line placement. $5-HT_3$ and dexamethasone. Moderately to highly emetogenic.

Fluorouracil 1000 mg/m²/day: IV continuous infusion on days 1–5.

Cisplatin 100 mg/m²: IV in 1000cc NS on day 2.

Major side effects: Neutropenia, thrombocytopenia, and anemia. Growth factor recommended. Mucositis and diarrhea severe and dose-limiting. Nephrotoxicity dose related, reduce risk with hydration. Decreases in Mg^{2+}, K^+, Ca^{2+}, Na^+, and Phos. Hyperpigmentation, photosensitivity, and nail changes. Hand-foot syndrome. Photophobia, increased lacrimation, acute and chronic conjunctivitis, blepharitis, and blurred vision.

Chair time: 1 hour on day1; 3 hours on day 2. Repeat every 21–28 days as tolerated or until disease progression.

BILIARY CANCER

Gemcitabine + Cisplatin[1,6]

Prechemo: CBC, Chem, LFTs, creatinine clearance, and CA 19-9.
5-HT$_3$ and dexamethasone 10–20 mg. Moderately to highly emetogenic.

Gemcitabine 1250 mg/m^2: IV in 250 cc NS on days 1 and 8.

Cisplatin 75 mg/m^2: IV in 1000 cc NS on days 1 and 15.

Side effects: Hypersensitivity reaction. Myelosuppression G-CSF recommended. Diarrhea and/or mucositis. Fever, malaise, chills, headache, and myalgias. Nephrotoxicity, neurotoxicity, electrolyte imbalance, elevation of serum transaminase and bilirubin levels. Pruritic, maculopapular skin rash, involving trunk and extremities. Edema. Alopecia. Ototoxicity.

Chair time: 3 hours on days 1 and 15; 1 hour on day 8. Repeat cycle every 21 days.

Gemcitabine + Capecitabine[1,7]

Prechemo: CBC, Chem, LFTs, creatinine clearance, and CA 19-9.

Premeds: Oral phenothiazine OR 5-HT$_3$ and dexamethasone 10 mg. Mildly to moderately emetogenic.

Gemcitabine 1000 mg/m^2: IV days 1 and 8 in 250 cc NS over 30 minutes.

Capecitabine 650 mg/m^2: PO BID on days 1–14. Contraindicated when creatinine clearance > 30 mL/min. Dose reduction to 75% with baseline creatinine clearance of 30–50 mL/min. Administer 30 minutes after a meal with plenty of water. Monitor international normalized ratios (INRs) with patients taking warfarin.

Side effects: Myelosuppression. Diarrhea and/or mucositis. Mild to moderate nausea and vomiting. Stomatitis. Fever, malaise, chills, headache, and myalgias. Elevation of serum transaminase and bilirubin levels. Modify capecitabine dose if hyperbilirubinemia occurs. Hand-foot syndrome. Pruritic, maculopapular skin rash.

Chair time: 1 hour on days 1 and 8. Repeat every 21 days until disease progression.

BLADDER CANCER

COMBINATION REGIMENS

Ifosfamide + Paclitaxel + Cisplatin (ITP)[1,8]

Prechemo: CBC, Chem, Mg^{2+}, 5-HT_3 and dexamethasone 10–20 mg in 100 cc of NS (days 1–3). Diphenhydramine 25–50 mg and an H_2 antagonist (day 1 only). Moderately to highly emetogenic.

Ifosfamide 1500 mg/m²: IV over 30 minutes on days 1, 2, and 3.

Paclitaxel 200 mg/m²: IV over 3 hours on day 1 (non-PVC tubing and containers and 0.22-micron inline filter).

Cisplatin 70 mg/m²: IV in 1000cc NS over 2 hours on day 1.

Side effects: Hypersensitivity reaction with paclitaxel. Myelosuppression G-CSF support recommended. Give paclitaxel before cisplatin to decrease severity of myelosuppression. Nausea and vomiting, acute or delayed. Mucositis and/or diarrhea common. Hemorrhagic cystitis dysuria and increased urinary frequency occurs with ifosfamide. Uroprotection with mesna and hydration mandatory. Decreases Mg^{2+}, K^+, Ca^{2+}, Na^+, and P. SIADH. Sensory neuropathy with numbness and paresthesias. Somnolence, confusion, depressive psychosis, or hallucinations. Alopecia. High-frequency hearing loss and tinnitus.

Chair time: 7 hours on day 1; 3 hours on days 2 and 3. Repeat every 21–28 days.

Gemcitabine + Cisplatin[1,9]

Prechemo: CBC, Chem, Mg^{2+}, and liver function tests (LFTs). 5-HT_3 and dexamethasone 10–20 mg. Moderately to highly emetogenic.

Gemcitabine 1000 mg/m²: IV over 30 minutes on days 1, 8, and 15.

Cisplatin 75 mg/m²: IV on day 1.

Side effects: Hypersensitivity reaction with cisplatin. Myelosuppression, with grade 3 and 4 thrombocytopenia more common in older patients. Nausea and vomiting, acute or delayed. Diarrhea and/or mucositis. Metallic taste. Flu-like syndrome. Nephrotoxicity with cisplatin.

Sensory neuropathy, dose related. Usually reversible. Decreased levels of Mg^{2+}, K^+, Ca^{2+}, Na^+, and P. SIADH. Elevated levels of serum transaminases and bilirubin. Pruritic, maculopapular skin rash, on trunk and extremities. Edema. Alopecia. High-frequency hearing loss and tinnitus.

Chair time: 3 hours on day 1; 1 hour on days 8 and 15. Repeat cycle every 28 days.

Methotrexate + Vinblastine + Doxorubicin + Cisplatin (MVAC)[1,10]

Prechemo: CBC, Chem, Mg^{2+}, multigated angiogram (MUGA). 5-HT$_3$ and dexamethasone 20 mg. Moderately to highly emetogenic.

Methotrexate 30 mg/m²: IV on days 1, 15, and 22.

Vinblastine 3 mg/m²: IV on days 2, 15, and 22. Potent vesicant.

Doxorubicin 30 mg/m²: IV on day 2. Potent vesicant.

Cisplatin 70 mg/m²: IV on day 2.

Side effects: Hypersensitivity reaction with cisplatin. Myelosuppression can be severe. Nausea and vomiting, acute or delayed. Mucositis can be severe. Constipation, abdominal pain, or paralytic ileus. Metallic taste. Cardiomyopathy with cumulative doses of doxorubicin >550 mg/m². Raynaud's syndrome seen with vinblastine. Acute renal failure, azotemia, urinary retention, and uric acid. Red-orange colored urine. Decreases Mg^{2+}, K^+, Ca^{2+}, Na^+, and P. SIADH. Pneumonitis, dose reduce doxorubicin with liver dysfunction. Hyperpigmentation, photosensitivity, and radiation recall occur. Alopecia. Peripheral sensory neuropathy, paresthesias. High-frequency hearing loss and tinnitus with cisplatin.

Chair time: 1 hour on days 1, 15, and 22; 3 hours on day 2. Repeat cycle every 28 days.

Cisplatin + Methotrexate + Vinblastine (CMV)[1,11]

Prechemo: CBC, Chem, Mg^{2+}, 5-HT$_3$ and dexamethasone 20 mg in 100 cc of NS. Moderately to highly emetogenic.

Cisplatin 100 mg/m²: IV on day 2 (give 12 hours after methotrexate).

Methotrexate 30 mg/m²: IV on days 1 and 8.

Vinblastine 4 mg/m²: IV on days 1 and 8. Potent vesicant.

Side effects: Hypersensitivity reaction with cisplatin. Myelosuppression can be severe. Nausea and vomiting, acute or delayed. Mucositis can be severe. Constipation, abdominal pain, or paralytic ileus. Metallic taste. Acute renal failure, azotemia, urinary retention, and uric acid nephropathy. Decreases Mg^{2+}, K^+, Ca^{2+}, Na^+, and P. SIADH. Pneumonitis. Rash, hyperpigmentation, photosensitivity, and radiation recall occur. Alopecia. Peripheral sensory neuropathy, paresthesias. High-frequency hearing loss and tinnitus with cisplatin.

Chair time: 1 hour on days 1 and 8; 3 hours on day 2. Repeat every 21 days.

Cyclophosphamide + Doxorubicin + Cisplatin (CISCA)[1,12]

Prechemo: CBC, Chem, Mg^{2+}. MUGA scan. 5-HT$_3$ and dexamethasone 20 mg. Moderately to severely emetogenic.

Cyclophosphamide 650 mg/m^2: IV on day 1.

Doxorubicin 50 mg/m^2: IV on day 1. Potent vesicant.

Cisplatin 100 mg/m^2: IV on day 2.

Side effects: Hypersensitivity reaction with cisplatin. Cyclophosphamide can cause rhinitis and irritation of nose and throat. Myelosuppression may be severe. Nausea and vomiting, acute or delayed. Stomatitis. Metallic taste. Pericarditis-myocarditis syndrome may occur acutely. With cumulative doses of doxorubicin (> 550 mg/m^2), cardiomyopathy may occur. Nephrotoxicity dose related with cisplatin; hemorrhagic cystitis, dysuria, and urinary frequency. Dose reduce in presence of liver dysfunction. Decreases Mg^{2+}, K^+, Ca^{2+}, Na^+, and P. SIADH. Hyperpigmentation, photosensitivity, and radiation recall occur. Complete alopecia. Peripheral sensory neuropathy dose-limiting toxicity. Paresthesias and numbness. High-frequency hearing loss and tinnitus with cisplatin.

Chair time: 2 hours on day 1; 3 hours on day 2. Repeat every 21–28 days.

Paclitaxel + Carboplatin[1,13]

Prechemo: CBC, Chem, Mg^{2+}. 5-HT$_3$ and dexamethasone 10–20 mg. Diphenhydramine 25–50 mg. Moderately to highly emetogenic.

Paclitaxel 225 mg/m^2: IV over 3 hours on day 1.

Carboplatin: AUC of 6 IV on day 1 (give 15 minutes after paclitaxel).

Side effects: Hypersensitivity reaction with paclitaxel. Increased risk of hypersensitivity to carboplatin in patients receiving more than seven courses of therapy. Myelosuppression cumulative and dose related. G-CSF support recommended. Nausea and vomiting, acute or delayed. Mucositis and/or diarrhea common. Nephrotoxicity symptomatic. Dose reduce with renal dysfunction. Decreases Mg^{2+}, K^+, Ca^{2+}, and Na^+. Sensory neuropathy with numbness and paresthesias; dose related, dose-limiting. Alopecia.

Chair time: 5 hours on day 1. Repeat cycle every 21 days until progression.

Cyclophosphamide + Doxorubicin + Cisplatin (CAP)[1,14]

Prechemo: CBC, Chem, Mg^{2+}. MUGA scan. 5-HT_3 and dexamethasone 10–20 mg. Moderately to highly emetogenic.

Cyclophosphamide 400 mg/m²: IV on day 1.

Doxorubicin 40 mg/m²: IV on day 1. Potent vesicant.

Cisplatin 75 mg/m²: IV over 1–3 hours on day 1.

Side effects: Hypersensitivity reaction with cisplatin. Cyclophosphamide can cause rhinitis and irritation of nose and throat. Myelosuppression dose related. Nausea and vomiting, acute or delayed. Mucositis. Metallic taste. Nephrotoxicity dose related with cisplatin, hemorrhagic cystitis, dysuria, and increased urinary frequency. Decreases Mg^{2+}, K^+, Ca^{2+}, Na^+, and P. Acutely, pericarditis or myocarditis can occur. With cumulative doses of doxorubicin (> 550 mg/m²), cardiomyopathy may occur. Peripheral sensory neuropathy dose-limiting with paresthesias and numbness. High-frequency hearing loss and tinnitus. Hyperpigmentation, photosensitivity, and radiation recall occur. Alopecia.

Chair time: 4 hours on day 1. Repeat cycle every 21 days.

Cisplatin + Methotrexate + Vinblastine + XRT (CMV + Radiation Therapy)[1,15]

Prechemo: CBC, Chem, Mg^{2+}. 5-HT_3 and dexamethasone 20 mg. Moderate to highly emetogenic.

Cisplatin 70 mg/m²: IV on day 2.

Methotrexate 30 mg/m²: IV on days 1, 15, and 22.

Vinblastine 3 mg/m²: IV on days 2, 15, and 22. Potent vesicant.

Repeat cycle every 28 days for two cycles. Radiation therapy given after two cycles of induction chemotherapy at a dose of 45 cGy in 180 cGy fractions combined with cisplatin 70 mg/m² on days 1 and 2 of radiation therapy.

Side effects: Hypersensitivity reaction with cisplatin. Myelosuppression can be severe. Nausea and vomiting, acute or delayed. Mucositis can be severe. Constipation, abdominal pain, or paralytic ileus. Metallic taste. Acute renal failure, azotemia, urinary retention, and uric acid nephropathy. Decreased Mg^{2+}, K^+, Ca^{2+}, Na^+, and P. SIADH. Pneumonitis. Rash, hyperpigmentation, photosensitivity, and radiation recall occur. Alopecia. Local tissue irritation to desquamation in radiation trials. Do not use oil-based lotions or creams in radiation field. Peripheral sensory neuropathy, paresthesias.

Chair time: 1 hour on days 1, 15, and 22; 3 hours on day 2. Repeat every 28 days for two cycles. Begin radiation therapy as described previously here.

SINGLE-AGENT REGIMENS

Gemcitabine[1,16]

Prechemo: CBC, Chem, and LFTs. Oral phenothiazine OR 5-HT$_3$ and dexamethasone 10 mg. Mildly to moderately emetogenic.

Gemcitabine 1200 mg/m^2: IV over 30 minutes on days 1, 8, and 15.

Side effects: Myelosuppression dose-limiting with grades 3 and 4 thrombocytopenia more common in older patients. Nausea and vomiting, diarrhea, mucositis. Flu-like syndrome. Mild dyspnea and drug induced pneumonitis. Transient elevation of serum transaminases and bilirubin. Pruritic, maculopapular skin rash, usually involving trunk and extremities. Edema. Alopecia is rare.

Chair time: 1 hour on days 1, 8, and 15. Repeat cycle every 28 days.

Paclitaxel

Prechemo: CBC, Chem, central line placement. 5-HT$_3$ and dexamethasone 10–20 mg in 100 cc of NS. Diphenhydramine 25–50 mg and H$_2$ antagonist. Mildly to moderately emetogenic.

Paclitaxel 250 mg/m^2: IV over 24 hours on day 1.[1,17]

OR

Paclitaxel 80 mg/m^2: IV weekly on day 1 for 3 weeks.[1,18,19,20]

Side effects: Hypersensitivity reaction. Myelosuppression dose-limiting G-CSF recommended. Mucositis and/or diarrhea. Nausea and vomiting. Sensory neuropathy with numbness and paresthesias, dose related and dose-limiting. More frequent with longer infusions and at higher doses. Transient elevations in serum transaminases, bilirubin, and alkaline phosphatase. Alopecia, total loss of body hair.

Chair time: 1 hour on day 1. Return day 2 to remove pump if 24-hour infusion. Repeat cycle every 28 days.

BONE METASTASIS

Zometa[1,21–25]

Pretreatment: Serum creatinine (check before each dose). Calculate baseline creatinine clearance. Calcium supplement 500 mg and vitamin D 400 IU PO daily. DO NOT give when treating hypercalcemia. Mildly to moderately emetogenic.

Zometa: 4 mg (adjusted for baseline creatinine clearance) in 100 cc of NS over a minimum of 15 minutes on day 1. Calculate patient's baseline creatinine clearance with the Cockcroft-Gault formula.

Side effects: Decreased renal function (increase of 0.5 mg/dL for patients with normal baseline creatinine or increase of 1.0 mg/dL for patients with an abnormal baseline creatinine). Hold for renal deterioration. Resume at the same dose when the creatinine within 10% of baseline value. Flu-like syndrome. Fever occurs in 44% of patients. Chills, bone pain, and/or arthralgias and myalgias. Nausea and vomiting. Diarrhea, constipation, abdominal pain, and anorexia. Not significant. Hypocalcemia, hypophosphatemia, hypomagnesemia, or increased blood urea nitrogen (BUN) and serum creatinine. Osteonecrosis of the jaw (ONJ). Dental visit recommended before starting. Seen more commonly when patient has a dental procedure. Discontinue therapy if osteonecrosis occurs.

Chair time: 15–30 minutes. Repeat every 3–4 weeks for multiple myeloma and solid tumor metastatic bone lesions. Hypercalcemia of malignancy every 7 days p.r.n.

Pamidronate[1,26]

Pretreatment: Serum creatinine clearance and BUN. Mild emetogenicity.

Pamidronate: 90 mg in 250 cc of NS or D5W IV over 2 hours for bone metastasis. Repeat cycle every 3–4 weeks.

OR

Pamidronate: 90 mg in 500 cc of NS or D5W over 4 hours for multiple myeloma. Repeat cycle every 4 weeks.

Side effects: Flu-like syndrome. Nausea, vomiting, abdominal discomfort, constipation, and anorexia rare. Hypocalcemia, hypercalcemia, hypokalemia, hypophosphatemia, hypomagnesemia, or increased BUN and serum creatinine levels. Renal dysfunction, renal failure. Use with extreme caution with renal impairment. Atrial fibrillation, tachycardia, hypertension, fluid overload. Infusion site reaction, pain at infusion site.

Chair time: 2–4 hours. Repeat cycle every 3–4 weeks.

BRAIN CANCER

ADJUVANT THERAPY
COMBINATION REGIMENS

Temozolomide + Radiation Therapy[1,27]

Prechemo: CBC, Chem, and LFTs. Oral 5-HT$_3$. Mild to moderately emetogenic.

Temozolomide 75 mg/m^2: PO daily for 6 weeks with radiation therapy, followed by **temozolomide 150 mg/m^2:** PO on days 1–5. If well tolerated, can increase dose to 200 mg/m^2 on days 1–5 (after radiation therapy) 5-, 20-, 100-, and 250-mg capsules. Take with full glass of water on an empty stomach.

Radiation therapy: 200 cGy/day for 5 days per week for total of 6 weeks.

Side effects: Myelosuppression dose-limiting toxicity. Older patients are at increased risk. Anemia. G-CSF not indicated. Nausea and vomiting. Diarrhea, constipation, and/or anorexia. Rash, itching, and alopecia. Fatigue, headache, ataxia, and dizziness.

Chair time: No chair time. Repeat maintenance dose every 28 days as tolerated or until disease progression.

Procarbazine + Lomustine + Vincristine (PCV)[1,28]

Prechemo: CBC, Chem, and LFTs. Oral 5-HT$_3$. Moderately to highly emetogenic.

Procarbazine 60 mg/m^2: PO on days 8–21. (50-mg capsules.)

Lomustine 130 mg/m^2: PO on day 1. (10-, 30-, and 100-mg capsules.) Take on empty stomach at bedtime.

Vincristine 1.4 mg/m^2: IV on days 8 and 29. Vesicant.

Food and drug interactions: Alcohol. Antabuse-like reaction if alcohol is consumed. Avoid foods containing high amounts of tyramine (dark beer, wine, cheese, bananas, yogurt, and pickled and smoked foods). CNS depressants: synergistic effect. Tricyclic antidepressants: results in CNS excitation.

Side effects: Myelosuppression with procarbazine dose-limiting toxicity. Delayed nadir, persists for 1–3 weeks. Nausea and vomiting dose-limiting. Constipation, abdominal pain, and paralytic ileus. Lethargy, depression, frequent nightmares, insomnia, nervousness, or hallucinations. Peripheral neuropathy with loss of deep-tendon reflexes, numbness, weakness, myalgias, cramping, and late, severe motor difficulties. Interstitial pneumonitis. Flu-like syndrome. Alopecia, pruritus, rash, and hyperpigmentation.

Chair time: 1 hour on days 8 and 29. Repeat cycle every 8 weeks for six cycles.

SINGLE-AGENT REGIMENS

BCNU (Carmustine)[1,29]

Prechemo: CBC, Chem, and LFTs. Pulmonary function tests. 5-HT$_3$ and dexamethasone 10–20 mg. Moderately to highly emetogenic.

BCNU 220 mg/m^2: IV in 100–250 cc of D5W/NS over 1–2 hours on day 1. Irritant.

OR

BCNU 75–100 mg/m^2: IV in 100–250 cc of D5W/NS over 1–2 hours on days 1 and 2.

Side effects: Myelosuppression delayed and cumulative. Cimetidine may increase myelosuppression. Severe nausea and vomiting. Interstitial lung disease and pulmonary fibrosis, cough, dyspnea, pulmonary infiltrates, and/or respiratory failure with cumulative doses > 1400 mg/m^2 or with a prior history of lung disease. Increased BUN usually reversible. Decreased kidney size, progressive azotemia, and renal failure. Transient elevations in serum transaminase within 1 week of therapy. Facial flushing and a burning sensation at the IV injection site. Skin contact with drug may cause brownish discoloration and pain. Infarcts of optic nerve fiber, retinal hemorrhage, and neuroretinitis with high-dose therapy.

Chair time: 3 hours on days 1 and 2. Repeat cycle every 6–8 weeks for 1 year.

ADVANCED DISEASE

COMBINATION REGIMENS

Procarbazine + Lomustine + Vincristine (PCV)[1,30]

Prechemo: CBC, Chem, and LFTs. Oral 5-HT$_3$. Moderate to highly emetogenic.

Procarbazine 75 mg/m^2: PO on days 8–21. (50-mg capsules.)

Lomustine 130 mg/m^2: PO on day 1. (10-, 30-, and 100-mg capsules.) Take on an empty stomach at bedtime.

Vincristine 1.4 mg/m^2: IV on days 8 and 29. Vesicant.

Drug and food interactions with procarbazine: Alcohol. Antabuse-like reaction if alcohol consumed. Avoid foods containing high amounts of tyramine (dark beer, wine, cheese, yogurt, and pickled and smoked foods). CNS depressants: synergistic effect. Tricyclic antidepressants: results in CNS excitation.

Side effects: Myelosuppression nadir is delayed, persists for 1–3 weeks. Nausea and vomiting dose-limiting. Constipation, abdominal pain, and paralytic ileus. Lethargy, depression, frequent nightmares, insomnia, nervousness, or hallucinations. Peripheral neuropathy with absent deep-tendon reflexes, numbness, weakness, myalgias, cramping, and later, severe motor difficulties. Flu-like syndrome. Alopecia, pruritus, rash, and hyperpigmentation.

Chair time: 1 hour on days 8 and 29. Repeat cycle every 8 weeks.

SINGLE-AGENT REGIMENS

BCNU (Carmustine)[1,29]

Prechemo: CBC, Chem, and LFTs. Pulmonary function tests. 5-HT$_3$ and dexamethasone 10–20 mg. Moderately to highly emetogenic.

BCNU 200 mg/m^2: IV in 100–250 cc of D5W/NS over 1–2 hours on day 1. Irritant.

Side effects: Myelosuppression delayed and cumulative. Cimetidine may increase Myelosuppression. Severe nausea and vomiting. Interstitial lung disease and pulmonary fibrosis, insidious cough, dyspnea, pulmonary infiltrates, and/or respiratory failure at cumulative doses of more than 1400 mg/m^2 or with a prior history of lung disease. Increased BUN, usually reversible. Decreased kidney size, progressive azotemia, and renal failure have occurred. Transient elevations in serum transaminase levels within 1 week of therapy. Facial flushing and a burning sensation at the IV injection site. Skin contact with drug may cause brownish discoloration and pain. Infarcts of optic nerve fiber, retinal hemorrhage, neuroretinitis associated with high-dose therapy.

Chair time: 3 hours on day 1. Repeat cycle every 6–8 weeks.

Procarbazine[1,31]

Prechemo: CBC, Chem, and LFTs. Oral 5-HT$_3$. Moderate to highly emetogenic.

Procarbazine 150 mg/m^2: PO daily divided into three doses. (50-mg capsules.)

Drug and food interactions: Alcohol. Antabuse-like reaction when alcohol consumed. Avoid foods containing high amounts of tyramine (dark beer, wine, cheese, brewer's yeast, chicken livers, and bananas). CNS depressants: synergistic effect with barbiturates, antihistamines, narcotics, hypotensive agents, and phenothiazines. Tricyclic antidepressants: results in CNS excitation, hypertension, tremors, palpitations, and in severe cases, hypertensive crisis and/or angina.

Side effects: Myelosuppression delayed and cumulative. Nausea and vomiting dose-limiting. Diarrhea rarely may require dose reduction. Lethargy, depression, frequent nightmares, insomnia, nervousness, or hallucinations. Peripheral neuropathy with absent deep-tendon reflexes, numbness, weakness, myalgias, cramping, severe motor difficulties. Foot drop and ataxia. Reversible when drug is discontinued. Flu-like syndrome. Alopecia, pruritus, rash, hyperpigmentation.

Chair time: No chair time. Repeat daily as tolerated or until disease progression.

Temozolomide[1,20,32]

Prechemo: CBC, Chem, and LFTs. Oral phenothiazine or 5-HT$_3$. Mild to moderately emetogenic.

Temozolomide 150 mg/m^2: PO on days 1–5. If well tolerated, may increase to 200 mg/m^2. (5-, 20-, 100-, and 250-mg capsules.) Take with full glass of water on an empty stomach.

Side effects: Myelosuppression dose-limiting toxicity. Older patients are at increased risk. Does not usually require G-CSF administration. Nausea and vomiting. Diarrhea, constipation, and/or anorexia. Rash, itching, and alopecia, fatigue, lethargy, headache, ataxia, and dizziness.

Chair time: No chair time. Repeat every 28 days as tolerated or until disease progression.

Irinotecan

Prechemo: CBC, Chem, 5-HT$_3$, and 10–20 mg of dexamethasone. Atropine 0.25–1.0 mg IV unless contraindicated. Moderate to highly emetogenic.

Irinotecan 125 mg/m^2: IV in 500 cc of D5W weekly for 4 weeks.[1,34]
OR

Irinotecan 350 mg/m²: IV in 500 cc of D5W over 90 minutes day 1 every 3 weeks. [1,33]

Side effects: Myelosuppression dose-limiting. G-CSF recommended. Antidiarrheal medicines required. Early diarrhea managed with atropine before therapy. Late diarrhea severe and should be treated aggressively with loperamide. Nausea and vomiting. Dyspnea to pulmonary infiltrates, fever, increased cough, decreased DLCO rare. Transient elevations in serum transaminases, alkaline, phosphatase, and bilirubin.

Chair time: 3 hours weekly for 4 weeks, repeat cycle every 6 weeks.
OR

3 hours day 1; repeat cycle every 3 weeks.

BREAST CANCER

NEOADJUVANT THERAPY

COMBINATION REGIMENS

Doxorubicin + Cyclophosphamide + Docetaxel (ACT)[1,35]

Prechemo: CBC, Chem, LFTs, and CA 27-29. MUGA scan. Dexamethasone 8 mg bid for 3 days, day before, day of, and day after treatment. 5-HT$_3$ (dexamethasone not necessary when taking oral dexamethasone). Moderately to highly emetogenic. (Optional diphenhydramine 25–50 mg and H$_2$ antagonist.

Doxorubicin 60 mg/m^2: IV push on day 1. Potent vesicant.

Cyclophosphamide 600 mg/m^2: IV in 500–1000 cc NS IV on day 1.

Docetaxel 100 mg/m^2: IV on day 1. Use non-PVC containers and tubing.

Side effects: Hypersensitivity reactions with docetaxel. Cyclophosphamide can cause rhinitis and irritation of nose and throat. Myelosuppression may be severe and dose-limiting. G-CSF recommended with first dose. Nausea and vomiting, acute or delayed. Stomatitis and diarrhea not dose-limiting. Acutely, pericarditis-myocarditis syndrome may occur. With cumulative doses >550 mg/m^2 of doxorubicin, cardiomyopathy may occur. Cyclophosphamide may increase the risk of doxorubicin-induced cardiotoxicity. Dose reduce with liver dysfunction. Peripheral neuropathy with sensory alterations and paresthesias. Dose reductions with grade 3 neuropathy, discontinue docetaxel for grade 4 neuropathy. Fluid retention syndrome: weight gain, peripheral and/or generalized edema, pleural effusion, and ascites. Hemorrhagic cystitis, dysuria, and urinary frequency. Red-orange discoloration of urine. Hyperpigmentation, photosensitivity, and radiation recall. Maculopapular rash and dry, itchy skin. Alopecia.

Chair time: 4 hours on day 1. Repeat every 21 days for four cycles followed by surgery.

ADJUVANT THERAPY

COMBINATION REGIMENS

Doxorubicin + Cyclophosphamide (AC)[1,36]

Prechemo: CBC, Chem, LFTs, and CA 27-29. MUGA scan. 5-HT$_3$ and dexamethasone 10–20 mg in 100 cc of NS. Moderately to highly emetogenic.

Doxorubicin 60 mg/m^2: IV push on day 1. Potent vesicant.

Cyclophosphamide 600 mg/m^2: IV in 500–1000 cc NS IV on day 1.

Side effects: Cyclophosphamide can cause rhinitis and irritation of nose and throat. Myelosuppression may be severe. G-CSF recommended. Nausea and vomiting, acute or delayed. Stomatitis and diarrhea not dose-limiting. Acutely, pericarditis-myocarditis syndrome may occur. With cumulative doses >550 mg/m^2 of doxorubicin, cardiomyopathy may occur. Cyclophosphamide may increase the risk of doxorubicin-induced cardiotoxicity. Dose reduce with liver dysfunction. Hemorrhagic cystitis, dysuria, and urinary frequency with cyclophosphamide. Red-orange discoloration of urine. Increased risk of secondary malignancy with cyclophosphamide. Hyperpigmentation, photosensitivity, and radiation recall occur. Complete alopecia. SIADH.

Chair time: 2 hours on day 1. Repeat cycle every 21 days for a total of four cycles.

Docetaxel + Doxorubicin + Cyclophosphamide (TAC)[1,37]

Prechemo: CBC, Chem, LFTs, and CA 27-29. MUGA. 5-HT$_3$ IV and diphenhydramine 25–50 mg and H$_2$ antagonist. Dexamethasone 8 mg bid for 3 days, starting the day before treatment. Moderately to highly emetogenic.

Doxorubicin 50 mg/m^2: IV Push on day 1. Potent vesicant.

Cyclophosphamide 500 mg/m^2: IV on day 1.

Docetaxel 75 mg/m^2: IV over 1 hour on day 1. Use non-PVC containers and tubing.

Side effects: Hypersensitivity reactions. Myelosuppression severe and dose-limiting G-CSF recommended. Nausea and vomiting acute or delayed. Stomatitis can be severe and diarrhea. Acute pericarditis-myocarditis. Cardiomyopathy with high cumulative doses of doxorubicin >550 mg/m^2. Cyclophosphamide may increase the risk of doxorubicin-induced cardiotoxicity. Use doxorubicin and docetaxel with caution in patients with abnormal liver function. Dose reduce with liver dysfunction. Peripheral neuropathy with sensory alterations and numbness. Fluid retention syndrome: weight gain, peripheral and/or generalized edema, pleural effusion, and ascites. Hemorrhagic cystitis, dysuria, and urinary frequency. Red-orange discoloration of urine. Hyperpigmentation, photosensitivity, and radiation recall. Maculopapular rash and dry, itchy skin. Complete alopecia.

Chair time: 3–4 hours on day 1. Repeat every 21 days for six cycles.

Docetaxel + Cyclophosphamide (TC)[1,38,39]

Prechemo: CBC, Chem, LFTs, and CA 27-29. 5-HT$_3$ IV and diphenhydramine 25–50 mg and H$_2$ antagonist. Dexamethasone 8 mg PO bid for 3 days, starting the day before treatment. Moderately to highly emetogenic.

Cyclophosphamide 600 mg/m²: IV on day 1.

Docetaxel 75 mg/m²: IV over 1 hour on day 1. Use non-PVC containers and tubing.

Side effects: Hypersensitivity reactions. Myelosuppression severe and dose-limiting G-CSF recommended. Nausea and vomiting acute or delayed. Stomatitis can be severe and diarrhea. Use docetaxel with caution in patients with abnormal liver function. Dose reduce with liver dysfunction. Peripheral neuropathy with sensory alterations and numbness. Fluid retention syndrome: weight gain, peripheral and/or generalized edema, pleural effusion, and ascites. Hemorrhagic cystitis, dysuria, and urinary frequency. Maculopapular rash and dry, itchy skin. Complete alopecia.

Chair time: 3 hours on day 1. Repeat every 21 days for six cycles.

Doxorubicin + Cyclophosphamide followed by Paclitaxel (AC followed by T)[1,40]

Prechemo: CBC, Chem, LFTs, and CA 27-29. MUGA scan. 5-HT$_3$ and dexamethasone 10–20 mg in 100 cc of NS. Add prior to paclitaxel: diphenhydramine 25–50 mg and H$_2$ antagonist. Moderately to highly emetogenic.

Doxorubicin 60 mg/m²: IV push on day 1. Potent vesicant.

Cyclophosphamide 600 mg/m²: IV in 500–1000 cc NS IV on day 1. Repeat cycle every 21 days for four cycles followed by:

Paclitaxel 175 mg/m²: IV over 3 hours on day 1. Use non-PVC containers and tubing with 0.22-micron inline filter.

Repeat cycle every 21 days for four cycles.

Side effects: Hypersensitivity reaction with paclitaxel. Cyclophosphamide can cause rhinitis and irritation of nose and throat. Myelosuppression dose-limiting. G-CSF recommended. Dose related sensory neuropathy with numbness and paresthesias. Nausea and vomiting acute or delayed. Mucositis and diarrhea not dose-limiting. Acutely, pericarditis-myocarditis syndrome may occur. With cumulative doses >550 mg/m² of doxorubicin, cardiomyopathy may occur. Cyclophosphamide may increase the risk of doxorubicin-induced cardiotoxicity. Dose reduce with liver dysfunction. Hemorrhagic cystitis, dysuria, and urinary frequency with cyclophosphamide. Red-orange discoloration of urine. SIADH. Hyperpigmentation, photosensitivity, and radiation recall occur. Complete alopecia.

Chair time: 2 hours on day 1 for AC, then 4–5 hours on day 1 for paclitaxel. Repeat AC every 21 days for a total of four cycles, followed by paclitaxel every 21 days for four cycles.

Doxorubicin + Cyclophosphamide followed by Paclitaxel + Trastuzumab (AC followed by T + Trastuzumab)[1,41]

Prechemo: CBC, Chem, LFTs, and CA 27-29. MUGA scan. FISH for HER2. 5-HT$_3$ and dexamethasone 20 mg in 100 cc of NS. Moderately to highly emetogenic.

Doxorubicin 60 mg/m²: IV push on day 1. Potent vesicant.

Cyclophosphamide 600 mg/m²: IV in 500–1000cc NS on day 1.

Repeat every 21 days for a total of four cycles, followed by four cycles paclitaxel + trastuzumab.

Premeds: 5-HT$_3$ and dexamethasone 10–20 mg. Moderately to highly emetogenic. Diphenhydramine 25–50 mg and H$_2$ antagonist.

Paclitaxel 80 mg/m²: IV over 1 hour on day 1.

Use non-PVC containers and tubing with 0.22-micron inline filter.

Trastuzumab 4 m/kg: Loading dose IV in 250 cc of NS over 90 minutes day 1 week 1 only. Then **trastuzumab 2 mg/kg** IV in 250 cc of NS over 30 minutes weekly. Repeat cycle weekly for 12 weeks, followed by:

Trastuzumab 2 m/kg: IV in 250 cc of NS over 30 minutes weekly for 40 weeks.

Side effects: Hypersensitivity reaction with paclitaxel. Hypersensitivity with trastuzumab: fever, chills, urticaria, flushing, fatigue, headache, bronchospasm, dyspnea, angioedema, and hypotension. Usually mild to moderate and most often in first dose trastuzumab only. Dose-limiting neutropenia with AC. G-CSF recommended. Dose related sensory neuropathy with numbness and paresthesias. Nausea and vomiting. Mucositis and diarrhea not dose-limiting. Acutely, pericarditis-myocarditis syndrome may occur. With cumulative doses >550 mg/m² of doxorubicin, cardiomyopathy may occur. Cyclophosphamide may increase risk of cardiotoxicity. Risk of cardiotoxicity with trastuzumab significantly increased when used in combination with anthracycline/cyclophosphamide regimen. Dose reduce with liver dysfunction. Hemorrhagic cystitis, dysuria, and urinary frequency with cyclophosphamide. Red-orange discoloration of urine. SIADH. Hyperpigmentation, photosensitivity, and radiation recall occur. Complete alopecia.

Chair time: 2 hours on day 1 for AC. 3 hours on day 1 for paclitaxel and trastuzumab, 1 hour for trastuzumab alone. Repeat AC every 21 days for a total of four cycles, followed by paclitaxel and trastuzumab weekly for 12 weeks, followed by trastuzumab weekly for 40 weeks.

Doxorubicin + Paclitaxel + Cyclophosphamide (A + T + C Dose-Dense Therapy)[1,42]

Prechemo: CBC, Chem, and CA 27-29. MUGA scan. 5-HT$_3$ and dexamethasone 10–20 mg. Moderately to highly emetogenic.

Doxorubicin 60 mg/m^2: IV push on day 1. Potent vesicant.

Repeat cycle every 2 weeks for four cycles, followed by:

Premeds: 5-HT$_3$ and dexamethasone 10–20 mg in 100 cc of NS. Diphenhydramine 25–50 mg and H$_2$ antagonist.

Paclitaxel 175 mg/m^2: IV over 3 hours on day 1.

Use non-PVC containers and tubing with 0.22-micron inline filter.

Repeat cycle every 2 weeks for four cycles, followed by:

Premeds: 5-HT$_3$ and dexamethasone 10–20 mg.

Cyclophosphamide 600 mg/m^2: IV in 500–1000 cc NS IV day 1.

Side effects: Hypersensitivity reaction to paclitaxel. Cyclophosphamide can cause rhinitis and irritation of nose and throat. Myelosuppression dose-limiting. G-CSF recommended. Nausea and vomiting, may be acute or delayed with cyclophosphamide. Mucositis and diarrhea seen. Acutely, pericarditis-myocarditis syndrome may occur. With cumulative doses >550 mg/m^2 of doxorubicin, cardiomyopathy may occur. Cyclophosphamide may increase risk of doxorubicin-induced cardiotoxicity. Dose reduce with liver dysfunction. Hyperpigmentation, photosensitivity, and radiation recall occur. Complete alopecia. Dose related sensory neuropathy with numbness and paresthesias. Hemorrhagic cystitis, dysuria, and urinary frequency with cyclophosphamide. Can be prevented with adequate hydration. Red-orange discoloration of urine.

Chair time: AC 1 hour every 2 weeks. Repeat cycle every 2 weeks for four cycles. Follow with paclitaxel 3–4 hours on day 1 every 2 weeks for 4 weeks, followed by cyclophosphamide 2 hours every 2 weeks for 4 weeks.

Cyclophosphamide + Doxorubicin + 5-Flourouracil (CAF)[1,43]

Prechemo: CBC, Chem, LFTs, and CA 27-29. MUGA scan. 5-HT$_3$ and dexamethasone 20 mg. Moderately to highly emetogenic.

Cyclophosphamide 600 mg/m^2: IV in 500–1000 cc NS IV on day 1.

Doxorubicin 60 mg/m^2: IV push on day 1. Potent vesicant.

5-Flourouracil 600 mg/m^2: IV push on day 1.

Side effects: Cyclophosphamide can cause rhinitis and irritation of nose and throat. Myelosuppression dose-limiting. G-CSF recommended. Nausea and vomiting, acute or delayed. Stomatitis and diarrhea can be severe and dose-limiting. Acutely, pericarditis-myocarditis syndrome may occur. With cumulative doses >550 mg/m² doxorubicin, cardiomyopathy may occur. Cyclophosphamide may increase the risk of doxorubicin-induced cardiotoxicity. Dose reduce with liver dysfunction. Hemorrhagic cystitis, dysuria, and urinary frequency with cyclophosphamide. Red-orange discoloration of urine. SIADH. Hyperpigmentation, photosensitivity, nail changes, and radiation recall occur. Complete alopecia. Hand-foot syndrome can be dose-limiting. Photophobia, increased lacrimation, acute and chronic conjunctivitis, blepharitis, and blurred vision.

Chair time: 2 hours on day 1. Repeat cycle every 21 days for six cycles.

Cyclophosphamide + Doxorubicin + 5-Flourouracil (CAF–Oral)[1,44]

Prechemo: CBC, Chem, LFTs, and CA 27-29. MUGA scan. 5-HT$_3$ and dexamethasone 20 mg on days 1 and 8. Oral 5-HT$_3$ or phenothiazine PO daily days 2–7 and 9–14. Moderately to highly emetogenic.

Cyclophosphamide 100 mg/m²/day: PO on days 1–14. (25- and 50-mg tablets.) Take with meals in morning or early afternoon to allow adequate excretion time.

Doxorubicin 30 mg/m²: IV on days 1 and 8. Potent vesicant.

5-Flourouracil 500 mg/m²: IV on days 1 and 8.

Side effects: Cyclophosphamide can cause rhinitis and irritation of nose and throat. Myelosuppression may be severe. G-CSF recommended. Nausea and vomiting, acute or delayed. Stomatitis and diarrhea can be severe and dose-limiting. Acutely, pericarditis-myocarditis syndrome may occur. With cumulative doses >550 mg/m² doxorubicin, cardiomyopathy may occur. Cyclophosphamide may increase the risk of doxorubicin-induced cardiotoxicity. Dose reduce with liver dysfunction. Hemorrhagic cystitis, dysuria, and urinary frequency with cyclophosphamide. Red-orange discoloration of urine. SIADH. Hyperpigmentation, photosensitivity, nail changes, and radiation recall occur. Complete alopecia. Hand-foot syndrome can be dose-limiting. Photophobia, increased lacrimation, acute and chronic conjunctivitis, blepharitis, and blurred vision.

Chair time: 1 hour on days 1 and 8. Repeat cycle every 28 days for six cycles.

Cyclophosphamide + Methotrexate + 5-Flourouracil (CMF-Bonadonna Regimen)[1,45]

Prechemo: CBC, Chem, LFTs, and CA 27-29. 5-HT$_3$ and dexamethasone 20 mg in 100 cc of NS on days 1 and 8. Oral 5-HT$_3$ or phenothiazine days 2–7 and 9–14. Moderately to highly emetogenic.

Cyclophosphamide 100 mg/m^2/day: PO on days 1–14. (25- and 50-mg tablets.) Take with meals in morning or early afternoon to allow adequate excretion time.

Methotrexate 40 mg/m^2: IV on days 1 and 8.

5-Flourouracil 600 mg/m^2: IV on days 1 and 8.

Side effects: Cyclophosphamide can cause rhinitis and irritation of nose and throat. Myelosuppression can be severe. Thrombocytopenia is less frequent, and anemia is mild. Nausea and vomiting. Mucositis and diarrhea can be severe, dose dependent. Acute renal failure, azotemia, urinary retention, and uric acid nephropathy have been observed with methotrexate. Hemorrhagic cystitis, dysuria, and urinary frequency with cyclophosphamide. SIADH. Photophobia, increased lacrimation, acute and chronic conjunctivitis, blepharitis, and blurred vision. Alopecia. Hyperpigmentation of nails and skin, banding of nails, and radiation recall may occur. Photosensitivity, sunburn-like rash. Hand-foot syndrome can be dose-limiting.

Chair time: 1 hour on days 1 and 8. Repeat cycle every 28 days for six cycles.

Cyclophosphamide + Methotrexate + 5-Flourouracil (CMF-IV Regimen)[1,46]

Prechemo: CBC, Chem, LFTs, and CA 27-29. 5-HT$_3$ and dexamethasone 20 mg. Moderately to highly emetogenic.

Cyclophosphamide 600 mg/m^2: IV in 500–1000 cc NS IV on day 1.

Methotrexate 40 mg/m^2: IV on day 1.

5-Flourouracil 600 mg/m^2: IV on day 1.

Side effects: Cyclophosphamide can cause rhinitis and irritation of nose and throat. Myelosuppression can be severe. Thrombocytopenia and anemia mild. Nausea and vomiting. Mucositis and diarrhea can be severe, dose dependent. Acute renal failure, azotemia, urinary retention, and uric acid nephropathy have been observed with methotrexate. Hemorrhagic cystitis, dysuria, and urinary frequency with cyclophosphamide. SIADH. Photophobia, increased lacrimation, acute and chronic conjunctivitis, blepharitis, and blurred vision. Alopecia. Hyperpigmentation of nails and skin, banding of nails, and radiation recall may occur. Photosensitivity, sunburn-like rash. Hand-foot syndrome can be dose-limiting.

Chair time: 2 hours on day 1. Repeat cycle every 21 days for six cycles.

Doxorubicin + CMF[1,47]

Prechemo: CBC, Chem, and CA 27-29. MUGA scan. 5-HT$_3$ and dexamethasone 10–20 mg. Moderately to highly emetogenic.

Doxorubicin 75 mg/m²: IV push on day 1. Potent vesicant.

Repeat cycle every 21 days for four cycles, followed by:

Premeds: 5-HT$_3$ and dexamethasone 20 mg.

Cyclophosphamide 600 mg/m²: IV in 500–1000cc NS on day 1.

Methotrexate 40 mg/m²: IV push on day 1.

5-Flourouracil 600 mg/m²: IV push on day 1.

Side effects: Cyclophosphamide can cause rhinitis and irritation of nose and throat. Myelosuppression may be severe. Nausea and vomiting. Mucositis and diarrhea can be severe, dose dependent. Acutely, pericarditis-myocarditis syndrome may occur. With cumulative doses >550 mg/m² of doxorubicin, cardiomyopathy may occur. Increased risk of cardiotoxicity when doxorubicin is given with cyclophosphamide. Acute renal failure, azotemia, urinary retention, and uric acid nephropathy have been observed with methotrexate. Hemorrhagic cystitis, dysuria, and urinary frequency with cyclophosphamide. SIADH. Photophobia, increased lacrimation, acute and chronic conjunctivitis, blepharitis, and blurred vision. Alopecia. Hyperpigmentation of nails and skin, banding of nails, and radiation recall may occur with 5-fluorouracil. Photosensitivity with a sunburn-like rash. Hand-foot syndrome can be dose-limiting.

Chair time: 1 hour on day 1 for doxorubicin. Repeat cycle every 21 days for four cycles, followed by 2 hours on day 1 for CMF every 21 days for eight cycles.

5-Fluorouracil + Epirubicin + Cyclophosphamide (FEC)[1,48]

Prechemo: CBC, Chem, LFTs, and CA 27-29. MUGA scan. 5-HT$_3$ and dexamethasone 20 mg. Moderately to highly emetogenic.

5-Flourouracil 500 mg/m²: IV on day 1.

Epirubicin 100 mg/m²: IV push on day 1. Vesicant.

Cyclophosphamide 500 mg/m²: IV in NS IV on day 1.

Side effects: Cyclophosphamide can cause rhinitis and irritation of nose and throat. Myelosuppression may be severe. Nausea and vomiting. Mucositis and diarrhea can be severe and dose-limiting. Cardiotoxicity is dose related, is cumulative, and may occur during or months to years after cessation of therapy. Cyclophosphamide may increase the risk of cardiotoxicity. Dose reduction is required in the presence of liver dysfunction. Hemorrhagic cystitis, dysuria, and urinary frequency, preventable with adequate hydration. Red-orange discoloration of urine. Epirubicin may cause "flare" reaction or streaking along vein during peripheral administration. If this occurs, slow drug administration time and flush more. Hyperpigmentation, photosensitivity, nail changes, and radiation recall occur. Complete alopecia. Hand-foot syndrome can be dose-limiting. SIADH. Photophobia, increased lacrimation, acute and chronic conjunctivitis, blepharitis, and blurred vision.

Chair time: 2 hours on day 1. Repeat cycle every 21 days for six cycles.

Cyclophosphamide + Methotrexate + 5-FU + Prednisone (CMFP) [1,49]

Prechemo: CBC, Chem, LFTs, and CA 27-29. 5-HT$_3$ and dexamethasone 20 mg on days 1 and 8. Oral 5-HT$_3$ or phenothiazine days 2–7 and 9–14. Moderately to highly emetogenic.

Cyclophosphamide 100 mg/m^2/day: PO on days 1–14. (25- and 50-mg tablets.) Take with meals in morning or early afternoon to allow adequate excretion.

Methotrexate 40 mg/m^2: IV push on days 1 and 8.

5-Flourouracil 600 mg/m^2: IV push on days 1 and 8.

Prednisone 20 mg: PO QID on days 1–7.

Side effects: Cyclophosphamide can cause rhinitis and irritation of nose and throat. Myelosuppression. Nausea and vomiting. Mucositis and diarrhea can be severe, dose dependent. Acute renal failure, azotemia, urinary retention, and uric acid nephropathy have been observed with methotrexate. Hemorrhagic cystitis, dysuria, and urinary frequency. Preventable with adequate hydration with cyclophosphamide. SIADH. Photophobia, increased lacrimation, acute and chronic conjunctivitis, blepharitis, and blurred vision. Alopecia. Hyperpigmentation of nails and skin, banding of nails, and radiation recall may occur. Photosensitivity, sunburn-like rash. Hand-foot syndrome can be dose-limiting. Steroid effect resulting in hyperglycemia, insomnia, emotional lability, agitation, fluid retention, and perceptual alterations related to cataracts or glaucoma with long-term use. Increased risk of secondary malignancies with cyclophosphamide.

Chair time: 1 hour on days 1 and 8. Repeat cycle every 28 days for six cycles.

SINGLE-AGENT REGIMENS

Tamoxifen (Nolvadex)

Pretreatment: CBC, Chem, LFTs, and CA 27-29. ER/PR testing.

Tamoxifen (Nolvadex) 20 mg: PO daily. (10- and 20-mg tablets) Monitor INR closely in patients taking warfarin; increases INR.

Side effects: Nausea and vomiting rarely observed. Tumor with bone pain, urinary retention, back pain with spinal cord compression and/or hypercalcemia. Deep vein thrombosis, pulmonary embolism, and superficial phlebitis. Fluid retention and peripheral edema. Menstrual irregularity, hot flashes, milk production in breasts, vaginal discharge, and bleeding. Increased incidence of endometrial hyperplasia, polyps, and endometrial cancer. Headache, lethargy, and dizziness occur rarely. Visual disturbances, including cataract, retinopathy, and decreased visual acuity. Mild, transient leukopenia and thrombocytopenia occur rarely. Elevations in serum triglyceride levels. Mildly emetogenic protocol.

Daily dosing for 5 years in ER+ tumors.

Anastrozole (Arimidex)[1,51]

Pretreatment: CBC, Chem, LFTs, and CA 27-29. ER/PR testing.

Anastrozole 1 mg: PO daily. (1-mg tablet.) Take with or without food, at approximately the same time of day

Side effects: Hot flashes and vaginal dryness. Thrombophlebitis is uncommon. Mild swelling of arms or legs. Mild nausea and vomiting. Mild constipation or diarrhea. Dry, scaling skin rash. Flu-like syndrome: fever, malaise, and myalgias. Arthralgias involve hands, knees, hips, lower back, and shoulders. Early morning stiffness. Headaches are mild, decreased energy and weakness.

Daily dosing for 5 years with ER+ tumors or with ER status unknown.

Tamoxifen + Letrozole[1,52]

Pretreatment: CBC, Chem, LFTs, and CA 27-29. ER/PR testing.

Tamoxifen 20 mg: PO daily. (10- and 20-mg tablets.)

Monitor INR closely in patients taking warfarin; increases INR.

Take daily for first 5 years, followed by:

Letrozol (Femara) 2.5 mg: PO daily. Food does not interfere with absorption.

Side effects: Tamoxifen: Nausea and vomiting rare. Tumor flare: increased bone pain, urinary retention, back pain with spinal cord compression and/or hypercalcemia. Deep vein thrombosis, pulmonary embolism, and superficial phlebitis are rare cardiovascular complications of tamoxifen therapy. Fluid retention and peripheral edema. Menstrual irregularity, hot flashes, milk production in breasts, vaginal discharge, and bleeding. Increased incidence of endometrial hyperplasia, polyps, and endometrial cancer. Headache, lethargy, and dizziness occur rarely. Visual disturbances, including cataract, retinopathy, and decreased visual acuity. Mild, transient leukopenia and thrombocytopenia. Elevations in serum triglyceride levels. **Letrozole:** Musculoskeletal pain (back, arms, legs) and arthralgias. Hot flashes. Thromboembolic events are rare and less common than with megestrol acetate. Chest pain reported in some patients. Mild nausea with vomiting and anorexia occurring less frequently. Mild constipation or diarrhea can also occur. Mild elevation in serum transaminase and serum bilirubin levels. Seen in patients with known metastatic disease in the liver.

Daily dosing with tamoxifien for 5 years followed by letrozole daily for 5 years.

Tamoxifen + Exemestane[1,53]

Pretreatment: CBC, Chem, LFTs, and CA 27-29. ER/PR testing.
Tamoxifen 20 mg: PO daily. (10- and 20-mg tablets.)
Monitor INR closely in patients taking warfarin; increases INR.
Daily for 2–3 years followed by:
Exemestane (Aromasin) 25 mg: PO daily for remainder of 5 years.
Side effects: Tamoxifen: Nausea and vomiting rare. Tumor flare: increased bone pain, urinary retention, back pain with spinal cord compression and/or hypercalcemia. Deep vein thrombosis, pulmonary embolism, and superficial phlebitis are rare cardiovascular complications of tamoxifen therapy. Fluid retention and peripheral edema. Menstrual irregularity, hot flashes, milk production in breasts, vaginal discharge, and bleeding. Increased incidence of endometrial hyperplasia, polyps, and endometrial cancer. Headache, lethargy, and dizziness occur rarely. Visual disturbances, including cataract, retinopathy, and decreased visual acuity. Mild, transient leukopenia and thrombocytopenia. Elevations in serum triglyceride levels. **Exemestane**: Hot flashes, increased sweating, and pain reported. Mild-to-moderate nausea, increased appetite, and weight gain reported. Depression and insomnia occurred in 13% and 11%, respectively. Headache and fatigue.

Daily dosing of tamoxifen for 2–3 years followed by daily exemestane for remainder of 5 years in ER + tumors.

METASTATIC BREAST CANCER

COMBINATION REGIMENS

Doxorubicin + Cyclophosphamide (AC)[1,36]

Prechemo: CBC, Chem, LFTs, and CA 27-29. MUGA. 5-HT$_3$ and dexamethasone 20 mg. Moderately to highly emetogenic.
Doxorubicin 60 mg/m^2: IV on day 1. Potent vesicant.
Cyclophosphamide 600 mg/m^2: IV on day 1.
Side effects: Cyclophosphamide can cause rhinitis and irritation of nose and throat. Myelosuppression may be severe. G-CSF recommended. Nausea and vomiting, acute or delayed. Stomatitis and diarrhea not dose-limiting. Pericarditis-myocarditis syndrome. With cumulative doses >550 mg/m^2 of doxorubicin, cardiomyopathy. Cyclophosphamide may increase risk of doxorubicin-induced cardiotoxicity. Dose reduce with liver dysfunction. Hemorrhagic cystitis, dysuria and urinary frequency with cyclophosphamide. Red-orange discoloration of urine. SIADH. Hyperpigmentation, photosensitivity, and radiation recall. Alopecia.
Chair time: 2 hours on day 1. Repeat every 21 days until progression.

Doxorubicin + Paclitaxel (AT)[1,54]

Prechemo: CBC, Chem, and CA 27-29. Central line placement. MUGA scan. 5-HT$_3$ and dexamethasone. Moderately to highly emetogenic. Diphenhydramine 25–50 mg and H$_2$ antagonist.
(1) Doxorubicin 50 mg/m^2: IV push on day 1. Potent vesicant.
Paclitaxel 150 mg/m^2: IV over 24 hours on day 1.
Repeat cycle every 21 days.
OR
(2) Doxorubicin 60 mg/m^2: IV on day 1. Potent vesicant.

33

Repeat cycle every 21 days up to a maximum of eight cycles, followed
by:

Paclitaxel 175 mg/m^2: IV on day 1.

Repeat cycle every 21 days until disease progression.

OR

(3) Paclitaxel 175 mg/m^2: IV on day 1.

Use non-PVC containers and tubing with 0.22-micron inline filter.

Repeat cycle every 21 days until disease progression, followed by:

Doxorubicin 60 mg/m^2: IV push on day 1. Potent vesicant.

Repeat cycle every 21 days up to a maximum of eight cycles.

Side effects: Hypersensitivity reaction with paclitaxel. Myelosuppression, dose-limiting. Use G-CSF support. Nausea and vomiting. Stomatitis not dose-limiting. Dose reduce doxorubicin with liver dysfunction.
Pericarditis-myocarditis. Cardiomyopathy with doses >550 mg/m^2 doxorubicin. Sensory neuropathy with numbness/paresthesias, dose related
and dose-limiting. Red-orange discoloration of urine. Hyperpigmentation, photosensitivity, and radiation recall. Alopecia.

Chair time: (1) 1 hour on day 1; repeat every 21 days. (2) 1 hour on
day 1; repeat every 21 days up to maximum of eight cycles and then 4
hours on day 1; repeat every 21 days until disease progression. (3) 4
hours on day 1; repeat every 21 days until disease progression, and then
chair time 1 hour on day 1, repeated every 21 days up to a maximum of
eight cycles.

Cyclophosphamide + Doxorubicin + 5-Flourouracil (CAF)[1,43]

Prechemo: CBC, Chem, LFTs, and CA 27-29. MUGA scan. HT$_3$ and
dexamethasone 20 mg. Moderately to highly emetogenic.

Cyclophosphamide 600 mg/m^2: IV in 500–1000 cc NS on day 1.

Doxorubicin 60 mg/m^2: IV push on day 1. Potent vesicant.

5-Flourouracil 600 mg/m^2: IV push on day 1.

Side effects: Cyclophosphamide can cause rhinitis and irritation of
nose and throat. Myelosuppression may be severe. G-CSF recommended. Nausea and vomiting, acute or delayed. Stomatitis and diarrhea
can be severe and dose-limiting. Pericarditis-myocarditis syndrome.
With cumulative doses >550 mg/m^2 of doxorubicin, cardiomyopathy.
Cyclophosphamide may increase the risk of doxorubicin-induced cardiotoxicity. Dose reduce doxorubicin with liver dysfunction. Hemorrhagic cystitis, dysuria, and urinary frequency. Red-orange discoloration
of urine. SIADH. Hyperpigmentation, photosensitivity, nail changes,
and radiation recall. Complete alopecia. Hand-foot syndrome can be
dose-limiting. Photophobia, increased lacrimation, acute and chronic
conjunctivitis, blepharitis, and blurred vision.

Chair time: 2 hours on day 1. Repeat cycle every 21 days until disease progression.

Cyclophosphamide + Epirubicin + 5-Fluorouracil (CEF)[1,55]

Prechemo: CBC, Chem, LFTs, and CA 27-29. MUGA scan. 5-HT$_3$ and dexamethasone 20 mg days 1 and 8. Oral 5-HT$_3$ or phenothiazine days 2–7 and 9–14. Moderately to highly emetogenic.

Cyclophosphamide 75 mg/m^2/day: PO days 1–14. (25- and 50-mg tablets.) Taken with meals in morning or early afternoon for adequate excretion time.

Epirubicin 60 mg/m^2: IV push on days 1 and 8. Vesicant.

5-Flourouracil 500 mg/m^2: IV on days 1 and 8.

Side effects: Cyclophosphamide can cause rhinitis and irritation of nose and throat. Myelosuppression may be severe. Nausea and vomiting. Mucositis and diarrhea severe and dose-limiting. Cardiotoxicity is dose related, is cumulative, and may occur during months to years after cessation of therapy. Cyclophosphamide may increase the risk of cardiotoxicity. Dose reduce with liver dysfunction. Hemorrhagic cystitis, dysuria, and urinary frequency. Red-orange discoloration of urine. Epirubicin may cause "flare" reaction or streaking along vein during peripheral administration. If occurs, slow drug administration and increase free-flowing IV. Hyperpigmentation, photosensitivity, nail changes, and radiation recall occur. Alopecia. Hand-foot syndrome can be dose-limiting. SIADH. Photophobia, increased lacrimation, acute and chronic conjunctivitis, blepharitis, and blurred vision.

Chair time: 1 hour on days 1 and 8. Repeat cycle every 28 days until progression.

Cyclophosphamide + Methotrexate + 5-Flourouracil (CMF-Bonadonna Regimen)[1,45]

Prechemo: CBC, Chem, LFTs, and CA 27-29. 5-HT$_3$ and dexamethasone 20 mg days 1 and 8. Oral 5-HT$_3$ or phenothiazine days 2–7 and 9–14. Moderately to highly emetogenic.

Cyclophosphamide 100 mg/m^2/day: PO on days 1–14. (25- and 50-mg tablets.) Taken with meals in morning or early afternoon for adequate excretion time.

Methotrexate 40 mg/m^2: IV on days 1 and 8.

5-Flourouracil 500 mg/m^2: IV on days 1 and 8.

Side effects: Rhinitis and irritation of nose and throat. Myelosuppression. Nausea and vomiting. Mucositis and diarrhea severe, dose dependent. Acute renal failure, azotemia, urinary retention, and uric acid nephropathy with methotrexate. Hemorrhagic cystitis, dysuria, and urinary frequency with cyclophosphamide. SIADH. Photophobia, increased lacrimation, acute and chronic conjunctivitis, blepharitis, and blurred vision. Alopecia. Hyperpigmentation of nails and skin, banding of nails, and radiation recall. Photosensitivity, sunburn-like rash. Hand-foot syndrome can be dose-limiting.

Chair time: 1 hour on days 1 and 8. Repeat every 28 days until disease progression.

Cyclophosphamide + Methotrexate + 5-Flourouracil (CMF IV Bolus)[1,46]

Prechemo: CBC, Chem, LFTs, and CA 27-29. 5-HT$_3$ and dexamethasone 20 mg. Moderately to highly emetogenic.

Cyclophosphamide 600 mg/m^2: IV on day 1.

Methotrexate 40 mg/m^2: IV on day 1.

5-Flourouracil 600 mg/m^2: IV on day 1.

Side effects: Rhinitis and irritation of nose and throat. Myelosuppression can be severe. Nausea and vomiting. Mucositis and diarrhea can be severe, dose dependent. Acute renal failure, azotemia, urinary retention, and uric acid nephropathy. Hemorrhagic cystitis, dysuria, and urinary frequency with cyclophosphamide. SIADH. Photophobia, increased lacrimation, acute and chronic conjunctivitis, blepharitis, and blurred vision. Complete alopecia. Hyperpigmentation of nails and skin, banding of nails, and radiation recall may occur. Photosensitivity, sunburn-like rash. Hand-foot syndrome, dose-limiting.

Chair time: 2 hours on day 1. Repeat every 21 days until disease progression.

Capecitabine + Docetaxel (XT)[1,56]

Prechemo: CBC, Chem, bilirubin, LFTs, creatinine clearance, and CA 27-29. Dexamethasone 8 mg PO bid the day before, the day of and day after treatment. Oral phenothiazine or 5-HT$_3$ days 1–14. Mildly emetogenic.

Capecitabine 1250 mg/m^2: PO bid on days 1–14. (May decrease dose to 850–1000 mg/m^2 PO bid to reduce the risk of toxicity without compromising efficacy.) 150- and 500-mg tablets. Taken within 30 minutes of a meal with plenty of water. May increase INR in patients taking warfarin.

Docetaxel 75 mg/m^2: IV 2500 cc NS on day 1. Use non-PVC containers and tubing.

Side effects: Hypersensitivity reactions with docetaxel. Myelosuppression, dose-limiting. G-CSF recommended. Nausea and vomiting. Diarrhea is common and can be severe. Stomatitis is common, can be severe. Peripheral neuropathy with sensory alterations are paresthesias and numbness. Fluid retention syndrome, weight gain, peripheral and/or generalized edema, pleural effusion, and ascites. Capecitabine contraindicated with baseline creatinine clearance < 30 mL/min. Dose reduction of 75% with baseline creatinine clearance of 30–50 mL/min. Hand-foot syndrome characterized by tingling, numbness, pain, erythema, dryness, rash, swelling, increased pigmentation, and/or pruritus of the hands and feet. Less frequent in reduced doses. Nail changes, rash, dry, pruritic skin seen. Alopecia. Blepharitis, tear-duct stenosis, acute and chronic conjunctivitis. Elevations in serum bilirubin, alkaline phosphatase, and hepatic transaminase (aspartate transaminase, alanine transaminase) levels. Dose modifications with hyperbilirubinemia.

Chair time: 2 hours on day 1. Repeat every 21 days until disease progression.

Capecitabine + Paclitaxel (XP)[1,57]

Prechemo: CBC, Chem, bilirubin, LFTs, creatinine clearance, and CA 27-29. 5-HT$_3$ and dexamethasone 10–20 mg. Diphenhydramine 25–50 mg and H$_2$ antagonist day 1. Oral phenothiazine or 5-HT$_3$ before capecitabine on days 2–14. Mildly emetogenic.

Capecitabine 825 mg/m²: PO bid on days 1–14. (150- and 500-mg tablets.) Taken within 30 minutes of a meal with plenty of water. May increase INR with warfarin.

Paclitaxel 175 mg/m²: IV over 3 hours on day 1. Use non-PVC containers and tubing with 0.22-micron inline filter.

Side effects: Hypersensitivity reaction with paclitaxel. Nausea and vomiting. Diarrhea and stomatitis can be severe. Elevations in serum bilirubin, alkaline phosphatase, and hepatic transaminase levels. Dose reduction with hyperbilirubinemia. Capecitabine contraindicated with baseline creatinine clearance < 30 mL/min. Dose reduction to 75% made with baseline creatinine clearance of 30–50 mL/min. Hand-foot syndrome tingling, numbness, pain, erythema, dryness, rash, swelling, increased pigmentation, and/or pruritus of the hands and feet. Alopecia. Myelosuppression, dose-limiting. G-CSF recommended. Sensory neuropathy with numbness and paresthesias, dose related. Myalgias and arthralgias. Blepharitis, tear-duct stenosis, acute and chronic conjunctivitis.

Chair time: 4 hours on day 1. Repeat every 21 days as tolerated or until disease progression.

Capecitabine + Vinorelbine (XN)[1,57]

Prechemo: CBC, Chem, bilirubin, LFTs, creatinine clearance, and CA 27-29. Oral phenothiazine or 5-HT$_3$ days 1–14. Mildly to moderately emetogenic.

Capecitabine 1000 mg/m²: PO bid on days 1–14. (150- and 500-mg tablets.) Taken within 30 minutes of a meal with plenty of water. May increase INR with warfarin.

Vinorelbine 25 mg/m²: IV on days 1 and 8. Vesicant. Dilute in syringe or IV bag to concentration of 1.5–3.0 mg/mL.

Side effects: Leukopernia is dose-limiting toxicity. Nausea and vomiting. Stomatitis and diarrhea can be severe. Elevations in LFT results. Capecitabine contraindicated with baseline creatinine clearance < 30 mL/min. Dose reduction of 75% with baseline creatinine clearance of 30–50 mL/min SIADH. Hand-foot syndrome can be dose-limiting. Alopecia. Neurotoxicity mild. Blepharitis, tear-duct stenosis, acute and chronic conjunctivitis.

Chair time: 1 hour on days 1 and 8. Repeat every 21 days until progression.

Docetaxel + Doxorubicin[1,58]

Prechemo: CBC, Chem, and CA 27-29. MUGA scan. Dexamethasone 8 mg PO bid for 3 days, the day before, day of, and day after treatment. HT₃ and dexamethasone 10–20 mg. Diphenhydramine 25–50 mg and H₂ antagonist. Moderately emetogenic.

Docetaxel 75 mg/m²: IV in 250 cc NS on day 1. Use non-PVC containers and tubing.

Doxorubicin 50 mg/m²: IV push on day 1. Potent vesicant.

Side effects: Hypersensitivity reaction with docetaxel. Myelosuppression, dose-limiting. G-CSF recommended. Nausea and vomiting. Stomatitis is not dose-limiting. Pericarditis-myocarditis syndrome. With high cumulative doses (>550 mg/m²) doxorubicin, cardiomyopathy. Peripheral neuropathy, paresthesias, and numbness. Fluid retention syndrome: weight gain, edema, pleural effusion, and ascites. Dose reduce doxorubicin with liver dysfunction. Red-orange discoloration of urine. Hyperpigmentation, nail changes, rash, dry, pruritic skin, photosensitivity, and radiation recall. Alopecia.

Chair time: 2 hours on day 1. Repeat every 21 days until disease progression.

5-Fluorouracil + Epirubicin + Cyclophosphamide (FEC-100)[1,59]

Prechemo: CBC, Chem, LFTs, and CA 27-29. MUGA scan. 5-HT₃ and dexamethasone 20 mg. Moderately to highly emetogenic.

5-Flourouracil 500 mg/m²: IV push on day 1.

Epirubicin 100 mg/m²: IV push on day 1. Vesicant.

Cyclophosphamide 500 mg/m²: in 500–1000 cc NS IV on day 1.

Side effects: Rhinitis and irritation of nose and throat. Myelosuppression may be severe. Nausea and vomiting. Mucositis and diarrhea dose-limiting. Cardiotoxicity is dose related, is cumulative, and may occur during months to years after cessation of therapy. Cyclophosphamide may increase the risk of cardiotoxicity. Dose reduction with liver dysfunction. Hemorrhagic cystitis, dysuria, and urinary frequency with cyclophosphamide. Red-orange discoloration of urine. Epirubicin may cause "flare" reaction or streaking along vein during peripheral administration. If occurs, slow drug administration time and increase rate of free-flowing IV. Hyperpigmentation, photosensitivity, nail changes, and radiation recall. Alopecia. Hand-foot syndrome dose-limiting. SIADH. Photophobia, increased lacrimation, conjunctivitis, and blurred vision.

Chair time: 2 hours on day 1. Repeat every 21 days until progression.

Paclitaxel + Vinorelbine[1,60]

Prechemo: CBC, Chem, and CA 27-29. 5-HT$_3$ and dexamethasone 10–20 mg. Diphenhydramine 25–50 mg H$_2$ antagonist. Mild to moderately emetogenic.

Paclitaxel 135 mg/m^2: IV over 3 hours on day 1; start 1 hour after vinorelbine. Use non-PVC containers and tubing with 0.22-micron inline filter.

Vinorelbine 30 mg/m^2: IV push over 20 minutes on days 1 and 8. Vesicant.

Dilute in syringe or IV bag to concentration of 1.5–3.0 mg/mL.

Side effects: Hypersensitivity reaction with paclitaxel and vinorelbine. Myelosuppression dose-limiting. G-CSF recommended. Nausea and vomiting. Stomatitis, constipation, diarrhea, and anorexia. Alopecia. Sensory neuropathy with numbness and paresthesias; dose related. Myalgias and arthralgias.

Chair time: 4 hours on day 1; 1 hour on day 8. Repeat every 28 days until disease progression.

Vinorelbine + Doxorubicin[1,61]

Prechemo: CBC, Chem, and CA 27-29. MUGA scan. 5-HT$_3$ and dexamethasone 10–20 mg. Moderately to highly emetogenic.

Vinorelbine 25 mg/m^2: IV push on days 1 and 8. Vesicant.

Dilute in syringe or IV bag to concentration of 1.5–3.0 mg/mL.

Doxorubicin 50 mg/m^2: IV push on day 1. Potent vesicant.

Side effects: Hypersensitivity reaction with vinorelbine. Myelosuppression may be severe. Nausea and vomiting. Stomatitis is mild to moderate. Constipation, diarrhea, and anorexia. Pericarditis-myocarditis syndrome. With cumulative doses >550 mg/m^2 of doxorubicin, cardiomyopathy. Mild to moderate neuropathy. Hyperpigmentation, photosensitivity and radiation recall. Alopecia.

Chair time: 1 hour on days 1 and 8. Repeat every 21 days until progression.

Trastuzumab + Paclitaxel

Prechemo: CBC, Chem, CA 27-29; HER-2 testing (FISH) preferred or (IHC) and MUGA scan. 5-HT$_3$ and dexamethasone 10–20 mg. Diphenhydramine 25–50 mg and H$_2$ antagonist. Mildly emetogenic protocol.

Trastuzumab 4 mg/kg: IV in 250 cc of NS over 90-minute loading dose, then:

Trastuzumab 2 mg/kg: IV in 250 cc of NS over 30 minutes weekly.

Paclitaxel 175 mg/m²: IV in 500 cc NS over 3 hours on day 1.

Repeat cycle every 21 days.[1,62]

OR

Trastuzumab 4 mg/kg: IV in 250 cc of NS over 90-minute loading dose, then:

Trastuzumab 2 mg/kg: IV in 250 cc of NS over 30 minutes weekly.

Paclitaxel 80 mg/m²: IV in 250 cc NS weekly. Use non-PVC containers and tubing with 0.22-micron inline filter.

Repeat cycle every 4 weeks. [1,63]

Side effects: Hypersensitivity reactions with either drug. Nausea and vomiting, mucositis, and diarrhea generally mild. Myelosuppression dose-limiting toxicity. G-CSF recommended. Pericarditis-myocarditis syndrome. With cumulative doses >550 mg/m² of doxorubicin, cardiomyopathy. Cough, dyspnea, pulmonary infiltrates, and/or pleural effusions. Dose related sensory neuropathy with numbness and paresthesias, dose-limiting. Myalgias and arthralgias. Alopecia.

Chair time: 5 hours on day 1 for cycle one only, 4 hours on day 1 for subsequent cycles; 1 hour for weeks 2 and 3. Repeat every 21 days OR 4 hours on day 1, 3 hours weekly thereafter. Repeat every 4 weeks.

Trastuzumab + Docetaxel[1,64]

Prechemo: CBC, Chem, and CA 27-29. HER-2 testing FISH preferred or IHC and MUGA scan. Dexamethasone 8 mg PO bid for 3 days, the day before, day of, and day after treatment. 5-HT$_3$ and dexamethasone 10–20 mg. Mildly emetogenic.

Trastuzumab 4 mg/kg: IV in 250 cc of NS over 90-minute loading dose day 1 first cycle only, then:

Trastuzumab 2 mg/kg: IV in 250 cc of NS over 30 minutes on days 1, 8, and 15.

Docetaxel 35 mg/m²: IV in 250 cc of NS over 1 hour days 1, 8, and 15. Use non-PVC containers and tubing.

Repeat cycle every 4 weeks.

Side effects: Hypersensitivity reactions with either drug. Nausea and vomiting. Mucositis and diarrhea. Dyspnea, edema, and reduced left ventricular function seen with trastuzumab. Cough, dyspnea, pulmonary infiltrates, and/or pleural effusions. Myelosuppression is dose-limiting toxicity. Dose-related sensory neuropathy with numbness and paresthesia. Edema, pleural effusion, and ascites. Alopecia. Nail changes, rash, and dry, pruritic skin. Hand-foot syndrome.

Chair time: 3 hours on days 1, 8 and 15. Repeat cycle every 4 weeks.

Gemcitabine + Paclitaxel[1,65]

Prechemo: CBC, Chem, LFTs, and CA 27-29. 5-HT_3 and dexamethasone 10–20 mg. Diphenhydramine 25–50 mg and H_2 antagonist. Mildly to moderately emetogenic.

Gemcitabine 1250 mg/m^2: IV in 250 cc NS over 30 minutes days 1 and 8.

Paclitaxel 175 mg/m^2: IV in 500 cc NS on day 1. Use non-PVC containers and tubing with 0.22-micron inline filter.

Side effects: Hypersensitivity reaction with paclitaxel. Myelosuppression is dose-limiting. G-CSF recommended. Mild dyspnea and drug induced pneumonitis. Nausea and vomiting, diarrhea, and mucositis. Sensory neuropathy with numbness and paresthesias, dose related and dose-limiting. Flu-like syndrome: fever, malaise, chills, headache, and myalgias. Transient elevation of serum transaminase and bilirubin levels. Edema occurs in some patients. Alopecia.

Chair time: 4 hours on day 1; 1 hour on day 8. Repeat every 21 days until disease progression.

Carboplatin + Paclitaxel[1,66]

Prechemo: CBC, Chem, Mg^{2+}, and CA 27-29. 5-HT_3 and dexamethasone 10–20 mg. Diphenhydramine 25–50 mg and H_2 antagonist. Mildly to moderately emetogenic protocol.

Paclitaxel 200 mg/m^2: IV in 500 cc NS over 3 hours on day 1. Use non-PVC containers and tubing with 0.22-micron inline filter.

Carboplatin AUC 6: IV in 500 cc NS on day 1: Give carboplatin after paclitaxel to decrease toxicities.

Side effects: Hypersensitivity reaction with paclitaxel, and increased risk of hypersensitivity in patients receiving more than seven courses of carboplatin therapy. Myelosuppression cumulative and dose related and dose-limiting. G-CSF recommended. Nausea and vomiting, acute or delayed. Mucositis and/or diarrhea. Transient elevations in serum transaminases, bilirubin and alkaline phosphatase. Decreases Mg^{2+}, K^+, Ca^{2+}, and Na^+. Sensory neuropathy with numbness and paresthesias; dose related and can be dose-limiting. Alopecia.

Chair time: 5 hours on day 1. Repeat every 21 days until progression.

Carboplatin + Docetaxel [1,67]

Prechemo: CBC, Chem, Mg^{2+}, and CA 27-29. Dexamethasone 8 mg PO bid day before, day of, and day after treatment. 5-HT$_3$ and dexamethasone 10–20 mg. Mildly to moderately emetogenic.

Docetaxel 75 mg/m^2: IV in 250 cc NS on day 1. Use non-PVC container and tubing.

Carboplatin AUC 6: IV in 500 cc NS on day 1.

Side effects: Hypersensitivity reaction docetaxel and increased risk in patients receiving more than seven courses of carboplatin. Myelosuppression dose related and can be dose-limiting. Nausea and vomiting. Decreases Mg^{2+}, K^+, Ca^{2+}, and Na^+. Neuropathy with numbness and paresthesia. Edema, pleural effusion, and ascites. Alopecia. Nail changes, rash, and dry, pruritic skin. Hand-foot syndrome.

Chair time: 3 hours on day 1. Repeat every 21 days until progression.

Ixabepilone (Ixempra) + Capecitabine [1,68]

Prechemo: CBC, Chem, bilirubin, LFTs, and CA 27-29. 5-HT$_3$ and dexamethasone 20. Diphenhydramine 25–50 mg and H_2 antagonist.

Ixabepilone 40 mg/m^2: IV over 3 hours on day 1.

Further dilute in lactated ringers to a final concentration of 0.2–0.6 mg/mL. 250-mL bag is usually sufficient. Use DEHP-free containers and tubing with 0.2–1.2 micron inline filter.

Capecitabine 1000 mg/m^2: PO bid on days 1–14. (150- and 500-mg tablets.) Administer with plenty of water within 30 minutes of a meal. Monitor INRs closely when taking warfarin, may increase INR.

Side effects: Patients with a history of a severe hypersensitivity reaction to agents containing Cremophorr EL or its derivatives should not be treated with Ixempra. Hypersensitivity reactions (flushing, rash, dyspnea, and bronchospasm) can occur. Myelosuppression dose dependent. Nausea, vomiting, diarrhea, stomatitis/mucositis, and anorexia common. Constipation, abdominal pain, and taste alterations. Combination capecitabine must not be given with AST or ALT >2.5 × upper normal limit (UNL< or bilirubin >1 × UNL. Nausea, vomiting, diarrhea, stomatitis/mucositis, and anorexia common. Peripheral neuropathy (burning sensation, hyperesthesia, paresthesia, discomfort, or neuropathic pain). Myalgias and arthralgias, fatigue, and asthenias. CYP3A4 inhibitors should be avoided. Grapefruit juice may also increase plasma concentrations. Palmar-plantar erythrodysesthesia (tingling, numbness, pain, erythema, dryness, rash, swelling, increased pigmentation, and/or pruritus of the hands and feet). Nail disorders, skin rash, and exfoliation. Contraindicated in patients with creatinine clearance >30 mL/min, dose reduce if creatinine clearance of 30–50 mL/min at baseline to 75% of total capecitabine dose. Use with caution with history of cardiac disease; discontinuation should be considered if cardiac ischemia or impaired cardiac function occurs. Blepharitis, tear-duct stenosis, acute and chronic conjunctivitis. Alopecia.

Chair time: 4 hours on day 1. Repeat every 21 days as tolerated or until progression.

Lapatinib (Tykerb) + Capecitabine (Xeloda)[1,69]

Pre-chemo: Baseline laboratory tests: CBC: CHEM, LFTs, creatinine clearance, and CA 27-29. HER-2 testing of tumor. FISH (preferred) or IHC, and MUGA scan. Oral phenothiazine or 5-HT3. Mildly to moderately emetogenic.

Lapatinib 1250 mg once daily. (250 mg tablets). Take all tablets at once; do not split the dose. Taken at least 1 hour before or 2 hours after a meal. Take at least 24 hours apart to reduce toxicity.

Capecitabine 2000 mg/m²: PO in 2 divided doses days 1–14. (150- and 500-mg tablets). Taken with food or within 30 minutes after food. May decrease to 850–1000 mg/m² PO bid on days 1–14 to reduce the risk of toxicity without compromising efficacy. Monitor INRs closely when taking warfarin; may increase INR.

Side effects: Drug interactions: Strong CYP3A4 inhibitors should be avoided. Grapefruit and pomegranate should be avoided. If CYP3A4 inhibitor is administered dose reduce to 500mg/day of lapatinib. Strong CYP3A4 inducers should be avoided or a dose increase made. Myelosuppression less frequent than with infusional 5-FU. Diarrhea common, can be severe. Nausea and vomiting. Stomatitis is sometimes severe. Anorexia and indigestion. Hand-foot syndrome (palmar-plantar erythrodysesthesia) commonly occurs. Blepharitis, tear-duct stenosis, acute and chronic conjunctivitis. Rash is common. Decrease tykerb dose to 750 mg/day in patients with severe hepatic impairment. Dose reduce capecitabine if hyperbilirubinemia occurs. Decreases in left ventricular ejection fraction with tykerb, prolongs the QT interval. Monitor ECG and electrolytes. Chest pain, EKG changes, and serum enzyme elevation occur rarely with capecitabine. Increased risk in patients with prior history of ischemic heart disease. Capecitabine is contraindicated with baseline creatinine clearance < 30 mL/min. Dose reduce to 75% of capecitabine with baseline creatinine clearance of 30–50 mL/min.

Chair time: No chair time. Repeat cycle every 21 days as tolerated or until disease progression.

Mitomycin + Vinblastine[1,70]

Prechemo: CBC, Chem, LFTs, creatinine clearance, and CA 27-29. Central line placement. 5-HT$_3$ and dexamethasone. Mildly to moderately emetogenic.

Mitomycin 20 mg/m²: IV bolus day 1. Potent vesicant.

Vinblastine 1.4–2.0 mg/m²: IV continuous infusion days 1–5. Vesicant.

Side effects: Myelosuppression dose-limiting and cumulative toxicity. Nausea and vomiting. Mucositis, constipation, abdominal pain, paralytic ileus. Anorexia and fatigue. Peripheral neuropathy paresthesias, paralysis, loss of deep-tendon reflexes, jaw pain, and autonomic nervous system dysfunction. Less commonly, cranial nerve paralysis, ataxia, cortical blindness, seizures, and coma. Alopecia.

Chair time: 1 hour day 1 and 30 minutes day 5. Repeat cycle every 6–8 weeks.

SINGLE-AGENT REGIMENS

Tamoxifen[1,71]

Pretreatment: CBC, Chem, LFTs, and CA 27-29. ER/PR testing.

Tamoxifen 20 mg: PO daily. (10- and 20-mg tablets.)

Monitor INR with warfarin; increases INR.

Side effects: Nausea and vomiting rarely observed. Tumor flair with bone pain, urinary retention, back pain with spinal cord compression, and/or hypercalcemia. Deep vein thrombosis, pulmonary embolism, and superficial phlebitis. Fluid retention and peripheral edema. Menstrual irregularity, hot flashes, milk production in breasts, vaginal discharge, and bleeding. Increased incidence of endometrial hyperplasia, polyps, and endometrial cancer. Headache, lethargy, and dizziness occur rarely. Visual disturbances, including cataract, retinopathy, and decreased visual acuity. Mild, transient leukopenia and thrombocytopenia occur rarely. Elevations in serum triglyceride levels. Mildly emetogenic protocol.

Chair time: No chair time. Daily dosing until disease progression.

Toremifene Citrate (Fareston)[1,72]

Pretreatment: CBC, Chem, LFTs, and CA 27-29. ER/PR testing, eye exam.

Toremifene citrate 60 mg: PO daily (60 mg tablets). Well absorbed after oral administration. Food does not interfere with absorption. Monitor INR closely in patients taking warfarin.

Side effects: Tumor flare reaction with bone and/or muscular pain, erythema, tumor pain, and transient increase in tumor size. Use with caution in the setting of brain and/or vertebral metastases. Toremifene is thrombogenic. Nausea and vomiting. Menstrual irregularity, hot flashes, sweating, milk production in breasts, vaginal discharge, and bleeding. Usually not severe enough to discontinue therapy. Hematologic: mild, transient leukopenia and thrombocytopenia rare. Increased risk of endometrial cancer. Cataract formation and xerophthalmia. Baseline and biannual eye exams are recommended. Rash alopecia and peripheral edema.

Chair time: No chair time. Daily dosing until disease progression.

Exemestane (Aromasin)[1,73]

Pretreatment: CBC, Chem, LFTs, and CA 27-29. ER/PR testing.
Exemestane 25 mg: PO daily. (25-mg tablet.) Take once daily after a meal.
Side effects: Hot flashes, increased sweating, and pain. Nausea, increased appetite, and weight gain. Depression and insomnia. Headache and fatigue. Mildly emetogenic protocol.
Chair time: No chair time. Daily until disease progression.

Anastrozole (Arimidex)[1,74]

Pretreatment: CBC, Chem, LFTs, and CA 27-29. ER/PR testing.
Anastrozole 1 mg: PO daily. (1-mg tablet.)
Take orally with or without food at approximately the same time daily.
Side effects: Hot flashes and vaginal dryness. Thrombophlebitis uncommon. Mild swelling of arms or legs. Nausea and vomiting. Mild constipation or diarrhea. Dry, scaling skin rash. Flu-like syndrome presents in the form of fever, malaise, and myalgias. Arthralgias involve hands, knees, hips, lower back, and shoulders. Early morning stiffness. Headaches are mild. Decreased energy and weakness. Mildly emetogenic protocol.
Chair time: No chair time. Daily dosing until disease progression.

Letrozole (Femara)[1,75]

Pretreatment: CBC, Chem, LFTs, and CA 27-29. ER/PR testing.
Letrozole 2.5 mg: PO daily. (2.5-mg tablets.)
Food does not interfere with oral absorption.
Side effects: Musculoskeletal pain (back, arms, legs) and arthralgias. Hot flashes. Thromboembolic events are rare. Chest pain reported in some patients. Nausea with vomiting and anorexia occurring less frequently. Mild constipation or diarrhea. Mild elevation in serum transaminase and serum bilirubin levels, especially with known metastatic disease in the liver. Headaches and fatigue are mild. Mildly emetogenic.
Chair time: No chair time. Daily dosing until disease progression.

Fulvestrant (Faslodex)[1,76]

Pretreatment: CBC, Chem, LFTs, and CA 27-29. ER/PR testing.
Fulvestrant 250 mg: IM on day 1. (250 mg per 5 mL and 125 mg per 2.5 mL prefilled syringes.) Administer slowly by IM injection (Z-track recommended) in one buttock (5 mL) or each buttock (2.5 mL).
Side effects: Back and bone pain, arthralgias. Hot flashes. Nausea, vomiting, and anorexia. Abdominal pain, constipation, and/or diarrhea. Mild headaches. Flu-like syndrome: fever, malaise, and myalgias. Injec-

tion site reactions with mild pain and inflammation that is usually transient. Dry, scaling skin rash. Mildly emetogenic protocol.
Chair time: Monthly injection until disease progression.

Megestrol (Megace)[1,77]

Pretreatment: CBC, Chem, LFTs, and CA 27-29. ER/PR testing.
Megestrol 40 mg: PO qid. (20- and 40-mg tablets.) 40 mg per mL suspension.
Side effects: Nausea and vomiting. Increased appetite with accompanying weight gain. Use with caution in patients with a history of either thromboembolic or hypercoagulable disorders. Increased incidence of thromboembolic events. Fluid retention. Hyperglycemia. Use with caution in patients with diabetes mellitus. Abnormal LFT results. Dose reduction with abnormal liver function. Breakthrough menstrual bleeding, hot flashes, sweating, and mood changes. Tumor flare reaction with bone and/or muscular pain, erythema, tumor pain, and transient increase in tumor size. Use with caution in the setting of brain and/or vertebral metastases. Mildly emetogenic protocol.
Chair time: No chair time. Daily dosing as tolerated or until progression.

Trastuzumab (Herceptin Weekly Dosing)[1,78]

Pretreatment: CBC, Chem, and CA 27-29; HER2 testing FISH (preferred) or IHC; MUGA scan. No premedication recommended. Mildly emetogenic.
Trastuzumab 4 mg/kg: IV in 250 cc of NS over 90-minute loading dose and then:
Trastuzumab 2 mg/kg: IV in 250 cc of NS over 30 minutes weekly.
Side effects: Infusion-related symptoms, fever, chills, urticaria, flushing, fatigue, headache, bronchospasm, dyspnea, angioedema, and hypotension. Usually mild to moderate in severity and seen most with initial dose. Nausea and vomiting and diarrhea, generally mild. Dyspnea, peripheral edema, and reduced left ventricular function. Increased risk when used in combination with anthracycline/cyclophosphamide regimen. Cardiac dysfunction reversible. Increased cough, dyspnea, rhinitis, sinusitis, pulmonary infiltrates, and/or pleural effusions.
Chair time: 2 hours on day 1 and 1 hour weekly thereafter. Weekly until progression.

Trastuzumab (Herceptin Every 3 Weeks)[1,79]

Pretreatment: CBC, Chem, and CEA. HER2 testing FISH (preferred) or IHC. MUGA scan. No premedication recommended. Mildly emetogenic.

Trastuzumab 8 mg/kg: IV in 250 cc of NS over 90-minute loading dose. (If patient has been on weekly trastuzumab without a break, loading dose is not necessary. Start with the 6m/kg dose.) Then:

Trastuzumab 6 mg/kg: IV in 250 cc of NS over 30 minutes every 3 weeks.

Side effects: Infusion related symptoms, fever, chills, urticaria, flushing, fatigue, headache, bronchospasm, dyspnea, angioedema, and hypotension. Usually mild to moderate in severity and seen most often with initial dose. Nausea and vomiting and diarrhea, generally mild. Dyspnea, peripheral edema, and reduced left ventricular function. Increased risk when used with anthracycline/cyclophosphamide regimen. Cardiac dysfunction reversible. Increased cough, dyspnea, rhinitis, sinusitis, pulmonary infiltrates, and/or pleural effusions.

Chair time: 2 hours on day 1 and 1 hour every 3 weeks thereafter. Repeat every 3 weeks until progression.

Capecitabine (Xeloda)[1,80]

Prechemo: CBC, Chem, bilirubin, LFTs, creatinine clearance, and CA 27-29. Oral phenothiazine or 5-HT$_3$. Mildly emetogenic.

Capecitabine 1250 mg/m²: PO bid for 2 weeks followed by a 1-week rest period. (Dose may be decreased to 850–1000 mg/m² PO bid on days 1–14, reducing the risk of toxicity without compromising efficacy). 150- and 500-mg tablets. Take within 30 minutes of a meal with plenty of water. Monitor INRs closely when taking warfarin; may increase INR.

Side effects: Myelosuppression. Nausea and vomiting, diarrhea. Hand-foot syndrome with tingling, numbness, pain, erythema, dryness, rash, swelling, increased pigmentation, and/or pruritus of the hands and feet. Blepharitis, tear-duct stenosis, and acute and chronic conjunctivitis. Elevations in serum bilirubin alkaline phosphatase and hepatic transaminases levels. Dose modifications if hyperbilirubinemia occurs. Capecitabine contraindicated with baseline creatinine clearance <30 mL/min. Dose reduction to 75% of capecitabine with baseline creatinine clearance of 30–50 mL/min.

Chair time: No chair time. Repeat cycle every 21 days until disease progression.

Docetaxel[1,81,82]

Prechemo: CBC, Chem, LFTs, and CA 27-29. Dexamethasone 8 mg bid day before, day of, and day after treatment. 5-HT$_3$ and 10- to 20-mg dexamethasone. Mildly to moderately emetogenic.

Docetaxel 100 mg/m²: IV in 2500 cc NS on day 1. Repeat cycle every 21 days.

OR

Docetaxel 35–40 mg/m^2: IV in 2500 cc NS weekly for 6 weeks. Repeat every 8 weeks. Use non-PVC containers and tubing.

Side effects: Hypersensitivity reactions. Myelosuppression. G-CSF recommended. Nausea and vomiting. Mucositis and diarrhea. Peripheral neuropathy with paresthesias. Fluid retention with weight gain, peripheral and/or generalized edema, pleural effusion, and ascites. Alopecia. Nail changes, rash, and dry, pruritic skin. Hand-foot syndrome.

Chair time: 2 hours on day 1. Repeat every 21 days for 8 weeks.

OR

Weekly for 6 weeks, repeat cycle every 8 weeks.

Paclitaxel[1,83,84]

Prechemo: CBC, Chem, Mg^{2+}, and CA 27-29. 5-HT$_3$ and dexamethasone 10–20 mg. Diphenhydramine 25–50 mg and H$_2$ antagonist. Mildly emetogenic.

Paclitaxel 175 mg/m^2: IV in 500 cc NS over 3 hours on day 1. Repeat cycle every 21 days.

OR

Paclitaxel 80–100 mg/m^2: IV in 500 cc NS weekly for 3 weeks. Repeat cycle every 4 weeks. Use non-PVC containers and tubing with 0.22-micron inline filter.

Side effects: Hypersensitivity reaction. Myelosuppression. Dose-limiting G-CSF recommended. Nausea and vomiting. Stomatitis. Sensory neuropathy with numbness and paresthesias, dose related. Arthralgias and myalgias. Transient elevations in serum transaminases, bilirubin, and alkaline phosphatase. Alopecia.

Chair time: 4 hours on day 1. Repeat every 21 days until progression.

OR

2 hours on day 1 for 3 weeks. Repeat every 4 weeks until progression.

Vinorelbine[1,85]

Prechemo: CBC, Chem, and CA 27-29. Oral phenothiazine or 5-HT$_3$. Mildly emetogenic.

Vinorelbine 30 mg/m^2: IV push on day 1. Dilute in syringe or IV bag to concentration of 1.5–3.0 mg/ml. Vesicant.

Side effects: Myelosuppression. Nausea and vomiting are mild. Stomatitis, constipation, diarrhea, and anorexia. Reduce by 50% if total bilirubin 2.1–3.0 mg/dL. If total bilirubin >3.0 mg/dL, reduce by 75%. Alopecia. Mild to moderate neuropathy with paresthesias.

Chair time: 1 hour on day 1. Repeat cycle weekly until progression.

Doxorubicin[1,86]

Prechemo: CBC, Chem, and CA 27-29. MUGA scan. 5-HT_3 and dexamethasone 10–20 mg. Mildly to moderately emetogenic.

Doxorubicin 20 mg/m^2: IV push on day 1 weekly. Potent vesicant.

Side effects: Myelosuppression may be severe. Nausea and vomiting. Dose reduce with liver dysfunction. Pericarditis-myocarditis syndrome. With cumulative doses >550 mg/m^2 of doxorubicin, cardiomyopathy. Red-orange discoloration of urine. Hyperpigmentation, photosensitivity, and radiation recall occur. Complete alopecia occurs with doses 50 mg/m^2.

Chair time: 1 hour on day 1. Repeat cycle weekly until progression.

Gemcitabine[1,87]

Prechemo: CBC, Chem, CA 27-29, and LFTs. Oral phenothiazine
OR
5-HT_3 and dexamethasone 10 mg. Mild to moderately emetogenic.

Gemcitabine 725 mg/m^2: IV over 30 minutes weekly for 3 weeks.

Side effects: Myelosuppression dose-limiting, with grades 3 and 4 thrombocytopenia more common in older patients. Nausea and vomiting, diarrhea, mucositis. Flu-like syndrome. Mild dyspnea and drug-induced pneumonitis. Transient elevation of serum transaminases and bilirubin. Pruritic, maculopapular skin rash, usually involving trunk and extremities. Edema. Alopecia is rare.

Chair time: 1 hour weekly for 3 weeks. Repeat cycle every 28 days.

Liposomal Doxorubicin (Doxil)[1,88]

Prechemo: CBC, Chem, and CA 27-29. MUGA scan. 5-HT_3 and dexamethasone 10–20 mg. Mild to moderately emetogenic.

Liposomal doxorubicin 45–60 mg/m^2: IV diluted in D5W on day 1.

Side effects: Infusion reaction: flushing, dyspnea, facial swelling, headache, back pain, tightness in the chest and throat, and/or hypotension. Myelosuppression, limiting. Nausea and vomiting. Stomatitis. Pericarditis-myocarditis syndrome. Cumulative doses >550 mg/m^2 of doxorubicin liposomal may cause cardiomyopathy. Red-orange discoloration of urine. Hand-foot syndrome with skin rash, swelling, erythema, pain, and /or desquamation. Hyperpigmentation of nails, skin rash, urticaria, and radiation recall occur. Alopecia.

Chair time: 2 hours on day 1. Repeat every 21–28 days until progression.

Paclitaxel Protein-Bound Particles for Injectable Suspension (Abraxane)[89,90]

Prechemo: CBC, Chem, and CA 27-29. 5-HT3 in 100 cc of NS.

Paclitaxel protein-bound particles for injectable suspension 260 mg/m^2: IV over 30 minutes every 3 weeks.

OR

Paclitaxel protein-bound particles for injectable suspension 100 mg/m^2: IV over 30 minutes weekly for 3 weeks or weekly.

Side effects: Hypersensitivity reactions rare. Myelosuppression, dose-limiting toxicity. Sensory neuropathy occurs frequently and is a cumulative effect. If grade 3 sensory neuropathy develops, hold until resolution to grade 1 or 2 followed by a dose reduction. Symptoms improve in about 22 days. Musculoskeletal: arthralgias/myalgias common. Nausea, vomiting, and diarrhea. Mucositis. Alopecia.

Chair time: 1 hour on day 1. Repeat every 21 days until progression.

OR

1 hour on day 1 for 3 weeks or weekly. Repeat cycle every 4 weeks.

Ixabepilone (Ixempra)[68]

Prechemo: CBC, Chem, bilirubin, LFTs, and CA 27-29. 5-HT$_3$ and dexamethasone. Diphenhydramine 25–50 mg and H$_2$ antagonist.

Ixabepilone 40 mg/m^2: IV over 3 hours on day 1.

Further dilute in lactated ringers to a final concentration of 0.2–0.6 mg/mL. 250-mL bag is usually sufficient. Use DEHP-free containers and tubing with 0.2–1.2 micron inline filter.

Side effects: Patients with a history of a severe hypersensitivity reaction to agents containing Cremophor EL or its derivatives should not be treated with Ixempra. Hypersensitivity reactions (flushing, rash, dyspnea, and bronchospasm). Myelosuppression dose dependent. Nausea, vomiting, diarrhea, stomatitis/mucositis, and anorexia common. Constipation, abdominal pain, and taste alterations. Nausea, vomiting, diarrhea, stomatitis/mucositis, and anorexia common. Peripheral neuropathy (burning sensation, hyperesthesia, paresthesia, discomfort, or neuropathic pain). Myalgias and arthralgias, fatigue and asthenias. CYP3A4 inhibitors should be avoided. Grapefruit juice may also increase plasma concentrations. Use with caution with history of cardiac disease. Discontinuation should be considered if cardiac ischemia or impaired cardiac function occurs. Alopecia.

Chair time: 4 hours on day 1. Repeat every 21 days as tolerated or until progression.

CANCER OF UNKNOWN PRIMARY

Paclitaxel + Carboplatin + Etoposide (PCE)[1,91]

Prechemo: CBC, Chem, Mg^{2+}. 5-HT$_3$ and dexamethasone 10–20 mg day 1. Diphenhydramine 25–50 mg and H$_2$ antagonist day 1. Oral phenothiazine or 5-HT$_3$ 30–60 minutes before etoposide on days 2–10. Mildly to moderately emetogenic.

Paclitaxel 200 mg/m²: IV in 2500 cc NS over 1 hour on day 1. Use non-PVC containers and tubing with 0.22-micron inline filter.

Carboplatin AUC 6: IV in 500 cc NS on day 1. Give carboplatin after paclitaxel to decrease toxicities.

Etoposide 50 mg alternating with 100 mg: PO days 1–10. (50- and 100-mg capsules.) Should be stored in the refrigerator.

Side effects: Hypersensitivity reaction paclitaxel and carboplatin: increased risk of hypersensitivity reactions in patients receiving more than seven courses of carboplatin therapy. Myelosuppression dose-limiting. G-CSF recommended. Nausea and vomiting may be acute or delayed. Oral etoposide has higher incidence of nausea/vomiting. Mucositis and/or diarrhea. Transient elevations in serum transaminases, bilirubin, and alkaline phosphatase. Electrolyte imbalance: decreases Mg^{2+}, K^+, Ca^{2+}, and Na^+. Sensory neuropathy with numbness and paresthesias, dose related and dose-limiting. Alopecia.

Chair time: 5 hours on day 1. Repeat every 21 days until progression.

Etoposide + Cisplatin (EP)[1,92]

Prechemo: CBC, Chem, Mg^{2+}. 5-HT$_3$ and dexamethasone 10–20 mg. Mild to moderately emetogenic.

Etoposide 100 mg/m²: IV in 2500 cc NS on days 1–5.

Cisplatin 100 mg/m²: IV in 500–1000 cc NS on day 1.

Side effects: Hypersensitivity reaction. Myelosuppression, dose-limiting toxicity. Nausea and vomiting, acute or delayed. Mucositis and diarrhea are rare. Metallic taste and anorexia. Nephrotoxicity dose related with cisplatin. Decreases Mg^{2+}, K^+, Ca^{2+}, and Na^+. SIADH. Peripheral sensory neuropathy with paresthesias and numbness. Ototoxicity. Alopecia.

Chair time: 3 hours on day 1 and 1 hour on days 2–5. Repeat cycle every 21 days.

Cisplatin + Etoposide + Bleomycin (PEB)[1,93]

Prechemo: CBC, Chem, Mg^{2+}. Baseline pulmonary function tests, chest x-ray before each cycle of therapy. 5-HT_3 and dexamethasone 10–20 mg. Acetaminophen 30 minutes before Bleomycin. Mildly to moderately emetogenic.

Cisplatin 20 mg/m²: IV in 500–1000 cc NS on days 1–5.

Etoposide 100 mg/m²: IV in 250 cc NS on days 1–5.

Bleomycin 30 units: IV on days 1, 8, and 15. Test dose of 2 units is recommended before first dose to detect hypersensitivity.

Side effects: Hypersensitivity reaction. Myelosuppression, dose-limiting. Nausea and vomiting, acute or delayed. Mucositis and diarrhea are rare. Metallic taste and anorexia. Pulmonary toxicity is dose-limiting in bleomycin. Usually presents as pneumonitis with cough, dyspnea, dry inspiratory crackles, and infiltrates on CXR. Nephrotoxicity is dose related with cisplatin. Decreases Mg^{2+}, K^+, Ca^{2+}, and Na^+. SIADH. Peripheral sensory neuropathy. Paresthesias and numbness. Ototoxicity. Alopecia.

Chair time: 4 hours on day 1, 1 hour on days 2–5, 8, and 15. Repeat every 21 days.

Gemcitabine + Carboplatin + Paclitaxel (GCP)[1,94]

Prechemo: CBC, Chem, Mg^{2+}, LFTs. 5-HT_3 and dexamethasone 10–20 mg. Diphenhydramine 25–50 mg H_2 antagonist. Mildly to moderately emetogenic.

Gemcitabine 1000 mg/m²: IV in 250 cc NS on days 1 and 8.

Carboplatin AUC 5: IV in 500 cc NS on day 1. Give carboplatin after paclitaxel to decrease toxicities.

Paclitaxel 200 mg/m²: IV in 500 cc NS over 3 hours on day 1.

Repeat cycle every 21 days for four cycles. Followed by:

Paclitaxel 70 mg/m²: IV in 250 cc NS over 1 hour on day 1 every week for 6 weeks with a 2-week rest. Repeat for a total of three cycles.

Use non-PVC containers and tubing with 0.22-micron inline filter.

Side effects: Hypersensitivity reaction with paclitaxel or carboplatin. Increased risk of hypersensitivity reactions in patients receiving more than seven courses of carboplatin therapy. Myelosuppression is cumulative, dose related and dose-limiting. G-CSF recommended. Nausea and vomiting, acute or delayed. Mucositis and diarrhea. Transient elevation of serum transaminase and bilirubin levels. Flu-like syndrome: fever, malaise, chills, headache, and myalgias. Decreases Mg^{2+}, K^+, Ca^{2+}, and Na^+. SIADH. Sensory neuropathy with numbness and paresthesias; dose related and can be dose-limiting. Pruritic, maculopapular skin rash, usually involving trunk and extremities. Edema. Alopecia.

Chair time: 5 hours on day 1 and 1 hour on day 8. Repeat every 21 days for four cycles. Then, 2 hours weekly for 6 weeks. Repeat every 8 weeks for three cycles.

CARCINOID TUMORS

COMBINATION REGIMENS

5-Fluorouracil + Streptozocin[1,95]

Prechemo: CBC, Chem, creatinine clearance. 5-HT$_3$ and dexamethasone 10–20 mg. Moderately to highly emetogenic.

Fluorouracil 400 mg/m²/day: IV push on days 1–5.

Streptozocin 500 mg/m²/day: IV over 1 hour days 1–5. Omit if creatinine clearance <60 mL/min. Give 1–2 L of hydration to avoid renal toxicity. Irritant.

Side effects: Renal dysfunction, dose-limiting with streptozocin. Myelosuppression mild. Nausea and vomiting. Hyperpigmentation, photosensitivity, and nail changes. Hand-foot syndrome, dose-limiting. Hypoglycemia or hyperglycemia. Photophobia, increased lacrimation, conjunctivitis, and blurred vision.

Chair time: 3 hours on days 1–5. Repeat cycle every 6 weeks.

Doxorubicin + Streptozocin[1,95]

Prechemo: CBC, Chem, CA 19-9, creatinine clearance. MUGA scan. 5-HT$_3$ and dexamethasone 10–20 mg. Moderately to highly emetogenic.

Doxorubicin 50 mg/m²: IV push on days 1 and 22. Potent vesicant.

Streptozocin 500 mg/m²/day: IV days 1–5. Omit if creatinine clearance <60 mL/min. Give with 1–2 liters of hydration to avoid renal toxicity. Irritant.

Side effects: Myelosuppression may be severe. Renal toxicity is dose-limiting with streptozocin. Nausea and vomiting. Stomatitis occurs in 10% of patients not dose-limiting. Pericarditis-myocarditis syndrome may occur acutely. Cumulative doses > 450 mg/m²of doxorubicin, cardiomyopathy. Hyperpigmentation, photosensitivity, and radiation recall. Alopecia. Hypoglycemia or hyperglycemia.

Chair time: 3 hours on days 1–5 and 1 hour on day 22. Repeat cycle every 6 weeks.

Cisplatin + Etoposide[1,96]

Prechemo: CBC, Chem, Mg^{2+}, central line placement. 5-HT_3 and dexamethasone 10–20 mg. Moderately to highly emetogenic.

Etoposide 130 mg/m²/day: IV continuous infusion on days 1–3.

Cisplatin 45 mg/m²/day: IV continuous infusion on days 2 and 3.

Side effects: Allergic reaction during rapid infusion of etoposide. Myelosuppression, dose-limiting. Nausea and vomiting, acute or delayed. Nephrotoxicity dose related. Decreases Mg^{2+}, K^+, Ca^{++}, Na^+, and P. Peripheral sensory. High-frequency hearing loss and tinnitus. Alopecia.

Chair time: 1 hour on days 1–3. Discontinue pump day 4. Repeat cycle every 21 days.

SINGLE-AGENT REGIMENS

Octreotide or Sandostatin LAR Depot (Octreotide Acetate Injectable Suspension)[1,97-99]

Prechemo: CBC, Chem, LFTs, thyroid function tests, 5-HIAA (urinary 5-hydroxyindole acetic acid). 5-HT_3 and dexamethasone 10–20 mg in 100 cc of NS. Mildly emetogenic.

Octreotide 150–250 mcg SC TID.

May change to long-acting depot if condition is already controlled on immediate-release preparation or after response to 2 weeks of immediate-release dosing.

OR

Sandostatin LAR 20–30 mg: IM 2-track method in gluteal muscle once per month.

Side effects: Transient hypoglycemia or hyperglycemia. Hypothyroidism. Nausea, vomiting, diarrhea, flatulence, and abdominal pain or discomfort. Rarely, lightheadedness, dizziness, fatigue, pedal edema, headache, facial flushing weakness. Pain at injection site with Sandostatin LAR depot.

Chair time: No chair time. Self administration of injections TID as tolerated. Sandostatin LAR, every 4-week appointments for IM injection.

CERVICAL CANCER

COMBINATION REGIMENS

Cisplatin + Radiation Therapy[1,100]

Prechemo: CBC, Chem, Mg^{2+}. 5-HT_3 and dexamethasone 10–20 mg. Moderately to highly emetogenic.

Radiation therapy: 1.8 to 2 cGy per fraction (total dose, 45 cGy).

Cisplatin 40 mg/m²: IV day 1 weekly (maximal dose is 70 mg/wk). Given 4 hours before radiation therapy on weeks 1–6.

Side effects: Myelosuppression. Nausea and vomiting, acute or delayed. Diarrhea can be severe. Nephrotoxicity dose related. Vigorous hydration before and after treatment required. Decreases Mg^{2+}, K^+, Ca^{2+}, Na^+, and P. Local tissue irritation progressing to desquamation can occur in radiation field. Do not use oil-based lotions or creams in radiation field. Alopecia. Peripheral sensory neuropathy, increased risk with cumulative doses. High-frequency hearing loss and tinnitus.

Chair time: 1–4 hours day 1 weekly for 6 weeks. May need more visits if patient needs hydration for nausea and vomiting.

Paclitaxel + Cisplatin[1,101]

Prechemo: CBC, Chem, Mg^{2+}. Central line placement. 5-HT_3 and dexamethasone 10–20 mg days 1 and 2. Diphenhydramine 25–50 mg and HT_2 antagonist (day 1 only). Moderately to highly emetogenic.

Paclitaxel 135 mg/m²: IV over 24 hours on day 1. Use non-PVC containers and tubing with 0.22-micron inline filter.

Cisplatin 75 mg/m²: IV in 1000 cc NS on day 2.

Side effects: Hypersensitivity reaction. Myelosuppression dose-limiting. G-CSF recommended. Nausea and vomiting, acute or delayed. Nephrotoxicity dose related. Decreases Mg^{2+}, K^+, Ca^{2+}, Na^+, and P. Sensory neuropathy with numbness and paresthesias, dose related. Alopecia.

Chair time: 1 hour on day 1 and 3 hours on day 2. Repeat every 21 days as tolerated or until progression.

Cisplatin + Topotecan[1,102]

Prechemo: CBC, Chem, Mg^{2+}. 5-HT$_3$ and dexamethasone 10–20 mg. Moderately to highly emetogenic.

Cisplatin 50 mg/m²: IV in 500–1000 cc NS over 1–3 hours on day 1.

Topotecan 0.75 mg/m²/day: IV in 100 cc NS on days 1–3.

Side effects: Myelosuppression dose-limiting. G-CSF recommended. Nausea and vomiting, acute or delayed. Diarrhea or constipation, abdominal pain. Dose reduce in patients with low protein and hepatic and renal dysfunction. Decreases Mg^{2+}, K^+, Ca^{2+}, Na^+, and P. Peripheral sensory neuropathy, paresthesias, and numbness—dose-limiting. High-frequency hearing loss and tinnitus. Alopecia.

Chair time: 3 hours on day 1 and 1 hour on days 2 and 3. Repeat cycle every 21 days.

Bleomycin + Ifosfamide + Mesna + Cisplatin (BIP)[1,103]

Prechemo: CBC, Chem, Mg^{2+}. Central line placement, pulmonary function tests (PFTs), chest x-ray study (CXR). 5-HT$_3$ and dexamethasone 10–20 mg. Acetaminophen 325–500 mg² PO before bleomycin. Moderately to highly emetogenic.

Bleomycin 30 units: IV over 24 hours on day 1. Test dose of 2 units SC or IM.

Ifosfamide 5000 mg/m²: IV over 24 hours on day 2.

Mesna 6000 mg/m²: IV over 36 hours on day 2.

Cisplatin 50 mg/m²: IV in 500–1000 cc NS infusion on day 2.

Side effects: Hypersensitivity reaction: Myelosuppression cumulative and dose-limiting. Nausea and vomiting acute or delayed. Mucositis and/or diarrhea. Pneumonitis with cough, rales, dyspnea, and infiltrates on CXR. Nephrotoxicity and/or hemorrhagic cystitis dose-limiting. Decreases Mg^{2+}, K^+, Ca^{2+}, Na^+, and P. Sensory neuropathy with numbness and paresthesias. Somnolence, confusion, depressive psychosis, or hallucinations (higher in patients with decreased renal function). Erythema, rash, striae, hyperpigmentation, vesiculation, hyperkeratosis, nail changes, skin peeling, macular rash, and urticaria. Alopecia.

Chair time: 1 hour on day 1 and 3 hours on day 2. Repeat cycle every 21 days.

Bleomycin + Ifosfamide + Mesna + Carboplatin (BIC)[1,104]

Prechemo: CBC, Chem, Mg^{2+}. Central line placement, pulmonary function tests (PFTs), chest x-ray study (CXR). 5-HT$_3$ and dexamethasone

10–20 mg. Acetaminophen 325–500 mg PO before Bleomycin. Moderately to highly emetogenic.

Bleomycin 30 units: IV over 10 minutes on day 1. Test dose of 2 units SC or IM.

Ifosfamide 2000 mg/m^2: IV in 1000 cc NS on days 1–3.

Mesna 400 mg/m^2: IV in 100 cc NS 15 minutes before and 4 and 8 hours after ifosfamide.

Carboplatin 200 mg/m^2: IV in 500 cc NS infusion over 30–60 minutes on day 1.

Side effects: Hypersensitivity reaction with bleomycin. Increased risk of hypersensitivity with carboplatin after seven doses. Myelosuppression cumulative and dose-limiting. Nausea and vomiting acute or delayed. Mild diarrhea. Pneumonitis with cough, rales, dyspnea, and infiltrates on CXR. Increased incidence in patients older than 70 years and with cumulative doses, 400 units. Nephrotoxicity and/or hemorrhagic cystitis. Decreases Mg^{2+}, K^+, Ca^{2+}, Na^+, and P. Sensory neuropathy with numbness. Somnolence, confusion, depressive psychosis, or hallucinations. Incidence higher with decreased renal function. Erythema, rash, striae, hyperpigmentation, vesiculation, hyperkeratosis, nail changes, skin peeling, macular rash, urticaria. Alopecia.

Chair time: 4 hours on day 1, 3 hours on days 2 and 3. Repeat every 21 days.

Cisplatin + 5-Fluorouracil[1,105]

Prechemo: CBC, Chem, Mg^{2+}. Central line placement. 5-HT$_3$ and dexamethasone 10–20 mg. Moderately to highly emetogenic.

Cisplatin 75 mg/m^2: IV in 1000 cc NS infusion on day 1.

5-Fluorouracil 1000 mg/m^2/day: IV continuous infusion days 2–5.

Side effects: Myelosuppression, dose related. Nausea and vomiting, acute or delayed. Mucositis and diarrhea, dose-limiting. Nephrotoxicity is dose related. Decreases Mg^{2+}, K^+, Ca^{2+}, Na^+, and P. Hyperpigmentation, photosensitivity, and nail changes may occur. Hand-foot syndrome dose-limiting. Photophobia, increased lacrimation, conjunctivitis, and blurred vision.

Chair time: 3 hours on day 1 and 1 hour on day 2. Repeat cycle every 21 days.

Cisplatin + Vinorelbine[1,106]

Prechemo: CBC, Chem, Mg^{2+}. 5-HT$_3$ and dexamethasone 10–20 mg. Moderately to highly emetogenic.

Cisplatin 80 mg/m^2: IV in 1000 cc NS on day 1.

Vinorelbine 25 mg/m²: IV push on days 1 and 8. Vesicant. Further dilute in syringe or IV bag to concentration of 1.5–3.0 mg/mL. Flush vein with at least 75–125 mL of IV fluid after drug infusion.

Side effects: Myelosuppression dose-limiting. Nausea and vomiting, acute or delayed. Constipation, diarrhea, stomatitis, and anorexia. Nephrotoxicity dose related. Decreases Mg^{2+}, K^+, Ca^{2+}, Na^+, and P. Alopecia. Jaw pain, myalgias, and arthralgias. Dyspnea and hypersensitivity reaction. Mild paresthesias.

Chair time: 3 hours on day 1 and 1 hour on day 8. Repeat cycle every 21 days.

Cisplatin + Irinotecan[1,107]

Prechemo: CBC, Chem, Mg^{2+}. 5-HT$_3$ and dexamethasone 10–20 mg. Atropine 0.25–1.0 mg IV unless contraindicated. Moderately to highly emetogenic.

Cisplatin 60 mg/m²: IV in 500–1000 cc NS over 1–3 hours on day 1.

Irinotecan 60 mg/m²: IV in 250–500 cc D5W on days 1, 8, and 15.

Side effects: Myelosuppression can be severe, dose-limiting toxicity. G-CSF recommended. Nausea and vomiting, acute or delayed. Diarrhea or constipation. Abdominal pain. Early diarrhea, managed with atropine before administration of irinotecan. Late diarrhea severe and should be treated aggressively. Consider Lomotil, Imodium, tincture of opium, and hydration. Dose reduce patients with low protein and hepatic and/or renal dysfunction. Decreases Mg^{2+}, K^+, Ca^{2+}, Na^+, and P. Peripheral sensory neuropathy, dose-limiting. Paresthesias and numbness. High-frequency hearing loss and tinnitus. Alopecia.

Chair time: 4 hours on day 1, 2 hours on days 8 and 15. Repeat every 28 days.

Mitomycin + Vincristine + Bleomycin + Cisplatin (MOBP)[1,108]

Prechemo: CBC, Chem, Mg^{2+}. Pulmonary function tests (PFTs), chest x-ray study (CXR). 5-HT$_3$ and dexamethasone 10–20 mg. Acetaminophen 325–500 mg PO before bleomycin. Moderately to highly emetogeni**Mitomycin 10 mg/m²:** IV push on day 1. Potent vesicant.

Vincristine 1 mg/m²: IV push on days 1, 8, 22, and 29. Not to exceed 2 mg. Vesicant.

Bleomycin 10 units: IV on days 1, 8, 15, and 22. Test dose of 2 units before the first dose to detect hypersensitivity.

Cisplatin 50 mg/m²: IV in 500–1000 cc NS on days 1 and 22.

Side effects: Allergic reaction: bleomycin. Myelosuppression, dose-limiting. Nausea and vomiting, acute or delayed. Mucositis is common. Constipation, abdominal pain, and paralytic ileus may occur with vincristine. Interstitial pneumonitis with bleomycin and mitomycin cough, dyspnea, pneumonia, pulmonary infiltrates on CXR. Nephrotoxicity secondary to cisplatin. Hemolytic-uremic syndrome, creatinine. Decreases Mg^{2+}, K^+, Ca^{2+}, Na^+, and P. Peripheral sensory neuropathy, dose-limiting. Alopecia, skin rash.

Chair time: 3 hours on day 1, 1 hour on days 8 and 15, and 3 hours on day 22. Repeat every 6 weeks.

SINGLE-AGENT REGIMENS

Cisplatin[1,109]

Prechemo: CBC, Chem, creatinine clearance. 5-HT$_3$ and dexamethasone 10–20 mg. Moderately to highly emetogenic.

Cisplatin 50–100 mg/m²: IV in 500–1000 cc NS over 1–3 hours on day 1.

Side effects: Myelosuppression can be severe and dose-limiting. Nausea and vomiting acute or delayed. Metallic taste to foods. Nephrotoxicity is dose related. Dose reduce with abnormal renal function. Decreases Mg^{2+}, K^+, Ca^{2+}, Na^+, and P. Peripheral sensory neuropathy, paresthesias and numbness, dose-limiting. High-frequency hearing loss and tinnitus. Alopecia.

Chair time: 3 hours on day 1. Repeat cycle every 21 days.

Docetaxel[1,110]

Prechemo: CBC, Chem, Mg^{2+}. Dexamethasone 8 mg PO bid day before, day of, and day after treatment. 5-HT$_3$ and dexamethasone 10–20 mg in 100 cc of NS. Moderately to highly emetogenic.

Docetaxel 100 mg/m²: IV in 250 cc NS on day 1. Use non-PVC containers and tubing.

Side effects: Hypersensitivity reactions. Myelosuppression. Nausea and vomiting. Mucositis and diarrhea. Peripheral neuropathy with sensory alterations and paresthesias. Weight gain, peripheral and/or generalized edema, pleural effusion, and ascites. Alopecia. Nail changes, rash, dry and pruritic skin. Hand-foot syndrome.

Chair time: 2 hours on day 1. Repeat cycle every 21 days.

Paclitaxel[1,111]

Prechemo: CBC, Chem, 5-HT$_3$, and dexamethasone 10–20 mg diphenhydramine 25–50 mg and H$_2$ antagonist. Mildly emetogenic.

Paclitaxel 175 mg/m²: IV in 500 cc NS over 3 hours on day 1. Use non-PVC containers and tubing with 0.22-micron inline filter.

Side effects: Hypersensitivity-reaction. Myelosuppression dose-limiting G-CSF recommended. Sensory neuropathy with numbness and paresthesias, dose related. Arthralgias and myalgias. Alopecia.

Chair time: 4–5 hours on day 1. Repeat cycle every 21 days as tolerated or until progression.

Irinotecan (weekly)[1,112]

Prechemo: CBC, Chem, 5-HT$_3$, and dexamethasone 10–20 mg in 100 cc of NS. Atropine 0.25–1.0 mg IV unless contraindicated. Moderately to highly emetogenic.

Irinotecan 125 mg/m^2: IV in 500 cc of D5W over 90 minutes.

Side effects: Early diarrhea can be managed with atropine before therapy. Late diarrhea can be severe and should be treated aggressively. Consider Lomotil, Imodium, tincture of opium, and hydration. Nausea and vomiting. Myelosuppression dose-limiting. G-CSF recommended. Alopecia.

Chair time: 3 hours weekly for 4 weeks. Additional days for hydration if patient has diarrhea. Repeat cycle every 6 weeks.

Vinorelbine[1,113]

Prechemo: CBC, Chem, LFTs. Oral phenothiazine or 5-HT$_3$ or 5-HT$_3$ and dexamethasone 10–20 mg. Mild to moderately emetogenic.

Vinorelbine 30 mg/m^2: IV weekly. Vesicant. Further dilute in syringe or IV bag to concentration of 1.5–3.0 mg/mL. Infuse over 6–10 minutes into sidearm port of free-flowing IV infusion. Use port closest to the IV bag, not to the patient. Flush vein with at least 75–125 mL of IV fluid after drug infusion.

Side effects: Myelosuppression, which can be severe. Nausea and vomiting. Stomatitis. Constipation, diarrhea, and anorexia. Alopecia. Mild to moderated paresthesias.

Chair time: 1 hour weekly. Repeat cycle weekly up to 12 cycles, to be followed by surgery or radiation.

Topotecan[1,114]

Prechemo: CBC, Chem, LFTs. 5-HT$_3$ and dexamethasone 10–20 mg. Mild to moderately emetogenic.

Topotecan 1.5 mg/m^2/day: IV in 100 cc NS days 1–5.

Side effects: Myelosuppression, dose-limiting. G-CSF recommended. Nausea and vomiting. Diarrhea, constipation, abdominal pain. Dose reduce with low protein and hepatic and renal dysfunction. Alopecia.

Chair time: 1 hour on days 1–5. Repeat every 21 days until progression.

COLORECTAL CANCER

NEOADJUVANT COMBINED MODALITY THERAPY

COMBINATION REGIMENS

5-Fluorouracil + Radiation Therapy (German AIO Regimen)[1,115]

Prechemo: CBC, Chem, CEA, LFTs. Central line placement. Oral phenothiazine or 5-HT$_3$ or 5-HT$_3$ and dexamethasone 10–20 mg. Mild to moderately emetogenic.

Fluorouracil 1000 mg/m^2/day: IV continuous infusion on days 1–5, weeks 1 and 5.

Radiation 180 cGy/day: 5 days per week (total dose 5040 cGy), followed by surgical resection and then adjuvant chemotherapy as follows:

5-FU 500 mg/m^2/day: IV for 5 days every 28 days for a total of four cycles.

Side effects: Myelosuppression, dose-limiting. Nausea and vomiting. Mucositis and diarrhea can be severe and dose-limiting. Local tissue irritation progressing to desquamation in radiation field can occur. Do not use oil-based lotions or creams in radiation field. Hyperpigmentation, photosensitivity, and nail changes may occur. Hand-foot syndrome can be dose-limiting. Photophobia, increased lacrimation, conjunctivitis, and blurred vision.

Chair time: 1 hour on day 1 & 5 weeks 1 and 5. During adjuvant therapy, 1 hour days 1 & 5, repeat every 28 days for four cycles.

Capecitabine + Radiation Therapy[1,116]

Prechemo: CBC, Chem, LFTs, CEA, creatinine clearance. Oral phenothiazine or 5-HT$_3$ or 5-HT$_3$ and dexamethasone 10–20 mg. Mild to moderately emetogenic.

Capecitabine 825 mg/m²: PO bid throughout the entire course of radiation therapy.

OR

Capecitabine 900–1000 mg/m²: PO bid on days 1–5 of each week of radiation therapy. Administer within 30 minutes of a meal with plenty of water. 150- and 500-mg tablets. Monitor INRs closely in patients taking warfarin, as may increase INR. Mildly to moderately emetogenic.

Radiation 180 cGy/day: 5 days per week (total dose 5040 cGy), followed by surgical resection and then adjuvant chemotherapy with 5-FU or 5-FU/LV for a total of four cycles.

Side effects: Nausea and vomiting. Diarrhea. Stomatitis can be severe. Local tissue irritation progressing to desquamation in radiation field. Do not use oil-based lotions or creams in radiation field. Hand-foot syndrome with tingling, numbness, pain, erythema, dryness, rash, swelling, increased pigmentation, and/or pruritus. Discontinue capecitabine at first sign of hand-foot syndrome. Contraindicated with creatinine clearance, 30 mL/min, dose reduce with creatinine clearance of 30–50 mL/min at baseline a dose reduction to 75. Blepharitis, tear-duct stenosis, acute and chronic conjunctivitis. Elevations in serum bilirubin alkaline phosphatase, and hepatic transaminase (SGOT, SGPT) levels. Dose reduce with hyperbilirubinemia.

ADJUVANT THERAPY

5-Fluorouracil + Leucovorin (Mayo Clinic Regimen)[1,117]

Prechemo: CBC, Chem, LFTs, CEA. Oral phenothiazine or 5-HT$_3$; or 5-HT$_3$ and dexamethasone 10–20 mg. Mild to moderately emetogenic.

Leucovorin 20 mg/m²/day: IV bolus on days 1–5. Administer before 5-FU.

5-Fluorouracil 425 mg/m²/day: IV push days 1–5.

Side effects: Myelosuppression dose related, dose-limiting. Nausea and vomiting. Mucositis and diarrhea can be severe and dose-limiting. Alopecia. Hyperpigmentation, photosensitivity, and nail changes may occur. Hand-foot syndrome with tingling, numbness, erythema, dryness, rash, swelling, or increased pigmentation of hands and/or feet can be dose-limiting. Photophobia, increased lacrimation, conjunctivitis, and blurred vision.

Chair time: 1 hour on days 1–5. Repeat cycle every 4–6 weeks for six cycles.

5-Fluorouracil + Leucovorin (Weekly Schedule/ High Dose)[1,118]

Prechemo: CBC, Chem, LFTs, CEA. Oral phenothiazine or 5-HT$_3$; or 5-HT$_3$ and dexamethasone 10–20 mg. Mildly to moderately emetogenic.
Leucovorin 500 mg/m^2: IV over 2 hours, weekly for 6 weeks. Give before 5-FU.
5-Fluorouracil 500 mg/m^2: IV push weekly for 6 weeks.
Side effects: Myelosuppression dose related, dose-limiting. Nausea and vomiting. Mucositis and diarrhea can be severe and dose-limiting. Alopecia. Hyperpigmentation, photosensitivity, and nail changes. Hand-foot syndrome characterized by tingling, numbness, erythema, dryness, rash, pruritus, swelling, or increased pigmentation of hands and/or feet, can be dose-limiting. Photophobia, increased lacrimation, conjunctivitis, and blurred vision.
Chair time: 2 hours weekly for 6 weeks. Repeat every 8 weeks for four cycles.

5-Fluorouracil + Leucovorin (Weekly Schedule/ Low Dose)[1,119]

Prechemo: CBC, Chem, CEA, LFTs. Oral phenothiazine or 5-HT$_3$; or 5-HT$_3$ and dexamethasone 10–20 mg. Mildly to moderately emetogenic.
5-Fluorouracil 500 mg/m^2: IV push weekly for 6 weeks.
Leucovorin 20 mg/m^2: IV push weekly for 6 weeks. Administered before 5-fluorouracil.
Side effects: Myelosuppression dose related, dose-limiting. Nausea and vomiting. Mucositis and diarrhea can be severe and dose-limiting. Alopecia. Hyperpigmentation, photosensitivity, and nail changes may occur. Hand-foot syndrome characterized by tingling, numbness, erythema, dryness, rash, swelling, or increased pigmentation of hands and/or feet can be dose-limiting. Photophobia, increased lacrimation, conjunctivitis, and blurred vision.
Chair time: 1 hour weekly for 6 weeks. Repeat every 8 weeks for four or six cycles.

Oxaliplatin + 5-Fluorouracil + Leucovorin (FOLFOX 4)[1,120]

Prechemo: CBC, Chem, LFTs, and CEA. Central line placement. 5-HT$_3$ and dexamethasone 10–20 mg. Moderately emetogenic.
Day 1: Oxaliplatin 85 mg/m^2: IV in 250–500 cc of D5W over 2 hours. Irritant but extravasations have resulted.
Leucovorin 200 mg/m^2: IV in 250–500 cc of D5W over 2 hours. Oxaliplatin and leucovorin are infused concurrently, in separate bags through a Y-site over 2 hours.

5-Fluorouracil 400 mg/m²: IV push over 2–4 minutes and then:

5-Fluorouacil 600 mg/m²: IV continuous infusion over 22 hours.

Day 2: Leucovorin 200 mg/m²: IV in 250–500 cc D5W or NS over 2 hours.

5-Fluorouracil 400 mg/m²: IV push over 2–4 minutes and then:

5-Fluorouracil 600 mg/m²: IV continuous infusion over 22 hours.

Day 3: Discontinue pump.

Side effects: Pharyngolaryngeal dysesthesia (sensation of discomfort or tightness in the back of the throat and inability to breathe), often precipitated by exposure to cold and characterized by dysesthesias, transient paresthesias or hypoesthesias of hands, feet, perioral area, and throat. Peripheral neuropathy with a cumulative dose of 800 mg/m² with paresthesias, dysesthesias, hypoesthesias. Nausea and vomiting. Diarrhea. Myelosuppression, mild to moderate. Delayed hypersensitivity reactions to Eloxatin™ may occur after 10–12 cycles.

Chair time: 3 hours on days 1 and 2 and 15 minutes on day 3. Repeat every 14 days for 12 cycles.

Capecitabine (Xeloda) [1,121]

Prechemo: CBC, Chem, LFTs, creatinine clearance, and CEA. Oral phenothiazine or 5-HT$_3$; or 5-HT$_3$. Mildly to moderately emetogenic.

Capecitabine 1250 mg/m²/day: PO bid on days 1–14.

Dose may be decreased to 850–1000 mg/m² PO bid on days 1–14 to reduce toxicities without compromising efficacy. 150- and 500-mg tablets. Administer within 30 minutes of a meal with plenty of water. Monitor INRs closely when taking warfarin; may increase INR.

Side effects: Nausea and vomiting. Diarrhea, stomatitis. Contraindicated with creatinine clearance <30 mL/min. Dose reduce with creatinine clearance of 30–50 mL/min at baseline to 75% of capecitabine. Hand-foot syndrome characterized by tingling, numbness, pain, erythema, dryness, rash, swelling, increased pigmentation, and/or pruritus of the hands and feet. Stop therapy at first signs of hand-foot syndrome or diarrhea. Blepharitis, tear-duct stenosis, acute and chronic conjunctivitis. Reduce does with elevations in serum bilirubin, alkaline phosphatase, or hepatic transaminase (SGOT, SGPT) levels.

Chair time: Repeat cycle every 21 days for a total of eight cycles.

METASTATIC DISEASE

COMBINATION REGIMENS

Irinotecan + 5-Fluorouracil + Leucovorin (IFL-Saltz Regimen)[1,122]

Prechemo: CBC, Chem, LFTs, and CEA. 5-HT$_3$ and dexamethasone 10–20 mg. Moderately to highly emetogenic. Atropine 0.25–1.0 mg IV unless contraindicated.

Irinotecan 125 mg/m²: IV in 500 cc of D5W over 90 minutes weekly for 4 weeks.

Leucovorin 20 mg/m²: IV push weekly for 4 weeks.

5-Fluorouracil 500 mg/m²: IV push weekly for 4 weeks.

Side effects: Acute diarrhea, can be managed with atropine before therapy. Late diarrhea can be severe, dose-limiting toxicity, and should be treated aggressively. Nausea and vomiting. Myelosuppression dose related, dose-limiting. Pulmonary toxicities ranging from transient dyspnea to pulmonary infiltrates, fever, and cough. Alopecia.

Chair time: 3 hours every week for 4 weeks. Repeat cycle every 6 weeks.

Irinotecan + 5-Fluorouracil + Leucovorin (IFL-Saltz Regimen) + Bevacizumab (BV)[1,123]

Prechemo: CBC, Chem, LFTs, CEA, urine test for protein baseline and periodically throughout treatment cycle 5-HT$_3$ and dexamethasone 10–20 mg. Atropine 0.25–1.0 mg IV unless contraindicated. Moderately to highly emetogenic.

Irinotecan 125 mg/m²: IV in 500 cc of D5W over 90 minutes weekly for 4 weeks.

Leucovorin 20 mg/m²: IV push weekly for 4 weeks.

Bevacizumab 5 mg/kg: IV every 2 weeks. Initial infusion 90 minutes. Second dose 60 minutes. Subsequent doses over 30 minutes. DO NOT administer perioperatively, as may inhibit wound healing.

Side effects: Infusion reaction with bevacizumab. Hypertension, hemostasis: thrombotic events. Nephrotic syndrome and proteinuria. Dipstick or urinalyses to detect proteinuria. Acute diarrhea managed with atropine therapy. Late diarrhea can be severe and should be treated aggressively. Initiate antidiarrheal protocol. Dose-limiting toxicity. Nausea and vomiting. Gastrointestinal perforation. Myelosuppression dose related, dose-limiting. Pulmonary toxicities ranging from transient dyspnea to pulmonary infiltrates, fever, and cough. Alopecia.

Chair time: 4 hours every week for 4 weeks. Repeat every 6 weeks.

Irinotecan + 5-Fluorouracil + Leucovorin (Modified IFL-Saltz Regimen)[1,124]

Prechemo: CBC, Chem, LFTs, and CEA. Oral phenothiazine or 5-HT$_3$; or 5-HT$_3$ and dexamethasone 10–20 mg. Atropine 0.25–1.0 mg IV unless contraindicated. Mild to moderately emetogenic

Irinotecan 125 mg/m^2: IV in 500 cc of D5W over 90 minutes weekly for 2 weeks.

Leucovorin 20 mg/m^2: IV push weekly for 2 weeks.

5-Fluorouracil 500 mg/m^2: IV push weekly for 2 weeks.

Side effects: Acute diarrhea, managed with atropine before therapy. Late diarrhea severe and should be treated aggressively. Initiate antidiarrheal protocol. Dose-limiting toxicity. Nausea and vomiting. Myelosuppression dose related, dose-limiting. Pulmonary toxicities, ranging from transient dyspnea to pulmonary infiltrates, fever, and cough. Alopecia.

Chair time: 3 hours every week for 2 weeks. Repeat every 3 weeks.

Irinotecan + 5-Fluorouracil + Leucovorin-(Douillard Regimen)[1,125]

Prechemo: CBC, Chem, LFTs, and CEA. Central line placement. 5-HT$_3$ and dexamethasone 10–20 mg. Atropine 0.25–1.0 mg IV unless contraindicated. Moderately to highly emetogenic.

Day 1: Irinotecan 180 mg/m^2: IV in 250–500 cc of D5W.

Leucovorin 200 mg/m^2: IV in 250–500 cc of D5W over 2 hours before 5-FU.

5-Fluorouracil 400 mg/m^2: IV bolus over 2–4 minutes.

5-Fluorouracil 600 mg/m^2: IV continuous infusion over 22 hours.

Day 2: Leucovorin 200 mg/m^2: IV in 250–500 cc of NS or D5W over 2 hours.

5-Fluorouracil 400 mg/m^2: IV bolus over 2–4 minutes.

5-Fluorouracil 600 mg/m^2: IV continuous infusion over 22 hours.

Day 3: Discontinue pump.

Side effects: Acute diarrhea, managed with atropine before therapy. Late diarrhea severe and should be treated aggressively. Initiate antidiarrheal protocol. Dose-limiting toxicity. Nausea and vomiting. Myelosuppression dose related, dose-limiting. Pulmonary toxicities ranging from transient dyspnea to pulmonary infiltrates, fever, and cough. Hand-foot syndrome characterized by tingling, numbness, pain, erythema, dryness, rash, swelling, increased pigmentation, and/or pruritus of the hands and feet. Blepharitis, tear-duct stenosis, acute and chronic conjunctivitis. Alopecia.

Chair time: 3 hours on days 1 and 2 and 15 minutes on day 3. Repeat every 2 weeks until disease progression.

Irinotecan + 5-Fluorouracil + Leucovorin (FOLFIRI Regimen)[1,126]

Prechemo: CBC, Chem, LFTs, and CEA. Central line placement. 5-HT$_3$ and dexamethasone 10–20 mg. Atropine 0.25–1.0 mg IV unless contraindicated. Moderately to highly emetogenic.

Day 1: Irinotecan 180 mg/m^2: IV in 250–500 cc of D5W over 90 minutes.

Leucovorin 200 mg/m^2: IV in 250–500 cc of D5W over 2 hours. Infuse during irinotecan therapy, before 5-FU infusion.

5-Fluorouracil 400 mg/m^2: IV bolus over 2–4 minutes.

5-Fluorouacil 2400 mg/m^2: IV continuous infusion over 46 hours.

Day 3: Discontinue pump.

Side effects: Acute diarrhea, managed with atropine before therapy. Late diarrhea severe and should be treated aggressively. Initiate antidiarrheal protocol. Dose-limiting toxicity. Nausea and vomiting. Myelosuppression dose related, dose-limiting. Pulmonary toxicities ranging from transient dyspnea to pulmonary infiltrates, fever, and cough. Alopecia. Hand-foot syndrome characterized by tingling, numbness, pain, erythema, dryness, rash, swelling, increased pigmentation, and/or pruritus of the hands and feet. Blepharitis, tear-duct stenosis, acute and chronic conjunctivitis.

Chair time: 3 hours on day 1 and 15 minutes on day 3. Repeat every 2 weeks.

Oxaliplatin + 5-Fluorouracil + Leucovorin (FOLFOX4)[1,127]

Prechemo: CBC, Chem, LFTs, and CEA. Central line placement. 5-HT$_3$ and dexamethasone 10–20 mg in D5W. Mild to moderately emetogenic.

Day 1: Oxaliplatin 85 mg/m^2: IV in 250–500 cc of D5W over 2 hours. Irritant, but extravasations have occurred.

Leucovorin 200 mg/m^2: IV in 250–500 cc of D5W. Oxaliplatin and leucovorin are infused concurrently in separate bags through a Y-site over 2 hours.

5-Fluorouracil 400 mg/m^2: IV bolus over 2–4 minutes.

5-Fluorouacil 600 mg/m^2: IV continuous infusion over 22 hours.

Day 2: Leucovorin 200 mg/m^2: IV in 250–500 cc of NS or D5W.

5-Fluorouracil 400 mg/m^2: IV bolus over 2–4 minutes.

5-Fluorouracil 600 mg/m^2: IV continuous infusion over 22 hours.

Day 3: Discontinue pump.

Side effects: Acute pharyngolaryngeal dysesthesia sensation of discomfort or tightness in the back of the throat and inability to breathe, often precipitated by exposure to cold and characterized by dysesthesias, transient paresthesias, or hypothesias of hands, feet, perioral area, and throat. Peripheral neuropathy with a cumulative dose of 800 mg/m^2. Paresthesias, dysesthesias, and altered proprioception. Nausea and vomiting. Diarrhea. Myelosuppression dose related, dose-limiting. Delayed hypersensitivity with oxaliplatin.

Chair time: 3 hours on days 1 and 2 and 15 minutes on day 3. Repeat every 2 weeks for 12 cycles.

Oxaliplatin + 5-Fluorouracil + Leucovorin (FOLFOX6)[1,128]

Prechemo: CBC, Chem, LFTs, and CEA. Central line placement. 5-HT$_3$ and dexamethasone 10–20 mg in D5W. Moderately to highly emetogenic.

Day 1: Oxaliplatin 100 mg/m^2: IV in 250–500 cc of D5W over 2 hours. Irritant, but extravasations have occurred.

Leucovorin 400 mg/m^2: IV in 250–500 cc of D5W. Oxaliplatin and leucovorin are infused concurrently in separate bags through a Y-site over 2 hours.

5-Fluorouracil 400 mg/m^2: IV bolus over 2–4 minutes.

5-Fluorouacil 2400 mg/m^2: IV continuous infusion over 46 hours.

Day 3: Discontinue pump.

Side effects: Acute pharyngolaryngeal dysesthesia sensation of discomfort or tightness in the back of the throat and inability to breathe, often precipitated by exposure to cold and characterized by dysesthesias, transient paresthesias, or hypoesthesias of hands, feet, perioral area, and throat. Peripheral neuropathy with a cumulative dose of 800 mg/m^2. Paresthesias, dysesthesias, altered proprioception. Nausea and vomiting. Diarrhea. Myelosuppression dose related, dose-limiting. Delayed hypersensitivity with oxaliplatin

Chair time: 3 hours on day 1 and 15 minutes on day 3. Repeat every 2 weeks for 12 weeks.

Oxaliplatin + 5-Fluorouracil + Leucovorin (FOLFOX7)[1,129]

Prechemo: CBC, Chem, LFTs, and CEA. Central line placement. 5-HT$_3$ and dexamethasone 10–20 mg in D5W. Moderately to highly emetogenic.

Day 1: Oxaliplatin 130 mg/m^2: IV in 250–500 cc of D5W over 2 hours. Irritant, but extravasations have occurred.

Leucovorin 400 mg/m^2: IV in 250–500-cc of D5W over 2 hours, oxaliplatin and leucovorin are infused concurrently in separate bags through a Y-site over 2 hours.

5-Fluorouacil 2400 mg/m^2: IV continuous infusion over 46 hours.

Day 3: Discontinue pump.

Side effects: Acute pharyngolaryngeal dysesthesia sensation of discomfort or tightness in the back of the throat and inability to breathe, often precipitated by exposure to cold and characterized by dysesthesias, transient paresthesias, or hypoesthesias of hands, feet, perioral area, and throat. Peripheral neuropathy with a cumulative dose of 800 mg/m². Paresthesias, dysesthesias, altered proprioception. Nausea and vomiting. Diarrhea. Myelosuppression dose related, dose-limiting. Delayed hypersensitivity with oxaliplatin.

Chair time: 3 hours on day 1 and 15 minutes on day 3. Repeat every 2 weeks for 12 weeks.

Cetuximab + Irinotecan[1,130]

Prechemo: CBC, Chem, electrolytes, LFTs. Diphenhydramine 50 mg. Moderately to highly emetogenic.

Cetuximab 400 mg/m²: IV over 2 hours week 1 only.

Cetuximab 250 mg/m²: IV over 1 hour weekly as maintenance dose. Administer through low-protein-binding 0.22-micron inline filter, followed by 1 hour of observation for infusion reactions.

Pre-meds for irinotecon: 5-HT₃ and dexamethasone 10–20 mg. Atropine 0.25–1.0 mg IV unless contraindicated.

Irinotecan 175 mg/m²: IV in 500 cc of D5W day 1 and every 3 weeks.

Side effects: Infusion reaction with erbitux. Severe allergic reactions with rapid onset of airway obstruction (bronchospasm, stridor, hoarseness), dyspnea, fever, chills, rash, itching, and/or hypotension require stop immediately and NOT started again. Mild or moderate infusion reactions, infusion rate permanently reduced by 50%. Acneform rash can be severe and require dose modification paronychial inflammation, especially in thumbs and great toes. Treat with topical antibiotic cream or oral antibiotics. Hypomagnesemia. Electrolyte replacement may be necessary. Acute diarrhea, managed with atropine before therapy. Late diarrhea severe and should be treated aggressively. Dose-limiting toxicity. Nausea and vomiting. Myelosuppression dose related, dose-limiting. Pulmonary toxicities ranging from transient dyspnea to pulmonary infiltrates, fever, and cough. Alopecia. Discontinue erbitux with interstitial pneumonitis with noncardiogenic pulmonary edema.

Chair time: 4 hours for first treatment with cetuximab and irinotecan, 1 hour for weekly cetuximab, and 3 hours for all other courses. Repeat every 21 days.

Capecitabine + Oxaliplatin (XELOX) or (Capox)[1,131]

Prechemo: CBC, Chem, LFTs, CEA, and creatinine clearance. 5-HT₃ and dexamethasone 10–20 mg in D5W. Moderately to highly emetogenic.

Oxaliplatin 130 mg/m²: IV in 250 cc of D5W over 2 hours on day 1.

Capecitabine 1000 mg/m²: PO bid on days 1–14. Administer within 30 minutes of a meal with plenty of water. 150- and 500-mg tablets. Monitor INRs closely in patients taking warfarin, as may increase INR.

Side effects: Acute pharyngolaryngeal dysesthesia sensation of discomfort or tightness in the back of the throat and inability to breathe, often precipitated by exposure to cold and characterized by dysesthesias, transient paresthesias, or hypothesias of hands, feet, perioral area, and throat. Peripheral neuropathy with a cumulative dose of 800 mg/m². Paresthesias, dysesthesias, altered proprioception. Nausea and vomiting. Diarrhea, stomatitis. Myelosuppression dose related, dose-limiting. Delayed hypersensitivity with oxaliplatin. Hand-foot syndrome. Blepharitis, tear-duct stenosis, acute and chronic conjunctivitis. Elevations in serum bilirubin alkaline phosphatase, and hepatic transaminases, SGOT, SGPT. Dose reduce with hyperbilirubinemia. Capecitabine contraindicated in patients with creatinine clearance, 30 mL/min. Baseline clearance of 30–50 mL/min dose reduce to 75%.

Chair time: 3 hours. Repeat cycle every 21 days until disease progression.

Capecitabine + Irinotecan (XELIRI)[1,132]

Prechemo: CBC, Chem, LFTs. Central line placement. 5-HT$_3$ and dexamethasone 10–20 mg. Moderately to highly emetogenic. Atropine 0.25–1.0 mg IV unless contraindicated.

Capecitabine 1000 mg/m²: PO bid days 1–14. Administer within 30 minutes of a meal with plenty of water. 150- and 500-mg tablets. Monitor INRs closely in patients taking warfarin, as may increase INR.

Irinotecan 200–250 mg/m²: IV in 250–500 cc of D5W over 90 minutes on day 1.

OR

Irinotecan 80 mg/m²: IV in 250 cc of D5W over 90 minutes on days 1 and 8.

Side effects: Nausea and vomiting diarrhea, dose-limiting. Stomatitis. Hand-foot syndrome. Myelosuppression. Elevations in serum bilirubin alkaline phosphatase, and hepatic transaminases, SGOT, SGPT. Dose reduce with hyperbilirubinemia. Capecitabine contraindicated in patients with creatinine clearance, 30 mL/min, Baseline clearance of 30–50 mL/min dose reduce to 75%. Blepharitis, tear-duct stenosis, acute and chronic conjunctivitis. Pulmonary toxicities ranging from transient dyspnea to pulmonary infiltrates, fever, and cough. Initiate antidiarrheal protocol.

Chair time: 2 hours. Repeat every 21 days as tolerated or until progression.

Oxaliplatin + Irinotecan (IROX Regimen)[1,133]

Prechemo: CBC, Chem, LFTs. 5-HT$_3$ and dexamethasone 10–20 mg in D5W. Moderately to highly emetogenic.

Oxaliplatin 85 mg/m²: IV in 250–500 cc of D5W on day 1.

Irinotecan 200 mg/m²: IV in 500 cc of D5W day 1.

Side effects: Acute pharyngolaryngeal dysesthesia sensation of discomfort or tightness in the back of the throat and inability to breathe, often precipitated by exposure to cold and characterized by dysesthesias, transient paresthesias or hypothesias of hands, feet, perioral area, and throat. Peripheral neuropathy with a cumulative dose of 800 mg/m². Paresthesias, dysesthesias, altered proprioception. Nausea and vomiting. Diarrhea. Myelosuppression dose related, dose-limiting. Delayed hypersensitivity with oxaliplatin. Initiate antidiarrheal.

Chair time: 4 hours on day 1. Repeat cycle every 3 weeks until progression.

5-Fluorouracil + Leucovorin (Mayo Clinic Regimen)[1,134]

Prechemo: CBC, Chem, LFTs, CEA. Oral phenothiazine or 5-HT$_3$ or 5-HT$_3$ and dexamethasone 10–20 mg. Mild to moderately emetogenic.

Leucovorin 20 mg/m²/day: IV push on days 1–5.

5-Fluorouracil 425 mg/m²/day: IV push 1 hour after leucovorin, days 1–5.

Side effects: Myelosuppression dose related, dose-limiting. Nausea and vomiting. Mucositis and diarrhea can be severe and dose-limiting. Pulmonary toxicities ranging from transient dyspnea to pulmonary infiltrates, fever, and cough. Alopecia. Hyperpigmentation, photosensitivity, and nail changes may occur. Hand-foot syndrome with tingling, numbness, erythema, dryness, rash, swelling, or increased pigmentation of hands and/or feet can be dose-limiting. Photophobia, increased lacrimation, conjunctivitis, and blurred vision.

Chair time: 1 hour on days 1–5. Repeat every 28 days for six cycles.

5-Fluorouracil + Leucovorin (Roswell Park Regimen/ High Dose)[1,135]

Prechemo: CBC, Chem, LFTs, CEA. Oral phenothiazine or 5-HT$_3$ or 5-HT$_3$ and dexamethasone 10–20 mg. Mild to moderately emetogenic.

Leucovorin 500 mg/m²: IV over 2 hours, weekly for 6 weeks.

5-Fluorouracil 500 mg/m²: IV push weekly for 6 weeks.

Side effects: Myelosuppression dose related, dose-limiting. Nausea and vomiting. Mucositis and diarrhea can be severe and dose-limiting. Alopecia. Hyperpigmentation, photosensitivity, and nail changes. Hand-foot syndrome characterized by tingling, numbness, erythema, dryness, rash, pruritus, swelling, or increased pigmentation of hands and/or feet can be dose-limiting. Photophobia, increased lacrimation, conjunctivitis, and blurred vision.

Chair time: 1 hour weekly for 6 weeks. Repeat every 8 weeks for four cycles.

5-Fluorouracil + Leucovorin + Bevacizumab[1,136]

Prechemo: CBC, Chem, LFTs, urine test for protein baseline and throughout treatment. 5-HT$_3$ and dexamethasone 10–20 mg. Moderately to highly emetogenic.

5-Fluorouracil 500 mg/m^2: IV push weekly for 6 weeks.

Leucovorin 500 mg/m^2: IV push weekly for 6 weeks.

Bevacizumab 5 mg/kg: IV in 100 cc NS every 2 weeks. Initial infusion 90 minutes; second dose 60 minutes, subsequent doses over 30 minutes. DO NOT administer perioperatively—may inhibit wound healing.

Side effects: Infusion reaction with bevacizumab. Hypertension, hemostasis: thrombotic events. Nephrotic syndrome and proteinuria. Dipstick or urinalyses to detect proteinuria. Diarrhea dose-limiting, antidiarrheal protocol. Nausea and vomiting. Gastrointestinal perforation. Hyperpigmentation, photosensitivity, and nail changes. Hand-foot syndrome dose-limiting. Photophobia, increased lacrimation, conjunctivitis, and blurred vision. Myelosuppression. Alopecia.

Chair time: 2 hours for 6 weeks. Repeat every 8 weeks.

Bevacizumab + IV 5-fluorouracil-based chemotherapy[1,136,140]

Prechemo: CBC, Chem, CEA, urine test for protein baseline and throughout treatment. Acetaminophen 1000 mg. Diphenhydramine 25–50 mg and H$_2$ antagonist only necessary with prior infusion reaction with bevacizumab.

Bevacizumab 5 mg/kg: IV every 2 weeks in combination with bolus IFL.

Bevacizumab 10 mg/kg: IV every 2 weeks in combination with FOL-FOX4. Initial infusion over 90 minutes; second dose over 60 minutes, subsequent doses over 30 minutes. DO NOT administer perioperatively—may inhibit wound healing.

Give with 5-fluorouracil based therapy. See specific protocol (IFL, FOLFOX)

Side effects: Myelosuppression mild. Infusion reaction with bevacizumab. Delayed wound healing. Hold 28 days prior to elective surgery; do not resume until fully healed (at least 28 days following major surgery). Wound dehiscence can result. Gastrointestinal perforation, fistulas, and/or intra-abdominal abscess; abdominal pain associated with

constipation, vomiting, and fever. Permanently discontinue bevacizumab if GI perforation occurs. Hypertension. Congestive heart failure, risk higher in patients who have received prior or concurrent
anthracyclines: cerebral infarction, transient ischemic attacks, myocardial infarction, angina, and a variety of other arterial thromboembolic
events. GI hemorrhage, subarachnoid hemorrhage, and hemorrhagic
stroke, or thrombocytopenia may occur. Reversible posterior leukoencephalopathy syndrome (RPLS), a rare but serious neurological disorder
characterized by: headache, seizure, lethargy, confusion, blindness, and
other visual and neurologic disturbances. RPLS can be confirmed by
magnetic resonance imaging (MRI). Symptoms usually resolve or improve within days. Discontinue bevacizumab for thromboembolic
events, serious hemorrhage, and RPLS. Nephrotic syndrome and proteinuria. Dipstick or urinalysis to detect proteinuria or use the protein-
to-creatinine (UPC) ratio to monitor. Hold for evidence of moderate to
severe proteinuria (2+ protein) and do 24-hour urine. Discontinue drug
with nephrotic syndrome. Abdominal pain, diarrhea, nausea, vomiting,
anorexia, stomatitis, constipation common. Diarrhea can be severe.
Upper respiratory infection, dyspnea. Exfoliative dermatitis.

Chair time: 90 minutes for first dose, 1 hour for second dose, 30 minutes for subsequent doses plus infusion time for 5-fluorouracil protocol.
Repeat cycle every 2 weeks.

5-Fluorouracil + Leucovorin (German Schedule/ Low Dose)[1,137]

Prechemo: CBC, Chem, LFTs, CEA. Oral phenothiazine or 5-HT$_3$ and
dexamethasone 10–20 mg. Mild to moderately emetogenic.
Leucovorin 20 mg/m^2: IV weekly for 6 weeks.
5-Fluorouracil 600 mg/m^2: IV weekly for 6 weeks.
Side effects: Myelosuppression dose related, can be dose-limiting.
Nausea and vomiting. Mucositis and diarrhea can be severe and dose-
limiting. Alopecia. Hyperpigmentation, photosensitivity, and nail
changes. Hand-foot syndrome characterized by tingling, numbness, erythema, dryness, rash, pruritus, swelling, or increased pigmentation of
hands and/or feet, can be dose-limiting. Photophobia, increased lacrimation, conjunctivitis, and blurred vision.
Chair time: 1 hour weekly for 6 weeks. Repeat every 8 weeks.

5-Fluorouracil + Leucovorin (de Gramont Regimen)[1,138]

Prechemo: CBC, Chem, LFTs, CEA. Oral phenothiazine or 5-HT$_3$; or
5-HT$_3$ and dexamethasone 10–20 mg. Mild to moderately emetogenic.
Leucovorin 200 mg/m^2: IV over 2 hours on days 1 and 2 before 5-FU.
5-Fluorouracil 400 mg/m^2: IV push.

5-Fluorouracil 600 mg/m²: IV continuous infusion over 22 hours on days 1 and 2.

Side effects: Myelosuppression dose related, can be dose-limiting. Nausea and vomiting. Mucositis and diarrhea can be severe and dose-limiting. Alopecia. Hyperpigmentation, photosensitivity, and nail changes. Hand-foot syndrome can be dose-limiting. Photophobia, increased lacrimation, conjunctivitis, and blurred vision.

Chair time: 2 hours on days 1 and 2, 15 minutes on day 3 to discontinue pump. Repeat every 2 weeks.

FOLFOX4 + Bevacizumab[1,139]

Prechemo: CBC, Chem, LFTs, CEA, and urine test for protein baseline and periodically throughout treatment. Central line placement. 5-HT₃ and dexamethasone 10–20 mg in D5W. Moderately emetogenic.

Bevacizumab 10 mg/kg: Every 2 weeks. Initial infusion 90 minutes; second dose 60 minutes, subsequent doses over 30 minutes. DO NOT administer perioperatively, as may inhibit wound healing.

Oxaliplatin 85 mg/m²: IV in 250–500 cc of D5W over 2 hours on day 1. Irritant, but extravasations have occurred.

Leucovorin 200 mg/m²: IV in 250–500-cc of D5W on days 1 and 2. Oxaliplatin and leucovorin are infused concurrently in separate bags through a Y-site over 2 hours.

5-Fluorouacil 400 mg/m²: IV bolus over 2–4 minutes followed by:

5-Fluorouacil 600 mg/m²: IV continuous infusion over 22 hours on days 1 and 2.

Day 3: Discontinue pump.

Side effects: Infusion reaction with bevacizumab. Hypertension, hemostasis: thrombotic events. Nephrotic syndrome and proteinuria. Dipstick or urinalysis to detect proteinuria. Acute pharyngolaryngeal dysesthesia sensation of discomfort or tightness in the back of the throat and inability to breathe. Often precipitated by exposure to cold and characterized by dysesthesias, transient paresthesias, or hypoesthesias of hands, feet, perioral area, and throat. Peripheral neuropathy, paresthesias, dysesthesias, altered proprioception. Nausea and vomiting. Diarrhea. Myelosuppression dose related, dose-limiting. Delayed hypersensitivity with oxaliplatin.

Chair time: 3 hours on days 1 and 2 and 15 minutes on day 3. Repeat every 2 weeks for 12 cycles.

Capecitabine + Oxaliplatin (XELOX) + Bevacizumab[1,140]

Prechemo: CBC, Chem, LFTs, CEA, and creatinine clearance. Urine test for protein baseline and periodically throughout treatment cycle. 5-HT₃ and dexamethasone 10–20 mg in D5W. Moderately to highly emetogenic.

Capecitabine 850 mg/m^2: PO bid on days 1–14. Administer within 30 minutes of a meal with plenty of water. 150 mg and 500 mg tablets. Monitor INRs closely when taking warfarin, as may increase INR.

Oxaliplatin 130 mg/m^2: IV in 250 cc of D5W over 2 hours on day 1.

Bevacizumab 7.5 mg/kg: Every 3 weeks. Initial infusion 90 minutes; second dose 60 minutes, subsequent doses over 30 minutes. DO NOT administer perioperatively, as may inhibit wound healing.

Side effects: Acute pharyngolaryngeal dysesthesia sensation of discomfort or tightness in the back of the throat and inability to breathe, often precipitated by exposure to cold and characterized by dysesthesias, transient paresthesias, or hypoesthesias of hands, feet, perioral area, and throat. Peripheral neuropathy, paresthesias, dysesthesias, altered proprioception. Nausea and vomiting. Diarrhea. Myelosuppression dose related, dose-limiting. Delayed hypersensitivity with oxaliplatin. Hand-foot syndrome. Blepharitis, tear-duct stenosis, acute and chronic conjunctivitis. Elevations in serum bilirubin alkaline phosphatase and hepatic transaminases, SGOT, SGPT. Dose reduce with hyperbilirubinemia. Capecitabine contraindicated in patients with creatinine clearance < 30 mL/min. For baseline clearance of 30–50 mL/min, dose reduce to 75%. Initiate antidiarrheal protocol.

Chair time: 3 hours. Repeat cycle every 21 days until progression.

Trimetrexate + 5-Fluorouracil + Leucovorin[1,141]

Prechemo: CBC, Chem, LFTs, CEA. Oral phenothiazine, or 5-HT$_3$ and dexamethasone 10–20 mg in D5W. Mild to moderately emetogenic.

Trimetrexate 110 mg/m^2: IV in 250 cc of D5W on day 1. Reconstitute with 2 mL of D5W or sterile water. Filter with a 0.22-micron filter before further dilution in D5W to a final concentration of 0.25–2.0 mg/mL. Inspect for cloudiness or precipitate.

Leucovorin 200 mg/m^2: IV on day 2, 24 hours after trimetrexate dose.

5-Fluorouracil 500 mg/m^2: IV push on day 2, immediately after leucovorin.

Leucovorin 15mg: PO every 6 hours for 7 doses, starting 6 hours after 5-fluorouracil.

Side effects: Myelosuppression dose-limiting toxicity. Nausea and vomiting. Mucositis and diarrhea can be severe and dose-limiting. Transient elevation in serum transaminase levels. Dyspnea may occur and can be severe. Hyperpigmentation, photosensitivity, and nail changes may occur. Hand-foot syndrome dose-limiting. Alopecia. Photophobia, increased lacrimation, conjunctivitis, and blurred vision.

Chair time: 1 hour weekly for 6 weeks. Repeat cycle every 8 weeks.

HEPATIC ARTERY INFUSION

Floxuridine[1,142]

Prechemo: CBC, Chem, LFTs, and CEA. Hepatic artery line for arterial infusion. Oral phenothiazine or 5-HT$_3$. H$_2$ antagonist antihistamine concurrently with intra-arterial infusion to prevent development of peptic ulcer disease. Mildly emetogenic.

Floxuridine 0.3 mg/kg/day: continuous HAI days 1–14.

Dexamethasone 20 mg: continuous HAI on days 1–14.

Heparin 50,000 units: continuous HAI on days 1–14.

Side effects: Nausea and vomiting. Anorexia, mild mucositis. Gastritis may occur, with abdominal cramping and pain. Duodenal ulcers may occur and lead to gastric outlet obstruction and vomiting. Chemical hepatitis may be severe, with increased alkaline phosphatase, liver transaminase, and bilirubin levels. Intra-arterial catheter problems: leakage, arterial ischemia or aneurysm, bleeding at catheter site, catheter occlusion, thrombosis or embolism of artery, vessel perforation or dislodged catheter, infection, and biliary sclerosis. Hand-foot syndrome. Erythema, dermatitis, pruritus, or rash. Somnolence, confusion, seizures, cerebellar ataxia, vertigo, nystagmus, depression, hemiplegia, hiccups, and lethargy. Blurred vision and rarely encephalopathy. Myelosuppression occurs rarely. Chest pain, electrocardiographic changes, and serum enzyme elevation occur rarely. Increased risk in patients with prior history of ischemic heart disease. Blepharitis, tear-duct stenosis, acute and chronic conjunctivitis. Fever malaise, catheter infections.

Chair time: 1 hour on days 1–14. Repeat every 14 days until disease progression. May require hospitalization for all or part of treatment.

SINGLE-AGENT REGIMENS

Capecitabine (Xeloda)[1,143]

Prechemo: CBC, Chem, LFTs, CEA, and creatinine clearance. Oral phenothiazine or 5-HT$_3$. Mild to moderately emetogenic.

Capecitabine 1250 mg/m^2/day: PO bid on days 1–14.

Dose may be decreased to 850–1000 mg/m^2 PO bid to reduce toxicities without compromising efficacy. 150- and 500-mg tablets. Administer within 30 minutes of a meal with plenty of water. Monitor INRs closely when taking warfarin, as may increase INR.

Side effects: Nausea and vomiting. Diarrhea, stomatitis. Contraindicated with creatinine clearance <30 mL/min. Dose reduce to 75% for baseline creatinine clearance of 30–50 mL/min. Hand-foot syndrome characterized by tingling, numbness, pain, erythema, dryness, rash, swelling, increased pigmentation, and/or pruritus of the hands and feet.

Stop therapy at first signs of hand-foot syndrome or diarrhea. Blepharitis, tear-duct stenosis, acute and chronic conjunctivitis. Reduce dose with elevations in serum bilirubin alkaline phosphatase and hepatic transaminase (SGOT, SGPT) levels.

Chair time: No chair time. Repeat cycle every 21 days for a total of eight cycles.

Irinotecan (CPT-11/Weekly Schedule)[1,144,145]

Prechemo: CBC, Chem, and CEA. 5-HT$_3$, and dexamethasone 10–20 mg. Atropine 0.25–1.0 mg IV unless contraindicated. Moderately to highly emetogenic.

Irinotecan 125 mg/m^2: IV in 500 cc of D5W over 90 minutes weekly for 4 weeks, repeat every 6 weeks.

OR

Irinotecan 125 mg/m^2: IV in 500 cc of D5W over 90 minutes weekly for 2 weeks, repeat every 3 weeks.

OR

Irinotecan 175 mg/m^2: IV in 500 cc of D5W over 90 minutes on days 1 and 10 every 3 weeks.

Side effects: Early diarrhea can be managed with atropine before therapy. Late diarrhea can be severe and should be treated aggressively. Consider Lomotil, Imodium, tincture of opium, and hydration. Nausea and vomiting. Myelosuppression, dose-limiting. G-CSF recommended. Pulmonary toxicities ranging from transient dyspnea to pulmonary infiltrates, fever, and cough. Alopecia.

Chair time: 3 hours every 3 weeks. Additional days for hydration if patient has diarrhea. Repeat as described above.

Irinotecan (CPT-11/Monthly Schedule)[1,146]

Prechemo: CBC, Chem, and CEA. 5-HT$_3$, and dexamethasone 10–20 mg in D5W. Atropine 0.25–1.0 mg IV unless contraindicated. Moderately to highly emetogenic.

Irinotecan 350 mg/m^2: IV in 500 cc of D5W over 90 minutes.

Side effects: Early diarrhea can be managed with atropine before therapy. Late diarrhea can be severe and should be treated aggressively. Consider Lomotil, Imodium, tincture of opium, and hydration. Nausea and vomiting. Myelosuppression, dose-limiting. G-CSF recommended. Pulmonary toxicities ranging from transient dyspnea to pulmonary infiltrates, fever, and cough.

Chair time: 3 hours every 3 weeks. Additional days for hydration if indicated.

Cetuximab (Erbitux) [1,147]

Prechemo: CBC, Chem, Mg^{2+}, LFTs, CEA, EGFR expression using immunohistochemistry. Diphenhydramine 50 mg. Mildly emetogenic.

Cetuximab 400 mg/m²: IV over 2 hours loading dose, week 1 only.

Cetuximab 250 mg/m²: IV over 1 hour weekly as maintenance dose. Maximum infusion rate 5 mL/min. Administer through low-protein-binding 0.22-micron inline filter. Observe for 1 hour after infusion for infusion reactions.

Side effects: Infusion reaction: severe allergic reactions should be stopped immediately and NOT started again. Mild or moderate infusion reactions infusion rate should be permanently reduced by 50%. Acneform rash can be severe and require dose modification. May be treated with topical antibiotic cream or oral antibiotics. Paronychial inflammation, especially in thumbs and great toes. Hypomagnesemia. Electrolyte replacement may be necessary. Closely monitor magnesium, potassium, and calcium levels. Nausea and vomiting. Interstitial pneumonitis with noncardiogenic pulmonary edema, drug should be discontinued if occurs.

Chair time: 2–3 hours, includes premeds, drug infusion, and 1-hour observation time. Repeat weekly as tolerated or until progression.

Panitumumab (Vectibix) [1,148]

Prechemo: CBC, Chem, Mg^{2+}, and CEA. EGFR expression using immunohistochemistry. Diphenhydramine 50 mg in 100 cc of NS.

Panitumumab 6 mg/Kg: IV over 1 hour every 14 days. Doses over 1000 mg should be administered over 90 minutes. Use low-protein-binding 0.2-micron or 0.22-micron inline filter. Final concentration should not exceed 10 mg/mL.

Side effects: Infusion reaction: immediately and permanently discontinue vectibix for severe reactions. Mild or moderate infusion reactions reduce infusion rate by 50% for the duration of that infusion. Acneform rash can be severe and require dose modification. Pruritus, erythema, rash, skin exfoliation, dry skin, and skin fissures. Treat with topical antibiotic cream or oral antibiotics. Sunlight can exacerbate skin reactions. Dose delay and dose reduction recommended for grade 3 or higher skin toxicities. Paronychial inflammation and other nail disorders. Conjunctivitis, ocular hyperemia, increased lacrimation, and eye/eyelid irritation. Hypomagnesemia may occur 6 or more weeks after treatment is initiated. In some patients, hypomagnesemia was associated with hypocalcemia. Electrolyte replacement may be necessary. Closely monitor magnesium and calcium levels. Diarrhea, stomatitis, and oral mucositis. Nausea and vomiting. Pulmonary fibrosis. Discontinue with interstitial lung disease, pneumonitis, or lung infiltrates.

Chair time: 2 hours. Repeat cycle every 14 days as tolerated or until progression.

5-Fluorouracil (Continuous Infusion)[1,149,150]

Prechemo: CBC, Chem, LFTs, and CEA. Central line placement. Oral phenothiazine or 5-HT$_3$; or 5-HT$_3$ and dexamethasone 10–20 mg. Mild to moderately emetogenic.

Fluorouracil 2600 mg/m²: IV over 24 hours weekly for 4 weeks.

OR

Fluorouracil 1000 mg/m²/day: IV continuous infusion on days 1–4.

Side effects: Myelosuppression dose related, dose-limiting. Nausea and vomiting. Mucositis and diarrhea can be severe and dose-limiting. Alopecia. Hyperpigmentation, photosensitivity, and nail changes. Hand-foot syndrome can be dose-limiting. Photophobia, increased lacrimation, conjunctivitis, and blurred vision.

Chair time: 1 hour weekly for 4 weeks. Repeat every 21–28 days.

ENDOMETRIAL CANCER

COMBINATION REGIMENS

Paclitaxel and Carboplatin[1,151]

Prechemo: CBC, Chem, Mg^{2+}. 5-HT_3 and dexamethasone 10–20 mg. Diphenhydramine 25–50 mg; H_2 antagonist. Moderately to highly emetogenic.

Paclitaxel 175 mg/m²: IV in 500 cc NS over 3 hours on day 1.

Carboplatin AUC of 5–7: IV in 500 cc NS on day 1. Give after paclitaxel to decrease toxicities.

Side effects: Hypersensitivity reaction with paclitaxel. Increased risk of carboplatin reaction in patients receiving more than seven courses of carboplatin therapy. Myelosuppression cumulative and dose related. G-CSF support recommended. Nausea and vomiting, acute or delayed. Mucositis and/or diarrhea common. Nephrotoxicity symptomatic. Dose reduce with renal dysfunction. Decreases Mg^{2+}, K^+, Ca^{2+}, and Na^+. Sensory neuropathy with numbness and paresthesias, dose related, dose-limiting. Alopecia.

Chair time: 5 hours on day 1. Repeat cycle every 28 days until progression.

Doxorubicin + Cyclophosphamide (AC)[1,152]

Prechemo: CBC, Chem, LFTs, and. MUGA. 5-HT_3 and dexamethasone 20 mg. Moderately to highly emetogenic.

Doxorubicin 60 mg/m²: IV push on day 1. Potent vesicant.

Cyclophosphamide 500 mg/m²: IV in 500 cc NS on day 1.

Side effects: Cyclophosphamide can cause rhinitis and irritation of nose and throat. Myelosuppression may be severe. G-CSF recommended. Nausea and vomiting, acute or delayed. Stomatitis and diarrhea not dose-limiting. Pericarditis-myocarditis syndrome. With cumulative doses >550 mg/m² of doxorubicin, cardiomyopathy. Cyclophosphamide may increase risk of cardiotoxicity. Dose reduce with liver dysfunction. Hemorrhagic cystitis, dysuria, and urinary frequency with cyclophosphamide. Red-orange discoloration of urine. SIADH. Hyperpigmentation, photosensitivity, and radiation recall. Alopecia.

Chair time: 2 hours on day 1. Repeat every 21 days until progression.

Doxorubicin + Cisplatin (AP)[1,153]

Prechemo: CBC, Chem, Mg^{2+}, MUGA scan. 5-HT_3 and dexamethasone 10–20 mg. Moderately to highly emetogenic.

Doxorubicin 50 mg/m²: IV push on day 1. Potent vesicant.

Cisplatin 50 mg/m²: IV in 500–1000 cc NS over 1–3 hours on day 1.

Side effects: Hypersensitivity reaction with cisplatin. Myelosuppression dose related. Nausea and vomiting, acute or delayed. Mucositis. Metallic taste. Nephrotoxicity dose related with cisplatin. Hemorrhagic cystitis, dysuria, and increased urinary frequency. Decreases Mg^{2+}, K^+, Ca^{2+}, Na^+, and P. Acutely, pericarditis or myocarditis can occur. Later, cardiomyopathy (congestive heart failure) may occur. Peripheral sensory neuropathy dose-limiting with paresthesias and numbness. High-frequency hearing loss and tinnitus. Hyperpigmentation, photosensitivity, and radiation recall occur. Alopecia.

Chair time: 4 hours on day 1. Repeat cycle every 21 days.

Doxorubicin + Paclitaxel (AT)[1,154]

Prechemo: CBC and Chem. Central line placement. MUGA scan. 5-HT_3 and dexamethasone 10–20 mg. Diphenhydramine 25–50 mg and H_2 antagonist. Moderately to highly emetogenic.

Doxorubicin 50 mg/m²: IV push on day 1. Potent vesicant.

Paclitaxel 150 mg/m²: IV over 24 hours on day 1. Use non-PVC containers and tubing with 0.22-micron inline filter.

Side effects: Hypersensitivity reaction with paclitaxel. Myelosuppression dose-limiting use G-CSF support. Nausea and vomiting. Stomatitis not dose-limiting. Dose reduce doxorubicin with liver dysfunction. Pericarditis-myocarditis. Cardiomyopathy with doses >550 mg/m² of doxorubicin. Sensory neuropathy with numbness/paresthesias, dose related and dose-limiting. Red-orange discoloration of urine. Hyperpigmentation, photosensitivity, and radiation recall. Alopecia.

Chair time: Chair time 4–5 hours day 1. Repeat cycle every 21 days.

Cisplatin + Doxorubicin + Paclitaxel[1,155]

Prechemo: CBC, Chem, LFTs, Mg^{2+}, and creatinine clearance. MUGA. 5-HT_3 and dexamethasone 10–20 mg. Moderately to highly emetogenic.

Cisplatin 50 mg/m²: IV in 500–1000 cc NS on day 1.

Doxorubicin 45 mg/m²: IV push on day 1. Potent vesicant.

Paclitaxel 160 mg/m²: IV in 500 cc NS over 3 hours on day 2. Use non-PVC containers and tubing with 0.22-micron inline filter.

Side effects: Hypersensitivity reaction. Myelosuppression severe, dose-limiting. G-CSF recommended. Sensory neuropathy dose-limiting toxicity, with peripheral sensory neuropathy. High-frequency hearing loss and tinnitus with cisplatin. Nausea and vomiting acute or delayed. Stomatitis. Cardiac: acutely, pericarditis-myocarditis syndrome. With high cumulative doses >550 mg/m² of doxorubicin, cardiomyopathy. Nephrotoxicity dose related with cisplatin. Red-orange discoloration of urine. Decreases Mg^{2+}, K^+, Ca^{2+}, $Na,^+$ and P. Hyperpigmentation, photosensitivity, and radiation recall. Alopecia.

Chair time: 3 hours on day 1 and 4 hours on day 2. Repeat cycle every 21 days.

Cyclophosphamide + Doxorubicin + Cisplatin (CAP)[1,156]

Prechemo: CBC, Chem, LFTs, Mg^{2+} and creatinine clearance. MUGA. 5-HT_3 and dexamethasone 10–20 mg. Moderately to highly emetogenic.

Cyclophosphamide 500 mg/m²: IV in 500 cc NS on day 1.

Doxorubicin 50 mg/m²: IV push on day 1. Potent vesicant.

Cisplatin 50 mg/m²: IV in 500–1000 cc NS over 1–3 hours on day 1.

Side effects: Myelosuppression dose related. G-CSF recommended. Nausea and vomiting, may be acute delayed. Mucositis. Red-orange discoloration of urine, dysuria, and increased urinary frequency. Adequately hydrate to decrease risk of nephrotoxicity and hemorrhagic cystitis. Decreases Mg^{2+}, K^+, Ca^{2+}, $Na,^+$ and P. Acutely, pericarditis-myocarditis syndrome. With high cumulative doses >550 mg/m² of doxorubicin, cardiomyopathy. Cyclophosphamide may increase the risk of cardiotoxicity. Sensory neuropathy. Paresthesias and numbness dose-limiting. Hyperpigmentation, photosensitivity, and radiation recall. Alopecia.

Chair time: 4 hours on day 1. Repeat cycle every 21 days.

SINGLE-AGENT REGIMENS

Doxorubicin[1,157]

Prechemo: CBC, Chem, MUGA scan. 5-HT_3 and dexamethasone 10–20 mg. Moderately emetogenic.

Doxorubicin 60 mg/m²: IV push on day 1. Potent vesicant.

Side effects: Myelosuppression may be severe. Nausea and vomiting. Dose reduce with liver dysfunction. Pericarditis-myocarditis syndrome. Cumulative doses >550 mg/m² of doxorubicin, cardiomyopathy. Red-orange discoloration of urine. Hyperpigmentation, photosensitivity, and radiation recall. Complete alopecia occurs with doses >50 mg/m^2.

Chair time: 1 hour on day 1. Repeat every 21 days.

Megestrol[1,158]

Pretreatment: CBC, Chem, and LFTs. Oral phenothiazine or 5-HT$_3$ PRN.

Megestrol 160 mg: PO daily. (20- and 40-mg tablets).

Side effects: Nausea and vomiting rarely observed. Increased appetite with accompanying weight gain. Use with caution with history of either thromboembolic or hypercoagulable disorders. Fluid retention. May exacerbate diabetes mellitus. Increased LFTs. Dose reduce with abnormal liver function. Breakthrough menstrual bleeding.

Chair time: No chair time. Daily PO dosing as tolerated or until progression.

Paclitaxel[1,159]

Prechemo: CBC, Chem, and Mg^{2+}. 5-HT$_3$ and dexamethasone 10–20 Mg. Diphenhydramine 25–50 mg and H$_2$ antagonist. Mildly emetigenic.

Paclitaxel 200 mg/m^2: IV in 500 cc NS over 3 hours on day 1. Reduce to 175m/m^2 for patients with prior pelvic radiation therapy. Use non-PVC containers and tubing with 0.22-micron inline filter.

Side effects: Hypersensitivity reaction. Myelosuppression dose-limiting G-CSF recommended. Nausea and vomiting. Stomatitis. Sensory neuropathy with numbness and paresthesias; dose related. Arthralgias and myalgias. Transient elevations in serum transaminases, bilirubin, and alkaline phosphatase. Alopecia.

Chair time: Chair time 4 hours on day 1. Repeat every 21 days as tolerated or until progression.

Topotecan[1,160]

Prechemo: CBC, Chem, and LFTs. 5-HT$_3$ and dexamethasone 10–20 mg. Moderately to highly emetigenic.

Topotecan 0.1 mg/m^2/day: IV on days 1–5. Reduce dose to 0.8 mg/m^2/day IV on days 1–3 in patients with prior radiation therapy.

Side effects: Myelosuppression dose-limiting toxicity. If severe neutropenia occurs, reduce dose by 0.25 mg/m^2/day or may use G-CSF. Nausea and vomiting dose related. Diarrhea, constipation, and abdominal pain. Dose reduce with low protein and hepatic and renal dysfunction. Microscopic hematuria. Alopecia.

Chair time: 1 hour days 1–5 or days 1–3. Repeat every 21 days.

Medroxyprogesterone[1,161]

Pretreatment: CBC, Chem, LFTs. Oral phenothiazine or 5-HT$_3$.

Medroxyprogesterone 200 mg: PO daily.

Side effects: Nausea and vomiting rarely observed. Use with caution with a history of thromboembolic or hypercoagulable disorders. Fluid retention. Increased LFTs.

Chair time: No chair time. Daily dosing as tolerated or until progression.

ESOPHAGEAL CANCER

COMBINATION REGIMENS

5-FU + Cisplatin + Radiation Therapy (Herskovic Regimen)[1,162]

Prechemo: CBC, Chem, and Mg^{2+}. Central line placement. 5-HT_3 and dexamethasone 10–20 mg. Moderately to highly emetogenic. Chemotherapy and radiation therapy given concurrently.

Fluorouracil 1000 mg/m²/day: IV continuous infusion on days 1–4.

Cisplatin 75 mg/m²/day: IV in 1000 cc NS on day 1. Repeat on weeks 1, 5, 8, and 11.

Radiation therapy: 200 cGy for 5 days per week (total dose 3000 cGy), followed by a boost to field of 2000 cGy.

Side effects: Hypersensitivity reactions with cisplatin. Bone marrow depression dose-limiting. Nausea and vomiting, acute or delayed. Mucositis and diarrhea can be severe and dose-limiting. Nephrotoxicity dose-limiting. Electrolyte imbalance. Decreases Mg^{2+}, K^+, Ca^{2+}, Na^+, and P. Local tissue irritation progressing to desquamation in radiation field. No oil-based lotions in radiation field. Hyperpigmentation, photosensitivity, and nail changes. Hand-foot syndrome can be dose-limiting. Photophobia, increased lacrimation, acute and chronic conjunctivitis, blepharitis, and blurred vision. Alopecia.

Chair time: 2 hours on days 1 of weeks 1, 5, 8, and 11.

5-FU + Cisplatin + Paclitaxel + Radiation Therapy (Hopkins/Yale Regimen)[1,163]

Prechemo: CBC, Chem, and Mg^{2+}. Central line placement. 5-HT_3 and dexamethasone 10–20 mg. Diphenhydramine 25–50 mg and H_2 antagonist. Moderately to highly emetogenic.

Preoperative Chemoradiation:

Fluorouracil 225 mg/m²/day: IV continuous infusion on days 1–30.

Cisplatin 20 mg/m²/day: IV in 500–1000 cc NS on days 1–5 and 26–30.

Radiation therapy 200 cGy/day: Total dose of 4400 cGy, followed by esophagectomy and then adjuvant chemotherapy in patients who had total gross removal of disease with negative margins.

Adjuvant Chemotherapy:

Paclitaxel 135 mg/m²: IV for 24 hours on day 1. Use non-PVC containers and tubing with 0.22-micron inline filter for administration.

Cisplatin 75 mg/m²: IV in 500–1000 c NS on day 2. Chemotherapy is given concurrently with radiation therapy.

Adjuvant chemotherapy is given 8–12 weeks after esophagectomy. Repeat cycle every 21 days for three cycles.

Side effects: Hypersensitivity reaction with paclitaxel. Myelosuppression cumulative, dose related, and dose-limiting. Nausea and vomiting acute or delayed. Mucositis and diarrhea severe and dose-limiting. Nephrotoxicity dose related. Provide adequate hydration to reduce risk. Decreases Mg^{2+}, K^+, Ca^{2+}, Na^+, and P. Local tissue irritation progressing to desquamation. Do not use oil-based lotions or creams in radiation field. Hand-foot syndrome can be dose-limiting. Sensory neuropathy with numbness and paresthesias; dose related. Alopecia.

Preoperative chemotherapy chair time: 2 hours on days 1–5 and 26–30.

Adjuvant therapy chair time: 1 hour on day 1 and 2 hours on day 2. Repeat every 21 days for three cycles.

METASTATIC DISEASE

5-FU + Cisplatin[1,164]

Prechemo: CBC, Chem, and Mg^{2+}. Central line placement. 5-HT$_3$ and dexamethasone 10–20 mg. Moderately to highly emetogenic.

Fluorouracil 1000 mg/m²/day: IV continuous infusion on days 1–5.

Cisplatin 100 mg/m²: IV on day 1 in 1000 cc NS.

Side effects: Myelosuppression G-CSF recommended. Mucositis and diarrhea, can be severe and dose-limiting. Nephrotoxicity. Electrolyte imbalance. Decreases Mg^{2+}, K^+, Ca^{2+}, Na^+, and P. Hyperpigmentation, photosensitivity, and nail changes. Hand-foot syndrome. Photophobia, increased lacrimation, acute and chronic conjunctivitis, blepharitis, and blurred vision.

Chair time: 3 hours on day 1, 1 hour on day 5. Repeat cycle on weeks 1, 5, 8, and 11.

Irinotecan + Cisplatin[1,165]

Prechemo: CBC, Chem, and Mg^{2+}. 5-HT_3 and dexamethasone 10–20 mg in D5W. Atropine 0.25–1.0 mg IV unless contraindicated. Moderately to highly emetogenic

Irinotecan 65 mg/m²: IV in 500 cc of D5W over 90 minutes weekly for 4 weeks.

Cisplatin 30 mg/m²: IV in 500–1000 cc NS weekly for 4 weeks.

Side effects: Early diarrhea, managed with atropine before therapy. Late diarrhea severe and should be treated aggressively. Nausea and vomiting. Myelosuppression can be dose-limiting. Nephrotoxicity dose related. Provide adequate hydration to reduce risk. Decreases Mg^{2+}, K^+, Ca^{2+}, Na^+, and P. Alopecia.

Chair time: 4 hours weekly for 4 weeks. Repeat every 6 weeks.

Paclitaxel + Cisplatin[1,166]

Prechemo: CBC, Chem, Mg^{2+}. Central line placement. 5-HT_3 and dexamethasone 10–20 mg. Diphenhydramine 25–50 mg and H_2 antagonist. Moderately to highly emetogenic.

Paclitaxel 200 mg/m²: IV over 24 hours on day 1. Use non-PVC containers and tubing with 0.22-micron inline filter.

Cisplatin 75 mg/m²: IV in 1000 cc NS on day 2.

Side effects: Hypersensitivity reaction. Myelosuppression dose-limiting. G-CSF recommended. Nausea and vomiting, acute and delayed. Stomatitis. Sensory neuropathy with numbness and paresthesias, dose related. Arthralgias and myalgias. Transient elevations in serum transaminases, bilirubin, and alkaline phosphatase. Nephrotoxicity dose related. Provide adequate hydration to reduce risk. Electrolyte imbalance. Decreases Mg^{2+}, K^+, Ca^{2+}, Na^+, and P. Sensory neuropathy with numbness and paresthesias, dose related. Alopecia.

Chair time: 1 hour on day 1 and 3 hours on day 2. Repeat every 21 days.

5-FU + Cisplatin + Definitive Radiation Therapy[1,167]

Prechemo: CBC, Chem, and Mg^{2+}. Central line placement. 5-HT_3 and dexamethasone 10–20 mg. Moderately to highly emetogenic. Chemotherapy and radiation therapy given concurrently.

Fluorouracil 1000 mg/m²/day: IV continuous infusion days 1–4, 29–32, 50–53, and 71–74.

Cisplatin 75 mg/m²: IV in 1000 cc NS on days 1, 29, 50, and 71.

External beam radiation therapy: 50 cGy at 1.8 cGy per day, 5 days per week.

Side effects: Hypersensitivity reactions. Myelosuppression cumulative and dose-limiting. Nausea and vomiting, acute or delayed. Mucositis and diarrhea, can be severe and dose-limiting. Nephrotoxicity dose related. Provide adequate hydration to reduce risk. Electrolyte imbalance. Decreases Mg^{2+}, K^+, Ca^{2+}, Na^+, and P. Local tissue irritation progressing to desquamation in radiation field. No oil-based lotions in radiation field. Hyperpigmentation, photosensitivity, and nail changes may occur. Hand-foot syndrome can be dose-limiting. Photophobia, increased lacrimation, acute and chronic conjunctivitis, blepharitis and blurred vision. Alopecia.

Chair time: 2 hours on days 1, 29, 50, and 71.

SINGLE-AGENT REGIMENS

Paclitaxel[1,168]

Prechemo: CBC, Chem, and Mg^{2+}. 5-HT$_3$ and dexamethasone 10–20mg. Diphenhydramine 25–50 mg and H_2 antagonist. Moderately to highly emetogenic.

Paclitaxel 250 mg/m²: IV over 24 hours on day 1. Use non-PVC containers and tubing with 0.22-micron inline filter.

Side effects: Hypersensitivity reaction. Myelosuppression dose-limiting G-CSF recommended. Nausea and vomiting. Stomatitis. Sensory neuropathy with numbness and paresthesias, dose related. Arthralgias and myalgias. Transient elevations in serum transaminases, bilirubin, and alkaline phosphatase. Alopecia.

Chair time: 1 hour. 1 hour for day 2 to discontinue pump. Repeat every 21 days.

GASTRIC CANCER

ADJUVANT THERAPY

Chemoradiation Therapy[1,169]

One cycle of chemotherapy administered as follows:

Prechemo: CBC, Chem, andMg^{2+}. Oral phenothiazine or 5-HT$_3$. Mildly to moderately emetogenic.

Fluorouracil 425 mg/m^2: IV push on days 1–5.

Leucovorin 20 mg/m^2: IV push on days 1–5. Chemoradiotherapy is then started 28 days after the start of the initial cycle of chemotherapy as follows:

Radiation therapy: 180 cGy/day to a total dose of 4,500 cGy starting on day 28.

Fluorouracil 400 mg/m^2: IV push on days 1–4 and days 23–25 of radiation therapy.

Leucovorin 20 mg/m^2: IV push on days 1–4 and days 23–25 of radiation therapy. Chemoradiotherapy is followed by two cycles of chemotherapy given 1 month apart as follows:

Fluorouracil 425 mg/m^2: IV push on days 1–5.

Leucovorin 20 mg/m^2: IV push on days 1–5.

Side effects: Myelosuppression can be dose-limiting. Nausea and vomiting, acute or delayed. Mucositis and diarrhea can be dose-limiting. Local tissue irritation progressing to desquamation in radiation field. No oil-based lotions in radiation field. Hyperpigmentation, photosensitivity, and nail changes may occur. Hand-foot syndrome can be dose-limiting. Photophobia, increased lacrimation, acute and chronic conjunctivitis, blepharitis, and blurred vision.

Chair time: 1 hour for chemotherapy for each visit.

COMBINATION REGIMENS

Docetaxel + Cisplatin + 5-FU (DCF)[1,170]

Prechemo: CBC, Chem, and Mg^{2+}. Central line placement. 5-HT_3 and dexamethasone 10–20 mg. Moderately to highly emetogenic.

Docetaxel 75 mg/m²: IV in 250 cc NS on day 1. Use non-PVC containers and tubing.

Cisplatin 75 mg/m²: IV in 1000 cc NS over 1–3 hours on day 1.

Fluorouracil 750 mg/m²/day: IV continuous infusion on days 1–5.

Side effects: Hypersensitivity reaction with docetaxel. Myelosuppression dose-limiting G-CSF recommended. Nausea and vomiting, acute or delayed. Stomatitis. Diarrhea can be dose-limiting. Nephrotoxicity is dose related. Provide adequate hydration to reduce risk. Sensory neuropathy with numbness and paresthesias, dose related. Arthralgias and myalgias. Transient elevations in serum transaminases, bilirubin, and alkaline phosphatase. Decreases Mg^{2+}, K^+, Ca^{2+}, Na^+, and P. Hyperpigmentation, photosensitivity, and nail changes may occur. Hand-foot syndrome can be dose-limiting. Photophobia, increased lacrimation, conjunctivitis, and blurred vision. Alopecia.

Chair time: 4 hours on day 1. Repeat cycle every 21 days.

5-FU + Cisplatin (CF)[1,170]

Prechemo: CBC, Chem, and Mg^{2+}. Central line placement. 5-HT_3 and dexamethasone 10–20 mg. Moderately to highly emetogenic.

Cisplatin 100 mg/m²: IV in 1000 cc NS over 1–3 hours on day 1.

Fluorouracil 1000 mg/m²/day: IV continuous infusion on days 1–5.

Side effects: Myelosuppression. Mucositis can be severe and dose-limiting. Nausea and vomiting, acute or delayed. Nephrotoxicity, dose related. Provide adequate hydration to reduce risk. Electrolyte imbalance: decreases Mg^{2+}, K^+, Ca^{2+}, Na^+, and P. Hyperpigmentation, photosensitivity, and nail changes. Hand-foot syndrome. Photophobia, increased lacrimation, acute and chronic conjunctivitis, blepharitis, and blurred vision.

Chair time: 3 hours on day 1. Repeat cycle every 28 days.

Etoposide + Doxorubicin + Cisplatin (EAP)[1,171]

Prechemo: CBC, Chem, Mg^{2+}, and MUGA scan. 5-HT_3 and dexamethasone 10–20 mg. Moderately to highly emetogenic.

Etoposide 120 mg/m²: IV in 250 cc NS over 30–60 minutes on days 4–6.

Doxorubicin 20 mg/m²: IV push on days 1 and 7. Potent vesicant.

Cisplatin 40 mg/m²: IV in 500–1000 cc NS over 1–3 hours on days 2 and 8.

Side effects: Hypersensitivity reaction with etoposide. Myelosuppression, dose-limiting G-CSF recommended. Nausea and vomiting, acute or delayed. Stomatitis. Sensory neuropathy with numbness and paresthesias, dose related. Arthralgias and myalgias. Transient elevations in serum transaminases, bilirubin, and alkaline phosphatase. Red-orange discoloration of urine. Nephrotoxicity dose related. Provide adequate hydration to reduce risk. Decreases Mg^{2+}, K^+, Ca^{2+}, Na^+, and P. Hyperpigmentation, radiation recall, and nail changes. Hypotension with rapid infusion of etoposide. Cardiomyopathy with high cumulative doses of doxorubicin.

Chair time: 1 hour on days 1, 4, 5, 6, and 7; 3 hours on days 2 and 8. Repeat cycle every 21–28 days.

Epirubicin + Cisplatin + Fluorouracil (ECF)[1,172]

Prechemo: CBC, Chem, LFTs, MUGA scan. 5-HT$_3$ and dexamethasone 20 mg. Moderately to highly emetogenic.

Epirubicin 50 mg/m²: IV push on day 1. Vesicant.

Cisplatin 60 mg/m²: IV in 500–1000 cc NS over 1–3 hours on day 1.

5-Flourouracil 200 mg/m²: IV continuous infusion for 21 days.

Side effects: Myelosuppression may be severe. Nausea and vomiting. Mucositis and diarrhea dose-limiting. Cardiotoxicity is dose related, is cumulative, and may occur during months to years after cessation of therapy with epirubicin. Dose reduce with liver dysfunction. Red-orange discoloration of urine. Epirubicin may cause "flare" reaction or streaking along vein during peripheral administration. Slow drug administration time and increase rate of free-flowing IV. Hyperpigmentation, photosensitivity, nail changes, and radiation recall. Hand-foot syndrome, dose-limiting. Photophobia, increased lacrimation, conjunctivitis, and blurred vision. Nephrotoxicity dose related, provide adequate hydration to reduce risk. Electrolyte imbalance: decreases Mg^{2+}, K^+, Ca^{2+}, Na^+, and P. Hand-foot syndrome can be dose-limiting. Alopecia.

Chair time: 3 hours on day 1 and 1 hour on day 8 & 15 for pump refill. Repeat every 21 days.

Etoposide + Leucovorin + Fluorouracil (ELF)[1,173]

Prechemo: CBC, Chem, and LFTs, 5-HT$_3$, and dexamethasone 20 mg. Moderately to highly emetogenic.

Etoposide 120 mg/m²: IV in 250 cc NS on days 1–3.

Leucovorin 300 mg/m²: IV on days 1–3.

5-Fluorouracil 500 mg/m²: IV push on days 1–3.

Side effects: Hypersensitivity reaction with etoposide. Myelosuppression dose-limiting. Nausea and vomiting. Mucositis and diarrhea can be severe and dose-limiting. Hypotension with rapid infusion of etoposide. Alopecia is dose dependent. Hyperpigmentation, photosensitivity, and nail changes. Hand-foot syndrome can be dose-limiting. Photophobia, increased lacrimation, conjunctivitis, and blurred vision.

Chair time: 1 hour on days 1–3. Repeat every 21–28 days as tolerated.

Irinotecan + Cisplatin (IP)[1,174]

Prechemo: CBC, Chem, Mg^{2+}, and LFTs. $5\text{-}HT_3$ and dexamethasone 20 mg in D5W. Atropine 0.25–1.0 mg IV unless contraindicated. Moderately to highly emetogenic.

Irinotecan 70 mg/m²: IV in 250–500 cc D5W on days 1 and 15.

Cisplatin 80 mg/m²: IV in 1000 cc NS over 1–3 hours on day 1.

Side effects: Myelosuppression can be severe, dose-limiting toxicity. Nausea and vomiting, acute or delayed. Diarrhea or constipation, abdominal pain, early diarrhea, managed with atropine before irinotecan. Late diarrhea severe and should be treated aggressively. Consider lomotil, Imodium, tincture of opium, and hydration. Dose reduce irinotecan for low protein and hepatic dysfunction. Dose reduce cisplatin for abnormal renal function. Nephrotoxicity dose related, provide adequate hydration to reduce risk. Decreases Mg^{2+}, K^+, Ca^{2+}, Na^+ and P. Peripheral sensory neuropathy, paresthesias, and numbness dose-limiting. Ototoxicity. Alopecia.

Chair time: 4 hours on day 1 and 2 hours on day 15. Repeat cycle every 28 days.

5-Fluorouracil + Doxorubicin + Mitomycin (FAM)[1,175]

Prechemo: CBC, Chem, LFTs, and MUGA scan. $5\text{-}HT_3$ and dexamethasone 20 mg. Moderately to highly emetogenic.

Fluorouracil 600 mg/m²: IV push on days 1, 8, 29, and 36.

Doxorubicin 30 mg/m²: IV push on days 1 and 29. Potent vesicant.

Mitomycin 10 mg/m²: IV push on day 1. Potent vesicant.

Side effects: Myelosuppression dose-limiting and cumulative. Nausea and vomiting. Mucositis and diarrhea can be severe and dose-limiting. Doxorubicin can cause cardiomyopathy with cumulative doses >450 mg/m². Hyperpigmentation, photosensitivity, radiation recall, and nail changes. Hand-foot syndrome can be dose-limiting. Photophobia, increased lacrimation, conjunctivitis, and blurred vision. Red-orange discoloration of urine. Hemolytic-uremic syndrome.

Chair time: 1 hour on days 1, 8, 29, and 36. Repeat cycle every 8 weeks.

5-Fluorouracil + Doxorubicin + Methotrexate (FAMTX)[1,176]

Prechemo: CBC, Chem, LFTs, MUGA scan. 5-HT$_3$ and dexamethasone 20 mg. Prehydration/posthydration: 1000 cc of 0.9% sodium chloride with two ampules of NaHCO$_3$. Moderately to highly emetogenic.

Fluorouracil 1500 mg/m^2: IV on day 1, starting 1 hour after MTX.

Leucovorin 15 mg/m^2: PO every 6 hours for 12 doses. Start 24 hours after MTX.

Leucovorin rescue: Must be given on time and should continue until MTX level is <50 nM.

Doxorubicin 30 mg/m^2: IV push on day 15. Potent vesicant.

Methotrexate 1500 mg/m^2: IV in 1000 cc NS over minimum of 3 hours on day 1.

High doses cross the blood-brain barrier; reconstitute with preservative-free 0.9% sodium chloride. Urine should be alkalized before and after administration to prevent crystallization in the kidneys.

Side effects: MTX may precipitate in renal tubules, causing acute renal tubular necrosis if urine pH > 7.0 is not maintained for 48–72 hours after administration. Myelosuppression dose-limiting and cumulative toxicity. Nausea and vomiting. Mucositis and diarrhea can be severe and dose-limiting. Red-orange discoloration of urine. Hyperpigmentation, photosensitivity, radiation recall, and nail changes. Hand-foot syndrome can be dose-limiting. Doxorubicin can cause cardiomyopathy at cumulative doses >450 mg/m^2. Photophobia, increased lacrimation, conjunctivitis, and blurred vision.

Chair time: 8 hours on day 1 and 1 hour on day 15. Repeat cycle every 28 days.

Fluorouracil + Doxorubicin + Cisplatin (FAP)[1,177]

Prechemo: CBC, Chem, LFTs, MUGA scan. 5-HT$_3$ and dexamethasone 20 mg. Moderately to highly emetogenic.

Fluorouracil 300 mg/m^2: IV push days 1–5.

Doxorubicin 40 mg/m^2: IV push on day. Potent vesicant.

Cisplatin 60 mg/m^2: IV in 500–1000 cc NS over 1–3 hours on day 1.

Side effects: Myelosuppression dose related. Nausea and vomiting may be acute or delayed. Mucositis and diarrhea can be severe and dose-limiting. Red-orange discoloration of urine. Doxorubicin can cause cardiomyopathy with cumulative doses, >450 mg/m^2. Nephrotoxicity is dose related, provide adequate hydration to reduce risk. Electrolyte imbalance: decreases Mg^{2+}, K^+, Ca^{2+}, Na^+, and P. Hyperpigmentation, radiation recall, photosensitivity, and nail changes. Hand-foot syndrome can be dose-limiting. Photophobia, increased lacrimation, conjunctivitis, and blurred vision.

Chair time: 3 hours on day 1 and 1 hour on days 2–5. Repeat cycle every 5 weeks.

Docetaxel + Cisplatin[1,178]

Prechemo: CBC, Chem, LFTs, MUGA scan. Dexamethasone 8 mg PO bid the day before the day of and the day after treatment. 5-HT_3. Moderately to highly emetogenic.

Docetaxel 85 mg/m²: IV in 250 cc NS on day 1. Use non-PVC containers and tubings.

Cisplatin 75 mg/m²: IV in 1000 cc NS over 1–3 hours on day 1.

Side effects: Hypersensitivity reaction. Myelosuppression dose related and dose-limiting. Nausea and vomiting may be acute or delayed. Nephrotoxicity dose related. Provide adequate hydration to reduce risk. Electrolyte imbalance: decreases Mg^{2+}, K^+, Ca^{2+}, Na^+, and P. Peripheral neuropathy. Alopecia. Nail changes.

Chair time: 4 hours on day 1. Repeat cycle every 21 days.

Docetaxel + Cisplatin + 5-FU (TCF)[1,179]

Prechemo: CBC, Chem, and LFTs. Central line placement. Dexamethasone 8-mg PO bid day before, day of, and day after treatment. 5-HT3. Moderately to highly emetogenic.

Docetaxel 75 mg/m²: IV in 250 cc NS on day 1. Use non-PVC containers and tubing.

Cisplatin 75 mg/m²: IV in 1000 cc NS on day 1.

Fluorouracil 750 mg/m²/day: IV continuous infusion on days 1–5.

Side effects: Hypersensitivity reaction with docetaxel and cisplatin. Myelosuppression dose related, dose-limiting. Nausea and vomiting acute or delayed. Mucositis and diarrhea can be severe and dose-limiting. Nephrotoxicity dose related and dose-limiting. Reduce risk with adequate hydration. Hemorrhagic cystitis. Fluid retention, weight gain, peripheral and/or generalized edema, pleural effusion and/or ascites. Dose-limiting peripheral sensory neuropathy. Paresthesias and numbness. Decreases Mg^{2+}, K^+, Ca^{2+}, Na^+, and Phos. Hyperpigmentation, photosensitivity, and nail changes. Hand-foot syndrome dose-limiting. Photophobia, increased lacrimation, conjunctivitis, and blurred vision.

Chair time: 4 hours on day 1. Repeat cycle every 21 days.

SINGLE-AGENT REGIMENS

5-Fluorouracil[1,180]

Prechemo: CBC, Chem, LFTs. Oral phenothiazide or 5-HT_3. Mild to moderately emetogenic.

5-Fluorouracil 500 mg/m²: IV push on days 1–5.

Side effects: Myelosuppression, dose related, dose-limiting. Nausea and vomiting. Mucositis and diarrhea can be severe and dose-limiting. Alopecia. Hyperpigmentation, photosensitivity, and nail changes may occur. Hand-foot syndrome can be dose-limiting. Photophobia, increased lacrimation, conjunctivitis, and blurred vision.

Chair time: 1 hour on days 1–5. Repeat cycle every 28 days.

Docetaxel[1,181]

Prechemo: CBC, Chem, and LFTs. Dexamethasone 8 mg PO bid day before, day of, and day after treatment. 5-HT$_3$ in 100cc NS. Moderately to highly emetogenic.

Docetaxel 100 mg/m²: IV in 250 cc NS on day 1. Repeat cycle every 21 days.

OR

Docetaxel 36 mg/m²: IV in 250 cc NS weekly for 6 weeks. Repeat every 8 weeks. Use non-PVC containers and tubing.

Side effects: Hypersensitivity reactions. Myelosuppression, G-CSF recommended. Nausea and vomiting. Mucositis and diarrhea. Peripheral neuropathy with paresthesias. Fluid retention with weight gain, peripheral and/or generalized edema, pleural effusion, and ascites. Alopecia. Nail changes, rash, and dry, pruritic skin. Hand-foot syndrome.

Chair time: 2 hours on day 1. Repeat cycle every 21 days.

OR

2 hours weekly for 6 weeks. Repeat cycle every 8 weeks.

GASTROINTESTINAL STROMAL TUMOR (GIST)

SINGLE-AGENT REGIMENS

Imatinib (Gleevec) [1,182]

Prechemo: CBC, Chem, LFTs, c-kit (CD117) expression. Oral phenothiazine or 5-HT₃. Mildly emetogenic.

Imatinib at 400 mg: PO per day. May increase dose to 600 or 800 mg
PO per day if no response. 800 mg dose is given 400 mg bid. 100- or
400-mg capsules. Taken with food and a large glass of water. Do NOT
take with grapefruit juice. Monitor INRs closely, inhibits metabolism
of warfarin.

Side effects: Nausea and vomiting, usually relieved when taken with
food. Diarrhea, or constipation seen. Myelosuppression. Hold for ANC
$<1.0 \times 10^9$/ L and platelets $<50 \times 10^9$/L. Hold until ANC >1500 and
platelets $>50,000$. Resume dose at 400 mg. If recurrence, decrease to
300 mg. Fluid retention, especially in older patients. Periorbital and
lower-extremity edema primarily seen, pleural effusions, ascites, rapid
weight gain, and pulmonary edema may develop. Hypokalemia. Muscle
cramps, arthralgias, headache, fatigue, and abdominal pain. Rash, treat
with systemic antihistamine, topical or systemic corticosteroid. Mild,
transient elevation in serum transaminase and bilirubin levels. Multiple
drug interactions with CYP3A4 pathway.

Chair time: No chair time. Daily as tolerated until disease progression.

Sunitinib (Sutent) [1,183]

Prechemo: CBC, Chem, with P, LFTs, and TFTs. Oral phenothiazine
or 5-HT₃.

Sunitinib 50 mg: PO per day, 4 weeks on 2 weeks off. (12.5-, 25-, and 50-mg capsules.) May be taken with or without food. Dose modification: increase or decrease by 12.5 mg based on individual safety and tolerance.

Side effects: Diarrhea, nausea and vomiting, stomatitis, constipation, and abdominal pain. Decreases in left ventricular ejection fraction dysfunction (LVEF). Monitor for signs and symptoms of congestive heart failure (CHF). Patients with cardiac history should have a baseline LVEF. Hypertension. Hemorrhagic events: epistaxis arthralgia, back pain, and myalgias. Acquired hypothyroidism. Multiple drug interactions: CYP3A4 pathway.

Chair time: No chair time. Daily for 4 weeks; repeat cycle every 6 weeks.

HEAD AND NECK CANCER

COMBINATION REGIMENS

Paclitaxel + Ifosfamide + Mesna + Cisplatin (TIP)[1,184]

Prechemo: CBC, Chem, and Mg^{2+}. 5-HT3 and dexamethasone 10–20 mg (days 1–3). Diphenhydramine 25–50 mg and H_2 antagonist (day 1 only). Moderately to highly emetogenic.

Paclitaxel 175 mg/m²: IV in 500 cc NS over 3 hours on day 1. Use non-PVC tubing and containers, and 0.22-micron inline filter.

Ifosfamide 1000 mg/m²: IV in 500 cc NS over 2 hours on days 1–3.

Mesna 400 mg/m²: IV in 100 cc NS over 15 minutes before ifosfamide.

Mesna 200 mg/m²: IV in 100 cc NS over 15 minutes 4 hours after ifosfamide mesna tablets may be given orally in a dosage equal to 40% of the ifosfamide dose.

Cisplatin 60 mg/m²: IV in 500–1000 cc NS over 1–2 hours on day 1.

Side effects: Hypersensitivity reaction with paclitaxel. Myelosuppression G-CSF support recommended. Give paclitaxel before cisplatin to decrease severity of myelosuppression. Nausea and vomiting, acute or delayed. Mucositis and/or diarrhea common. Hemorrhagic cystitis dysuria and increased urinary frequency occurs with ifosfamide. Uroprotection with mesna and hydration mandatory. Decreases Mg^{2+}, K^+, Ca^{2+}, Na^+, and P. SIADH. Sensory neuropathy with numbness and paresthesias. Somnolence, confusion, depressive psychosis, or hallucinations. High-frequency hearing loss and tinnitus. Alopecia.

Chair time: 7 hours on day 1 and 3 hours on days 2 and 3. Repeat every 21–28 days.

Docetaxel + Cisplatin + 5-FU (TPF)[1,185]

Prechemo: CBC, Chem, and Mg^{2+}. Central line placement. 5-HT3. Dexamethasone 8-mg PO bid day before, day of, and day after docetaxel. Moderately to highly epometogenic.

Docetaxel 75 mg/m²: IV in 250 cc NS on day 1. Use non-PVC containers and tubing.

Cisplatin 75–100 mg/m²: IV in 1000 cc NS over 24 hours on day 1.

Fluorouracil 1000 mg/m²/day: IV continuous infusion on days 1–4.

Side effects: Hypersensitivity reaction: with docetaxel and cisplatin. Myelosuppression, dose related and dose-limiting. Nausea and vomiting acute or delayed. Mucositis and diarrhea can be severe and dose-limiting. Nephrotoxicity, dose related and dose-limiting. Reduce risk with adequate hydration. Hemorrhagic cystitis. Fluid retention weight gain, peripheral and/or generalized edema, pleural effusion, and/or ascites. Dose-limiting peripheral sensory neuropathy. Paresthesias and numbness. Decreases Mg^{2+}, K^+, Ca^{2+}, Na^+, and Phos. Hyperpigmentation, photosensitivity, and nail changes. Hand-foot syndrome dose-limiting. Photophobia, increased lacrimation, conjunctivitis, and blurred vision. Alopecia.

Chair time: 3 hours on day 1. Repeat cycle every 21 days.

Paclitaxel + Ifosfamide + Mesna + Carboplatin (TIC)[1,186]

Prechemo: CBC, Chem, BUN, creatinine clearance, and Mg^{2+}. 5-HT3 and dexamethasone 10–20 mg (days 1–3). Diphenhydramine 25–50 mg and H_2 antagonist (day 1 only). Moderately to highly emetogenic.

Paclitaxel 175 mg/m²: IV in 500 cc NS over 3 hours on day 1. Use non-PVC tubing and containers and 0.22-micron inline filter.

Ifosfamide 1000 mg/m²: IV in 500 cc NS over 2 hours on days 1–3.

Mesna 400 mg/m²: IV in 100 cc NS over 15 minutes before ifosfamide.

Mesna 200 mg/m²: IV in 100 cc NS over 15 minutes for 4 hours after ifosfamide.

Carboplatin AUC 6: IV in 500 cc NS on day 1. Give after paclitaxel to decrease toxicity.

Side effects: Hypersensitivity reaction: paclitaxel and carboplatin. Increased risk of carboplatin reaction after more than seven doses of carboplatin. Myelosuppression, dose-limiting. G-CSF recommended. Nausea and vomiting acute or delayed. Mucositis and/or diarrhea. Nephrotoxicity dose-limiting toxicity. Reduce risk with adequate hydration. Hemorrhagic cystitis. Decreases Mg^{2+}, K^+, Ca^{2+}, Na^+, and Phos. Dose-limiting peripheral sensory neuropathy. Paresthesias and numbness are cumulative. Somulence, confusion, depressive psychosis, or hallucinations. Alopecia.

Chair time: 7 hours on day 1; 4 hours on days 2 and 3. Repeat cycle every 21–28 days.

Paclitaxel + Carboplatin[1,187]

Prechemo: CBC, Chem, and Mg^{2+}. $5-HT_3$ and dexamethasone 10–20 mg in 100 cc of NS. Diphenhydramine 25–50 mg and H_2 antagonist in 100 cc of NS. Mildly to moderately emetogenic protocol.

Paclitaxel 175 mg/m²: IV in 500 cc NS over 3 hours on day 1. Use non-PVC containers and tubing with 0.22-micron inline filter.

Carboplatin AUC 6: IV in 500 cc NS on day 1. Give after paclitaxel to decrease toxicities.

Side effects: Hypersensitivity reaction with paclitaxel or carboplatin. Increased risk of carboplatin reaction in patients receiving more than seven courses of carboplatin therapy. Myelosuppression cumulative and dose related and dose-limiting. G-CSF recommended. Nausea and vomiting acute or delayed. Mucositis and/or diarrhea. Transient elevations in serum transaminases, bilirubin, and alkaline phosphatase. Decreases Mg^{2+}, K^+, Ca^{2+}, and Na^+. Sensory neuropathy with numbness and paresthesias. Dose related and can be dose-limiting. Alopecia.

Chair time: 5 hours on day 1. Repeat cycle every 21 days until disease progression.

Paclitaxel + Cisplatin[1,188]

Prechemo: CBC, Chem, and Mg^{2+}. 5-HT3 and dexamethasone 10–20 mg in (days 1 and 2). Diphenhydramine 25–50 mg and H_2 antagonist (day 1 only). Moderately to highly emetogenic.

Paclitaxel 175 mg/m²: IV in 500 cc NS over 3 hours on day 1. Use non-PVC containers and tubing with a 0.22-micron inline filter.

Cisplatin 75 mg/m²: IV in 500–1000 cc NS day 2.

Side effects: Hypersensitivity reaction with paclitaxel or cisplatin. Myelosuppression, cumulative, dose related, and dose-limiting. G-CSF recommended. Nausea and vomiting acute or delayed. Mucositis and/or diarrhea. Metallic taste to food and loss of appetite. Nephrotoxicity dose related, reduce risk with hydration. Decreases in Mg^{2+}, K^+, Ca^{2+}, Na^+, and Phos. Dose-limiting peripheral sensory neuropathy. Paresthesias and numbness is cumulative. Alopecia.

Chair time: 5 hours on days 1 and 2. Repeat cycle every 21 days until progression.

5-FU + Cisplatin (PF)[1,189]

Prechemo: CBC, Chem, and Mg^{2+}. Central line placement. $5-HT_3$ and dexamethasone 10–20 mg. Moderately to highly emetogenic.

Cisplatin 100 mg/m²: IV on day 1 in 1000 cc NS.

Fluorouracil 1000 mg/m²/day: IV continuous infusion on days 1–5.

Side effects: Neutropenia, thrombocytopenia, and anemia. Growth factor recommended. Mucositis and diarrhea, severe and dose-limiting. Nephrotoxicity dose related, reduce risk with hydration. Decreases in Mg^{2+}, K^+, Ca^{2+}, Na^+, and Phos. Hyperpigmentation, photosensitivity, and nail changes. Hand-foot syndrome. Photophobia, increased lacrimation, acute and chronic conjunctivitis, blepharitis, and blurred vision. Alopecia.

Chair time: 3 hours on day 1. Repeat cycle every 21–28 days.

Cisplatin + Fluorouracil + Leucovorin (PFL)[1,190]

Prechemo: CBC, Chem, and Mg^{2+}. Central line placement. 5-HT_3 and dexamethasone 10–20 mg. Moderately to highly emetogenic.

Cisplatin 100 mg/m²: IV in 1000 cc NS on day 1 in 1000 cc NS.

Fluorouracil 800 mg/m²/day: IV continuous infusion on days 1–5.

Leucovorin 50 mg/m²: PO every 6 hours on days 1–5.

Side effects: Myelosuppression, G-CSF recommended. Mucositis and diarrhea, severe and dose-limiting. Nephrotoxicity dose related, reduce risk with hydration. Decreases in Mg^{2+}, K^+, Ca^{2+}, Na^+, and Phos. Hyperpigmentation, photosensitivity, and nail changes. Hand-foot syndrome. Photophobia, increased lacrimation, acute and chronic conjunctivitis, blepharitis, and blurred vision.

Chair time: 3 hours on day 1. Repeat cycle every 21 days.

Cisplatin + Fluorouracil + Radiation Therapy (PF-Larynx Preservation)[1,191]

Prechemo: CBC, Chem, and Mg^{2+}. Central line placement. 5-HT_3 and dexamethasone 10–20 mg. Moderately to highly emetogenic.

Cisplatin 100 mg/m²: IV on day 1.

Fluorouracil 1000 mg/m²/day: IV continuous infusion days 1–5.

Radiation therapy: 6600–7600 cGy in 180 to 200 cGy fractions.

Side effects: Hypersensitivity reactions, myelosuppression. Nausea and vomiting, acute or delayed. Mucositis and diarrhea can be severe. Nephrotoxicity dose related, reduce risk with hydration. Decreases in Mg^{2+}, K^+, Ca^{2+}, Na^+, and Phos. Local tissue irritation progressing to desquamation in radiation field. No oil-based lotions in radiation field. Hyperpigmentation, photosensitivity, and nail changes may occur. Hand-foot syndrome can be dose-limiting. Photophobia, increased lacrimation, acute and chronic conjunctivitis, blepharitis, and blurred vision. Alopecia.

Chair time: 2 hours on day 1 of each cycle. Repeat cycle every 21–28 days for three cycles.

Concurrent Chemoradiation Therapy for Laryngeal Preservation[1,192]

Prechemo: CBC, Chem, and Mg^{2+}. Central line placement. 5-HT_3 and dexamethasone 10–20 mg. Moderately to highly emetogenic.

Cisplatin 100 mg/m²/day: IV in 1000 cc on days 1, 22, and 43.

Radiation therapy: 7000 cGy in 200 cGy fractions.

Side effects: Hypersensitivity reactions, myelosuppression. Nausea and vomiting, acute or delayed. Mucositis and diarrhea can be severe. Nephrotoxicity dose related, reduce risk with hydration. Decreases in Mg^{2+}, K^+, Ca^{2+}, Na^+, and Phos. Alopecia. Local tissue irritation progressing to desquamation in radiation field. No oil-based lotions in radiation field.

Chair time: 2 hours on days 1, 22, and 43.

Chemoradiotherapy for Nasopharyngeal Cancer[1,193]

Prechemo: CBC, Chem, and Mg^{2+}. Central line placement. 5-HT_3 and dexamethasone 10–20 mg. Moderately to highly emetogenic.

Cisplatin 100 mg/m²: IV in 1000 cc NS on days 1, 22, and 43 during radiation.

Radiation therapy: 7000 cGy in 180–200 cGy fractions.

At the completion of chemoradiotherapy, chemotherapy is administered as follows:

Cisplatin 80 mg/m²: IV in 1000 cc NS on day 1.

Fluorouracil 1000 mg/m²/day: IV continuous infusion on days 1–4. Repeat cycle every 28 days for a total of three cycles.

Side effects: Hypersensitivity reactions, myelosuppression. Nausea and vomiting, acute or delayed. Mucositis and diarrhea can be severe. Nephrotoxicity dose related, reduce risk with hydration. Decreases in Mg^{2+}, K^+, Ca^{2+} Na^+, and Phos. Local tissue irritation progressing to desquamation in radiation field. No oil-based lotions in radiation field. Hyperpigmentation, photosensitivity, and nail changes may occur. Hand-foot syndrome can be dose-limiting. Photophobia, increased lacrimation, acute and chronic conjunctivitis, blepharitis, and blurred vision. Alopecia.

Chair time: 2 hour on days 1, 22, and 43 during radiation therapy. Then, 2 hours day 1 after radiation therapy. Repeat cycles every 28 days for a total of three cycles.

Carboplatin + Fluorouracil[1,194]

Prechemo: CBC, Chem, and Mg^{2+}. 5-HT3 and dexamethasone 10–20mg. Moderately to highly emetogenic.

Carboplatin 300–400 mg/m²: IV in 500 cc NS on day 1.

Fluorouracil 600 mg/m²: IV push on day 1.

Side effects: Hypersensitivity reactions carboplatin, increased risk after seven cycles of carboplatin. Myelosuppression, dose related and dose-limiting. Anemia with prolonged treatment. Nausea and vomiting acute or delayed. Mucositis and diarrhea can be severe and dose-limiting. Nephrotoxicity is less common than with cisplatin and is rarely symptomatic. Decreases in Mg^{2+}, K^+, Ca^{2+}, Na^+, and Phos. Hyperpigmentation, photosensitivity, and nail changes may occur. Hand-foot syndrome can be dose-limiting. Photophobia, increased lacrimation, conjunctivitis, and blurred vision. Alopecia.

Chair time: 2 hours on day 1. Repeat the cycle every 21 days.

Vinorelbine + Cisplatin (VP)[1,195]

Prechemo: CBC, Chem, and Mg^{2+}. 5-HT3 and dexamethasone 10–20 mg. Moderately to highly emetogenic.

Vinorelbine 25 mg/m²: IV on days 1 and 8. Vesicant.

Further dilute in syringe or IV bag to concentration of 1.5–3.0 mg/mL. Infuse diluted drug IV over 6–10 minutes into sidearm port of free-flowing IV infusion. Use port closest to the IV bag, not to the patient. Flush with at least 75–125 mL of IV fluid after administration.

Cisplatin 80 mg/m²: IV in 1000 cc NS over 1–2 hours day 1.

Side effects: Myelosuppression dose related and can be dose-limiting. Nausea and vomiting acute or delayed. Constipation, diarrhea, stomatitis, and anorexia. Nephrotoxicity is dose related. Decreases in Mg^{2+}, K^+, Ca^{2+}, Na^+, and Phos. Peripheral sensory neuropathy, paresthesias, and numbness—can be dose-limiting. High-frequency hearing loss and tinnitus. Alopecia.

Chair time: 3 hours on day 1 and 1 hour on day 8. Repeat the cycle every 21 days.

SINGLE-AGENT REGIMENS

Docetaxel[1,196]

Prechemo: CBC, Chem, and LFTs. Dexamethasone 8-mg PO bid day before, day of, and day after treatment. 5-HT$_3$. Mildly to moderately emetogenic.

Docetaxel 100 mg/m²: IV on day 1. Use non-PVC containers and tubing.

Side effects: Hypersensitivity reactions. Myelosuppression. G-CSF recommended. Nausea and vomiting. Mucositis and diarrhea. Peripheral neuropathy with paresthesias. Fluid retention with weight gain, peripheral and/or generalized edema, pleural effusion, and ascites. Nail changes, rash, and dry, pruritic skin. Hand-foot syndrome. Alopecia.

Chair time: 2 hours on day 1. Repeat cycle every 21 days.

Paclitaxel[1,197]

Prechemo: CBC, Chem, and Mg^{2+}. Central line placement for continuous infusion dosing. 5-HT_3 and dexamethasone 10–20 mg. Diphenhydramine 25–50 mg and H_2 antagonist. Mildly to moderately emetogenic.

Paclitaxel 250 mg/m²: IV over 24 hours on day 1. Repeat every 21 days.

OR

Paclitaxel 137–175 mg/m²: IV in 500 cc NS over 3 hours on day 1. Repeat every 21 days. Use non-PVC containers and tubing with 0.22-micron inline filter.

Side effects: Hypersensitivity reaction. Myelosuppression, dose-limiting. G-CSF recommended. Nausea and vomiting. Stomatitis. Sensory neuropathy with numbness and paresthesias, dose related. Arthralgias and myalgias. Transient elevations in serum transaminases, bilirubin, and alkaline phosphatase. Alopecia.

Chair time: 1 hour for continuous infusion on day 1 and d/c pump on day 2.

OR

4 hours on day 1 for 3-hour infusion. Repeat either cycle every 21 days.

Methotrexate[1,198]

Prechemo: CBC, Chem, and Mg^{2+}. Oral phenothiazine or 5-HT3. Mildly to moderately emetogenic.

Methotrexate 40 mg/m²: IV or IM weekly.

Side effects: Myelosuppression, can be dose-limiting toxicity. Mild nausea and vomiting. Mucositis can be dose-limiting. Acute renal failure, azotemia, urinary retention, and uric acid nephropathy. Poorly defined pneumonitis characterized by fever, cough, and interstitial pulmonary infiltrates. Pruritus and urticaria may occur. Photosensitivity, sunburn-like rash, and radiation recall. Alopecia and dermatitis are uncommon.

Chair time: 1 hour weekly as tolerated or until progression.

Vinorelbine[1,199]

Prechemo: CBC, Chem. Oral phenothiazine or 5-HT_3.

Vinorelbine 30 mg/m²: IV push weekly. Vesicant.

Further dilute in syringe or IV bag to concentration of 1.5–3.0 mg/mL. Infuse diluted drug IV over 6–10 minutes into sidearm port of free-flowing IV infusion, either peripheral or via central line. Use port closest to the IV bag, not to the patient. Flush with at least 75–125 mL of IV fluid after administration.

Side effects: Myelosuppression. Nausea and vomiting are mild. Stomatitis, constipation, diarrhea, and anorexia. Reduce dose by 50% if total bilirubin is 2.1–3.0 mg/dL. If total bilirubin >3.0 mg/dL, reduce by 75%. Mild to moderate neuropathy with paresthesias, constipation. Alopecia.

Chair time: 1 hour on day 1. Weekly as tolerated or until disease progression.

Capecitabine (Xeloda)[1,200]

Prechemo: CBC, Chem, bilirubin, LFTs, creatinine clearance. Oral phenothiazine or 5-HT$_3$. Mildly to moderately emetogenic.

Capecitabine 1000 mg/m²/day: PO bid for 14 days followed by a 7-day rest period. Dose may be decreased to 850–1000 mg/m² PO bid on days 1–14 to reduce the risk of toxicity without compromising efficacy. 150- and 500-mg tablets. Taken within 30 minutes of a meal with plenty of water. Monitor INRs closely when taking warfarin, may increase INR.

Side effects: Myelosuppression. Nausea and vomiting, diarrhea. Hand-foot syndrome with tingling, numbness, pain, erythema, dryness, rash, swelling, increased pigmentation, and/or pruritus of the hands and feet. Blepharitis, tear-duct stenosis, acute and chronic conjunctivitis. Elevations in serum bilirubin alkaline phosphatase and hepatic transaminases levels. Dose modifications if hyperbilirubinemia occurs. Contraindicated with baseline creatinine clearance <30 mL/min. Dose reduction to 75% with baseline creatinine clearance of 30–50 mL/min.

Chair time: No chair time. Repeat every 21 days until progression.

HEPATOCELLULAR CANCER

SINGLE-AGENT REGIMENS

Doxorubicin[1,201]

Prechemo: CBC, Chem. MUGA scan. 5-HT$_3$ and dexamethasone 10–20 mg. Mildly to moderately emetogenic.
Doxorubicin 20–30 mg/m^2: IV push on day 1 weekly. Potent vesicant.
Side effects: Myelosuppression may be severe. Nausea and vomiting. Dose reduce with liver dysfunction. Pericarditis-myocarditis syndrome. With cumulative doses >450 mg/m^2 of doxorubicin, cardiomyopathy. Red-orange discoloration of urine. Hyperpigmentation, photosensitivity, and radiation recall occur. Complete alopecia occurs with doses >50 mg/m^2.
Chair time: 1 hour on day 1. Repeat cycle weekly until progression.

Cisplatin[1,202]

Prechemo: CBC, Chem, and Mg^{2+}. 5-HT3 and dexamethasone 10–20 mg. Moderately to highly emetogenic.
Cisplatin 80 mg/m^2: IV in 1000 cc NS over 1–3 hours on day 1.
Side effects: Myelosuppression dose related. Nausea and vomiting, acute or delayed. Metallic taste of foods and loss of appetite. Nephrotoxicity dose related, reduce risk with hydration. Decreases in Mg^{2+}, K$^+$, Ca^{2+},Na$^+$, and Phos. Dose-limiting peripheral sensory neuropathy. Paresthesias and numbness are cumulative. High-frequency hearing loss and tinnitus. Alopecia.
Chair time: 2 hours on day 1. Repeat cycle every 28 days.

Capecitabine (Xeloda)[1,203]

Prechemo: CBC, Chem, bilirubin, LFTs, and creatinine clearance. Oral phenothiazine or 5-HT$_3$. Mildly to moderately emetogenic.

Capecitabine 1000 mg/m²/day: PO bid for 2 weeks followed by a 1-week rest period. Dose may be decreased to 850–1000 mg/m² PO bid to reduce the risk of toxicity without compromising efficacy. 150- and 500-mg tablets. Taken within 30 minutes of a meal with plenty of water. Monitor INRs closely when taking warfarin, may increase INR.

Side effects: Myelosuppression. Nausea and vomiting, diarrhea. Hand-foot syndrome with tingling, numbness, pain, erythema, dryness, rash, swelling, increased pigmentation, and/or pruritus of the hands and feet. Blepharitis, tear-duct stenosis, acute and chronic conjunctivitis. Elevations in serum bilirubin alkaline phosphatase, and hepatic transaminases levels. Dose modifications if hyperbilirubinemia occurs. Capecitabine contraindicated with baseline creatinine clearance <30 mL/min. Dose reduction to 75% of capecitabine with baseline creatinine clearance of 30–50 mL/min.

Chair time: No chair time. Repeat very 21 days until disease progression.

KAPOSI'S SARCOMA

COMBINATION REGIMENS

Bleomycin + Vincristine (BV)[1,204]

Prechemo: CBC, Chem. Pulmonary function tests (PFTs) and chest x-ray (CXR). Tylenol or *Tylenol*™ ES, two tablets orally 30 minutes before treatment. Oral 5-HT3 if prior nausea exhibited (phenothiazines enhances activity of bleomycin). Mildly emetogenic.

Bleomycin 10 units/m²: IV over 10 minutes on days 1 and 15. Test dose with first dose.

Vincristine 1.4mg/m²: IV push on days 1 and 15. (Maximum dose 2 mg).Vesicant.

Side effects: Hypersensitivity reaction: fever and chills. Pulmonary toxicity is dose-limiting in bleomycin. Myelosuppression is mild. Nausea with or without vomiting usually mild. Constipation, abdominal pain, and paralytic ileus are common. A prophylactic bowel regimen for constipation is recommended. Peripheral neuropathies with absent deep-tendon reflexes, numbness, weakness, myalgias, cramping, and late severe motor difficulties. Impotence may result, secondary to nerve damage. Skin changes with or without rash and nail changes or loss. Alopecia.

Chair time: 1 hour days 1 and 15. Repeat cycle every 2 weeks.

Doxorubicin + Bleomycin + Vinblastine (ABV)[1,205]

Prechemo: CBC, Chem. MUGA. CXR baseline. Pulmonary function tests. Tylenol or *Tylenol*™ ES, two tablets orally 30 minutes before treatment. Bleomycin. 5-HT3 and dexamethasone 10–20 mg. Moderately to highly emetogenic.

Doxorubicin 40 mg/m²: IV push day 1. Potent vesicant.

Bleomycin 15 units/m²: IV over 10 minutes on days 1 and 15. A test dose of 2 units is recommended before the first dose to detect hypersensitivity.

Vinblastine 6 mg/m²: IV push on day 1. Vesicant.

Side effects: Hypersensitivity reaction bleomycin: fever and chills. Pulmonary toxicity is dose-limiting in bleomycin. Myelosuppression is mild. Nausea with or without vomiting. Stomatitis. Constipation, abdominal pain, and paralytic ileus are common. A prophylactic bowel regimen for constipation is recommended. Peripheral neuropathies with absent deep-tendon reflexes, numbness, weakness, myalgias, cramping, and late severe motor difficulties. Impotence may result, secondary to nerve damage. Red-orange discoloration of urine. Cardiotoxicity: acutely, myocarditis or subsequently, cardiomyopathy. Skin changes with or without rash and nail changes or loss. Alopecia.

Chair time: 1 hour days 1 and 15. Repeat cycle every 28 days.

SINGLE-AGENT REGIMENS

Liposomal Daunorubicin (DaunoXome)[1,206]

Prechemo: CBC, Chem. MUGA scan at baseline, at 320 mg/m^2 cumulative dose and every 160 mg/m^2 dose thereafter. Central line placement. 5-HT3 and Dexamethasone 10–20 mg. Mild to moderately emetogenic.

Liposomal daunorubicin 40 mg/m^2: IV over 1 hour on day 1. Vesicant. Further dilute drug in D5W to a final concentration of 1 mg/mL.

Side effects: Infusion reaction usually occurs within first 5 minutes of infusion. Myelosuppression can be severe. G-CSF may be needed. Mucositis and diarrhea are common but not dose-limiting. Dose reduction required for abnormal liver function. Acute, pericarditis and/or myocarditis, EKG changes, or arrhythmias. CHF with cumulative doses >320 mg/m^2. Folliculitis, seborrhea, and dry skin. Alopecia.

Chair time: 2 hours on day 1. Repeat cycle every 14 days.

Liposomal Doxorubicin (Doxil)[1,207]

Prechemo: CBC, Chem. MUGA scan. 5-HT3 and dexamethasone 10–20 mg. Mild to moderately emetogenic.

Liposomal doxorubicin 20 mg/m^2: IV on day 1. Irritant. Dilute doses up to 90 mg in 250 cc of D5W, 500-mL D5W doses >90 mg. Initial rate of 1 mg/mL if no reaction increase rate to complete administration in 1 hour.

Side effects: Infusion reaction. May administer corticosteroids or diphenhydramine before rechallenging, or have patient take steroids for 24 hours prior to the next administration. Myelosuppression. Dose-limiting toxicity in the treatment of HIV-infected patients. Nausea and vomiting. Stomatitis. Diarrhea. Red-orange discoloration of urine. Acute pericarditis and/or myocarditis, EKG changes, or arrhythmias. Not dose related. With high cumulative doses, >550 mg/m^2, cardiomyopathy may occur. Hand-foot syndrome with skin rash, swelling, erythema, pain, and/or desquamation, dose related. Hyperpigmentation of nails, skin rash, urticaria, and radiation recall. Alopecia.

Chair time: 2 hours on day 1. Repeat cycle every 21 days.

Paclitaxel (Taxol)[1,208,209]

Prechemo: CBC, Chem. 5-HT$_3$ and dexamethasone 10–20 mg in 100 cc of NS Diphenhydramine 25–50 mg and H$_2$ antagonist. Mildly to moderately emetogenic.

Paclitaxel 135 mg/m^2: IV in 500 cc NS over 3 hours on day 1. Repeat cycle every 21 days.

OR

Paclitaxel 100 mg/m^2: IV in 500 cc NS on day 1. Repeat cycle every 2 weeks.

Use non-PVC containers and tubing with 0.22-micron inline filter.

Side effects: Hypersensitivity reaction. Myelosuppression, dose-limiting G-CSF recommended. Nausea and vomiting. Stomatitis. Sensory neuropathy with numbness and paresthesias, dose related and dose-limiting. Arthralgias and myalgias. Transient elevations in serum transaminases, bilirubin, and alkaline phosphatase. Alopecia.

Chair time: 4 hours on day 1. Repeat cycle every 21 days.

OR

2 hours on day 1. Repeat cycle every 2 weeks.

Interferon α-2a[1,210,211]

Prechemo: CBC, Chem, LFTs. Oral phenothiazine or 5-HT3. Acetaminophen. Moderately to highly emetogenic.

Interferon α-2a 36-million IU/m^2: SC or IM, daily for 8–12 weeks.

OR

Interferon α-2b 30-million IU/m^2: SC or IM three times weekly.

Side effects: Flu-like syndrome: fever, chills, headache, myalgias, and arthralgias. Managed with acetaminophen and increased oral fluid intake. Myelosuppression. Nausea, diarrhea, and vomiting. Anorexia cumulative and dose-limiting. Taste alteration and xerostomia. Mild proteinuria and hypocalcemia. Mild transient elevations in serum transaminases. Dose-dependent toxicity with pre-existing liver abnormalities. Dry skin, pruritus, and irritation at injection. Retinopathy with cotton-wool spots and small hemorrhages. Usually asymptomatic and resolves when drug discontinued. Alopecia is partial.

Chair time: 1 hour on day 1 for self-injection teaching.

LEUKEMIA: ACUTE LYMPHOCYTIC LEUKEMIA (ALL)

LINKER REGIMEN[1,212,213]

INDUCTION THERAPY

Prechemo: CBC, Chem, LFTs, and renal function tests, central line placement, EKG, and MUGA. Bone marrow biopsy at baseline, day 14 and day 28. $5-HT_3$ and dexamethasone 10–20 mg. Diphenhydramine 25–50 mg and H_2 antagonist. Highly emetogenic.

Daunorubicin 50 mg/m²: IV push every 24 hours on days 1–3. Vesicant.

Vincristine 2 mg: IV push on days 1, 8, 15 and 22. Vesicant.

Prednisone 60 mg/m²: PO divided into three doses on days 1–28.

L-Asparaginase 6000 units/m²: IM on days 17–28.

If bone marrow on day 14 is positive for residual leukemia, Daunorubicin 50 mg/m²: IV push on day 15.

If bone marrow on day 28 is positive for residual leukemia, Daunorubicin 50 mg/m²: IV push on days 29 and 30.

Vincristine 2 mg: IV push on days 29 and 36.

Prednisone 60 mg/m²: PO on days 29–42.

L-Asparaginase 6000 units/m²: IM on days 29–35.

Side effects: Anaphylactic reaction with asparaginase, seen in 20% to 30% of patients. Incidence increases with subsequent doses. Myelosuppression. Nausea and vomiting, anorexia, and mucositis. Constipation, paralytic ileus. Dose reduce with impaired renal functions. Acute myocarditis or pericarditis, CHF with cumulative doses daunorubicin >550mg/m². Daily weights. Lethargy, drowsiness, and somnolence with asparaginase. Peripheral neuropathy: absent deep-tendon reflexes, numbness, weakness, myalgias, jaw pain, diplopia, vocal cord paralysis, and metallic taste. Discoloration of urine pink to red, red-orange. Tumor lysis syndrome 1–5 days after initiation of treatment. Radiation recall, sun sensitivity, and alopecia.

Chair time: 2 hours on days 1–3, 8, 15, 17–36. May require hospitalization. Repeat until remission (usually two to three cycles), then follow with consolidation therapy.

CONSOLIDATION THERAPY

Treatment A (cycles 1, 3, 5, and 7) alternating with
Treatment B (cycles 2, 4, 6, and 8) followed by
Treatment C (cycle 9)

Prechemo: CBC, Chem, LFTs, and renal function tests central line placement, EKG, and MUGA if cardiac changes with induction therapy. Bone marrow biopsy to demonstrate remission.

Treatment Cycle A (cycles 1, 3, 5, and 7)

5-HT3 and dexamethasone 10–20 mg. Highly emetogenic.
Daunorubicin 50 mg/m^2: IV push days 1 and 2. Vesicant.
Vincristine 2 mg: IV push on days 1 and 8. Vesicant.
Prednisone 60 mg/m^2: PO in three divided doses on days 1–14.
L-Asparaginase 12,000 U/m^2: IM on days 2, 4, 7, 9, 11, and 14.

Treatment B (cycles 2, 4, 6, and 8)

Teniposide (Vumon) 165 mg/m^2: IV over 30–60 minutes days 1, 4, 8, and 11. Requires non-DEHP containers and tubing.
Cytarabine (Ara-C) 300 mg/m^2: IV in 500 cc NS on days 1, 4, 8, and 11.

Treatment C (cycle 9)

Methotrexate 690 mg/m^2: IV over 42 hours.
Leucovorin 15 mg/m^2: IV over 15 minutes every 6 hours for 12 doses stating at 42 hours. Continue until MTX levels fall below 5×10^{-8}.
Side effects: Hypersensitivity/anaphylactic reactions: occurs in 20% to 30% of patients receiving L-asparaginase; incidence increases with subsequent doses. Can also occur with teniposide infusion. Dose reduce drugs with impaired liver or renal functions. Myelosuppression dose-limiting. Nausea and vomiting, anorexia, mucositis, and stomatitis. Constipation, paralytic ileus with vincristine. Acute myocarditis or pericarditis, CHF with cumulative doses daunorubicin >550 mg/m^2. Daily weights. Lethargy, drowsiness, and somnolence with asparaginase. Peripheral neuropathy: absent deep-tendon reflexes, numbness, weakness, myalgias, jaw pain, diplopia, vocal cord paralysis, and metallic taste. Discoloration of urine pink to red, red-orange. Tumor lysis

syndrome 1–5 days after initiation of treatment. Acute cerebral dysfunction with paresis, aphasia, behavioral abnormalities, and seizures with high-dose methotrexate therapy. Azotemia, urinary retention, and uric acid nephropathy with high-dose methotrexate. Radiation recall, sun sensitivity, and alopecia.

Chair time: Treatment A: 2 hours on days 1, 2, 4, 7–9, 11, and 14; Treatment B: 3 hours on days 1, 4, 8, and 11. Treatment C: 1 hour day 1. May require hospitalization.

MAINTENANCE THERAPY

Prechemo: CBC, Chem, LFTs, and renal function tests. Bone marrow biopsy.

Methotrexate 20 mg/m^2: PO weekly (5-, 7.5-, 10-, 12.5-, and 15-mg tablets). Take at the same time each week.

6-Mercaptopurine 75 mg/m^2: PO daily (50-mg tablets). Take on an empty stomach; continue for a total of 30 months for complete response. Anticoagulant effects of Coumadin™ are inhibited. Monitor PT/INR.

Side effects: Myelosuppression. Dose-limiting. Nausea and vomiting, anorexia, mucositis, and stomatitis.

CNS PROPHYLAXIS

Cranial irradiation 1800 rad in 10 fractions over 12–14 days.

Methotrexate 12 mg: IT (intrathecal) weekly for 6 weeks. **Use preservative-free solution only.** Begin within 1 week of complete response. In patients with documented CNS involvement at time of diagnosis, intrathecal chemotherapy should begin during induction chemotherapy.

Methotrexate 12 mg: IT weekly for 10 doses. **Use preservative-free solution only.**

Cranial irradiation 2800 rad.

Side effects: Myelosuppression. Dose-limiting. Nausea and vomiting, anorexia. CNS changes due to IT MTX: Dizziness, malaise, and blurred vision. May increase CSF pressure. Keep patient supine for at least 1 hour after IT injection to prevent headache. Brain XRT after MTX can result in neurologic changes. Sensory neuropathy: loss of vibratory sensation, unsteady gate may occur.

Chair time: 1–2 hours weekly for 10 weeks.

LARSON REGIMEN[1,214]

Prechemo: CBC, Chem, LFTs, and RFTs. Bone marrow biopsy, central line placement, EKG, and MUGA. 5-HT3 and dexamethasone 20 mg

IV infusion days. 5-HT3 PO as neede all other days. Moderately to highly emetogenic.

INDUCTION THERAPY (WEEKS 1–4)

Cyclophosphamide 1200 mg/m^2: IV in 500–1000 cc NS over 1–2 hours on day 1.

Daunorubicin 45 mg/m^2: IV push on days 1–3. Vesicant.

Vincristine 2 mg: IV push on days 1, 8, 15, and 22. Vesicant.

Prednisone 60 mg/m^2/day: PO on days 1–21. (5-, 10-, 20-, and 50-mg tablets. Take in the morning with food.)

L-Asparaginase 6000 IU/m^2: SC on days 15, 18, 22, and 25.

EARLY INTENSIFICATION (WEEKS 5–12)

Methotrexate 15 mg: IT (intrathecal) on day 1. **Use preservative-free solution only.**

Cyclophosphamide 1000 mg/m^2: IV in 500–1000 cc NS over 2 hours on day 1.

6-Mercaptopurine 60 mg/m^2/day: PO on days 1–4 and 8–11. (50-mg tablets.) Take on an empty stomach.

Cytarabine (Ara-C) 75 mg/m^2: IV in 500 cc NS on days 1–14.

Vincristine 2 mg: IV push on days 15 and 22. Vesicant.

L-Asparaginase: 6000 IU/m^2: SC on days 15, 18, 22, and 25.

Repeat the early intensification cycle once.

CNS PROPHYLAXIS AND INTERIM MAINTENANCE (WEEKS 13–25)

Cranial irradiation 2400 cGy: Days 1–12.

Methotrexate 15 mg: IT on days 1, 8, 15, 22, and 29. **Use preservative-free solution only.**

6-Mercaptopurine 60 mg/m^2/day: PO on days 1–70. (50-mg tablets.) Take on an empty stomach.

Methotrexate 20 mg/m^2: PO on days 36, 43, 50, 57, and 64. (5-, 7.5-, 10-, 12.5-, and 15-mg tablets.) Take at the same time each week.

LATE INTENSIFICATION (WEEKS 26–33)

Doxorubicin 30 mg/m^2: IV push on days 1, 8, and 15. Potent vesicant.

Vincristine 2 mg: IV push on days 1, 8, and 15. Vesicant.

Dexamethasone 10 mg/m^2/day: PO on days 1–14. (4-mg tablets.) Take in the morning with food.

Cyclophosphamide 1000 mg/m^2/day: In 1000 cc NS over 2 hours on day 29.

6-Thioguanine 60 mg/m^2/day: PO on days 29–42. (40-mg tablets.) Take on an empty stomach.

Cytarabine (Ara-C) 75 mg/m^2: IV in 500 cc NS on days 29, 32, and 36–39.

PROLONGED MAINTENANCE

Continue until 24 months after diagnosis.

Vincristine 2 mg: IV push on day 1. Vesicant.

Prednisone 60 mg/m^2/day: PO on days 1–5. (5-, 10-, 20-, and 50-mg tablets.) Take in the morning with food.

Methotrexate 20 mg/m^2: PO on days 1, 8, 15, and 22. (5-, 7.5-, 10-, 12.5-, and 15-mg tablets.) Take at the same time each week.

6-Mercaptopurine 80 mg/m^2/day: PO on days 1–28. (50-mg tablets.) Take on an empty stomach. Repeat maintenance cycle every 28 days.

Side effects: Hypersensitivity/anaphylactic reactions: occurs in 20% to 30% of patients receiving L-asparaginase; incidence increases with subsequent doses. Dose reduce with impaired liver or renal functions. Myelosuppression dose-limiting. Nausea and vomiting, anorexia. Mucositis and stomatitis. Constipation, paralytic ileus with vincristine. Acute myocarditis or pericarditis, CHF with cumulative doses daunorubicin>550 mg/m^2 or doxorubicin >450 mg/m^2. Daily weights. Lethargy, drowsiness, and somnolence with asparaginase. Peripheral neuropathy: absent deep-tendon reflexes, numbness, weakness, myalgias, jaw pain, diplopia, vocal cord paralysis, and metallic taste. Discoloration of urine pink to red, red-orange. Tumor lysis syndrome 1–5 days after initiation of treatment. Acute cerebral dysfunction with paresis, aphasia, behavioral abnormalities, and seizures with high-dose methotrexate therapy. Azotemia, urinary retention, and uric acid nephropathy with high-dose methotrexate. Radiation recall, sun sensitivity, and alopecia.

Chair time: Induction therapy: 1–3 hours per visit, weeks 1–4. Early intensification: 1–3 hours per visit, repeat cycle one time at 28 days. CNS prophylaxis: 2 hours per visit, weeks 13–25. Late intensification: 1–3 hours per visit, weeks 25–33. Prolonged maintenance: 1 hour per visit, continue until 24 months after diagnosis. May require hospitalization.

HYPER-CVAD REGIMEN[1,215]

Prechemo: CBC, Chem, LFTs, and renal function test, lumbar puncture (if symptomatic), central line placement, EKG, and MUGA scan. Bone marrow biopsy with cytogenetics, immunophenotyping, or cytochemistry; HLA typing (in patients considering BMT) and donor search if indicated; FLT3 mutation evaluation. Repeat bone marrow biopsy 7–14 days after chemotherapy (7 days after last dose of G-CSF 7 to document remission). 5-HT_3 and dexamethasone 10–20 mg. Diphenhydramine 25–50 mg and H_2 antagonist. Highly emetogenic.

INDUCTION THERAPY

Cyclophosphamide 300 mg/m²: IV in 500 cc NS over 3 hours every 12 hours for six doses on days 1–3.

Mesna 600 mg/m²: IV over 24 hours on days 1–3 ending 6 hours after the last dose of cyclophosphamide.

Vincristine 2 mg: IV push on days 4 and 11. Vesicant.

Doxorubicin 50 mg/m²: IV push on day 4. Potent vesicant.

Dexamethasone 40 mg: PO or IV on days 1–4 and 11–14. (5-, 10-, 20-, and 50-mg tablets.) Take in the morning with food.

Alternate cycles every 21 days with the following:

HIGH-DOSE METHOTREXATE/CYTARABINE

Methotrexate 200 mg/m²: IV in 500–1000 cc NS over 2 hours, followed by:

Methotrexate 800 mg/m²: IV in 500–1000 cc NS over 24 hours on day 1.

Leucovorin 15 mg: IV in 100 cc NS over 15 minutes every 6 hours for 8 doses, starting 24 hours after the completion of methotrexate infusion.

Cytarabine 3000 mg/m²: IV in 1000 cc NS over 2 hours every 12 hours for four doses days 2–3.

Methylprednisolone 50 mg: IV bid on days 1–3.

Chair time: Alternate four cycles of hyper-CVAD with four cycles of high-dose methotrexate and cytarabine therapy every 3 to 4 weeks.

CNS PROPHYLAXIS

Methotrexate 12 mg: IT (intrathecal) on day 2. **Use preservative-free solution only.**

Cytarabine 100 mg: IT on day 8. **Use preservative-free solution only**.

Repeat with each cycle of chemotherapy, depending on the risk of CNS disease.

Side effects: Myelosuppression dose-limiting toxicity. Dose adjust for elevated renal of hepatic function. Nausea and vomiting, anorexia, and stomatitis. Acute, pericarditis, or myocarditis. CHF with cumulative doxorubicin doses >450 mg/m². Discoloration of urine from pink to red. Cerebellar toxicity, including nystagmus, dysarthria, ataxia, slurred speech, or difficulty with fine-motor coordination, lethargy, or somnolence with high doses methotrexate and cytarabine. Observe neurologic status, handwriting, or gait before and during cytarabine therapy. Rapidly rising creatinine caused by tumor lysis syndrome or neurotoxicity should discontinue the high-dose cytarabine, treat with hydration and allopurinol. Saline or steroid drops to both eyes may be indicated for 24 hours after completion of high cytarabine. Maculopapular rash, total alopecia.

SUPPORTIVE CARE

Recommended as part of treatment plan.

Ciprofloxacin 500 mg PO bid; fluconazole: 200 mg/day PO; acyclovir: **200 mg PO bid.** G-CSF: 10 mg/kg/day starting 24 hours after the end of chemotherapy (day 5 of hyper-CVAD therapy and day 4 of high-dose methotrexate and cytarabine therapy).

Chair time: Varies. May require hospitalization, daily CBC.

SINGLE-AGENT REGIMENS

Clofarabine[1,216]

Prechemo: CBC, Chem, LFTs, and RFTs (dose reduce with impaired functions), central line placement. Bone marrow biopsy before and after therapy. 5-HT$_3$ and dexamethasone 10–20 mg. Diphenhydramine 25–50 mg and H$_2$ antagonist. Highly emetogenic.

Clofarabine 52 mg/m^2: IV over 2 hours daily for 5 days with continuous IV fluids throughout the dosing course.

Side effects: Myelosuppression dose-limiting. Febrile neutropenia common. Infections include bacteremia, cellulitis, herpes simplex, oral candidiasis, pneumonia, sepsis, and staphylococcal infections. Dehydration, hypotension, and capillary leak syndrome. Tumor lysis syndrome. Use allopurinol and adequate hydration to prevent renal toxicities. Nausea and vomiting. Anorexia and diarrhea or constipation. Hepatotoxicity and jaundice. Maculopapular rash, with or without fever, myalgias, bone pain, occasional chest pain, conjunctivitis, and malaise (cytarabine syndrome) may occur 6–12 hours after administration; corticosteroids used to treat/prevent syndrome. Mucosal inflammation and ulceration of anus/rectum may occur. Edema, fatigue, lethargy and pain: fatigue 36%, hand-foot syndrome. Alopecia.

Chair time: 3 hour on days 1–5, may require hospitalization. Repeat cycle every 2–6 weeks after recovery of all baseline organ functions.

LEUKEMIA: ACUTE LYMPHOCYTIC LEUKEMIA: RELAPSED OR REFRACTORY PH + ALL

SINGLE-AGENT REGIMENS

Imatinib (Gleevec) [1,217]

Prechemo: CBC, Chem, renal and liver functions. Bone marrow biopsy. Prochlorperazine or 5-HT$_3$ PO daily prn. Mildly to moderately emetogenic.

Imatinib 600 mg: Per day. (100- and 400-mg tablets.)

Taken with food and a large glass of water. Do NOT take with grapefruit juice. Monitor INRs closely if taking warfarin; inhibits metabolism of warfarin.

Side effects: Nausea and vomiting, usually relieved when taken with food. Diarrhea and constipation. Myelosuppression. Hold for ANC <1.0 × 10^9/ L and platelets <50 × 10^9/L. Hold until ANC ≥1500 and platelets >50,000. Resume dose at 400 mg; if recurrence, decrease to 300 mg. Fluid retention especially in older patients. Periorbital and lower-extremity edema primarily. Pleural effusions, ascites, rapid weight gain, and pulmonary edema may develop. Hypokalemia. Muscle cramps, arthralgias, headache, fatigue, and abdominal. Rash, treat with systemic antihistamine, topical or systemic corticosteroid. Mild, transient elevation in serum transaminase and bilirubin levels. Multiple drug interactions with CYP3A4 pathway.

Chair time: No chair time. Treatment continues as long as patient derives benefit from drug.

LEUKEMIA: ACUTE MYELOGENOUS LEUKEMIA (AML)

INDUCTION REGIMENS

Ara-C 1 Daunorubicin (7 1 3)1,218

Prechemo: CBC, Chem, LFTs, and renal function tests (dose reduce with impaired functions), EKG, and MUGA. Bone marrow biopsy. Central line placement, 5-HT$_3$ and dexamethasone 10–20 mg. Diphenhydramine 25–50 mg and H$_2$ antagonist. Highly emetogenic.

Cytarabine 100 mg/m^2/day: IV continuous infusion on days 1–7.

Daunorubicin 45mg/m^2: IV push on days 1–3. Vesicant.

Side effects: Myelosuppression, dose-limiting. Nausea,vomiting anorexia, mucositis and diarrhea, not dose-limiting. Tumor lysis syndrome 1–5 days after initiation of treatment; treat with hydration and allopurinol. Electrolytes, Cr, BUN, uric acid, and PO$_4$ daily to evaluate tumor lysis. Acute pericarditis, and/or myocarditis. CHF dose of daunorubicin >550 mg/m^2. Red-orange discoloration of urine. Cerebellar toxicity, including seizures, nystagmus, dysarthria, ataxia, slurred speech, or difficulty with fine-motor coordination, lethargy, or somnolence. Conjunctivitis, treat with corticosteroid eye drops. Hyperpigmentation of nails, skin rash, and urticaria. Radiation recall, photosensitivity. Alopecia.

Chair time: 1 hour on days 1–3; 30 minutes for pump refill day 3. Cycle does not repeat. May require hospitalization.

Ara-C + Idarubicin[1,219]

Prechemo: CBC, Chem, LFTs, and renal function tests (dose reduce with impaired functions), EKG, and MUGA. Bone marrow biopsy. Central line placement, 5-HT$_3$ and dexamethasone 10–20 mg. Diphenhydramine 25–50 mg and H$_2$ antagonist. Highly emetogenic.

Idarubicin 12mg/m^2: IV push vesicant on days 1–3.

Cytarabine 100 mg/m²/day: IV continuous infusion on days 1–7.
OR
Cytarabine 25 mg/m²: IV push. Irritant, followed by:
Cytarabine 200 mg/m²/day: IV continuous infusion on days 1–5. Irritant.
Side effects: Myelosuppression, dose-limiting. Nausea and vomiting. Anorexia, stomatitis, mucositis, and diarrhea common. Tumor lysis syndrome 1–5 days after initiation of treatment; treat with hydration and allopurinol. Electrolytes, Cr, BUN, uric acid, and PO₄ daily to evaluate tumor lysis. Acute pericarditis, and/or myocarditis. Cumulative doses of 150 mg/m² idarubicin associated with decreased LVEF. Cerebellar toxicity, including seizures, nystagmus, dysarthria, ataxia, slurred speech, difficulty with fine-motor coordination, lethargy, or somnolence with high-dose cytarabine. Conjunctivitis, treat with corticosteroid eye drops. Red-orange discoloration of urine. Maculopapular rash 6–12 hours after infusion. Alopecia.
Chair time: 1 hour on days 1–3; 30 minutes for pump refill day 3. Repeat cycle until remission (usually two to three cycles). May require hospitalization.

Ara-C + Doxorubicin[1,220]

Prechemo: CBC, Chem, LFTs, and renal function tests (dose reduce with impaired functions) EKG, and MUGA. Central line placement. Bone marrow biopsy, with cytogenetics, immunophenotyping, or cytochemistry. HLA typing (in patients considering BMT) and donor search if indicated. FLT3 mutation evaluation, lumbar puncture, if symptomatic. 5-HT₃ and dexamethasone 10–20 mg. Diphenhydramine 25–50 mg and H₂ antagonist. Highly emetogenic.
Cytarabine 100 mg/m²/day: IV continuous infusion on days 1–7.
Doxorubicin 30 mg/m²: IV push on days 1–3. Vesicant.
Side effects: Myelosuppression, dose-limiting. Daily CBC during chemotherapy and then every other day until WBCs >500 per mcl, platelet transfusions as indicated. Tumor lysis syndrome 1–5 days after initiation of treatment; treat with hydration and allopurinol. Electrolytes, Cr, BUN, uric acid, and PO₄ daily to evaluate tumor lysis. Nausea and vomiting, anorexia; stomatitis, mucositis, and diarrhea. Acute pericarditis, and/or myocarditis. CHF when dose of doxorubicin >450 mg/m². Discoloration of urine from pink to red. Hemorrhagic cystitis, preventable with appropriate hydration. At high doses of cytarabine cerebellar toxicity, including nystagmus, dysarthria, ataxia, slurred speech, difficulty with fine-motor coordination, lethargy, or somnolence. Conjunctivitis, treat with corticosteroid eye drops. Hyperpigmentation of nails, skin rash, and urticaria. Radiation recall. Total alopecia.
Chair time: 1 hour on days 1–3 and 30 minutes for pump refill day 3.

CONSOLIDATION REGIMENS

Ara-C + Daunorubicin (5 + 2)[1,221]

Prechemo: CBC, Chem, LFTs, and renal function tests (dose reduce with impaired functions), EKG, and MUGA. Bone marrow biopsy. Central line placement, 5-HT3, and dexamethasone 10–20 mg. Diphenhydramine 25–50 mg and H2 antagonist. Highly emetogenic.

Cytarabine 100 mg/m^2/day: IV continuous infusion on days 1–5.

Daunorubicin 45 mg/m^2: IV push on days 1 and 2. Vesicant.

Side effects: Myelosuppression, dose-limiting. Daily CBC during chemotherapy and then every other day until WBCs >500 per mcl, platelet transfusions as indicated. Nausea and vomiting, anorexia, stomatitis, mucositis, and diarrhea. Acute pericarditis, and/or myocarditis. CHF when dose of daunorubicin >550 mg/m^2. Discoloration of urine from pink to red. Hemorrhagic cystitis, preventable with appropriate hydration. At high doses of cytarabine cerebellar toxicity, including nystagmus, dysarthria, ataxia, slurred speech, difficulty with fine-motor coordination, lethargy, or somnolence. Conjunctivitis, treat with corticosteroid eye drops. Hyperpigmentation of nails, skin rash, and urticaria. Radiation recall. Total alopecia.

Chair time: 2 hours on days 1–2 and 30 minutes for pump refill day 3. Given once after an induction regimen has been used.

Ara-C + Idarubicin[1,221]

Prechemo: CBC, Chem, LFTs, and renal function tests (dose reduce with impaired functions), EKG, and MUGA. Bone marrow biopsy. Central line placement, 5-HT$_3$, and dexamethasone 10–20 mg. Diphenhydramine 25–50 mg and H$_2$ antagonist. Highly emetogenic.

Cytarabine 100 mg/m^2/day: IV continuous infusion on days 1–5. Irritant.

Idarubicin 13 mg/m^2: Slow IV push on days 1 and 2. Vesicant.

Side effects: Myelosuppression, dose-limiting. Nausea and vomiting. Anorexia, stomatitis, mucositis, and diarrhea common. Acute pericarditis and/or myocarditis. Idarubicin cumulative doses of 150 mg/m^2 associated with decreased LVEF. Red-orange discoloration of urine. Cerebellar toxicity, including seizures, nystagmus, dysarthria, ataxia, slurred speech, difficulty with fine-motor coordination, lethargy, or somnolence with high-dose cytarabine. Conjunctivitis, treat with corticosteroid eye drops. Maculopapular rash 6–12 hours after infusion. Alopecia.

Chair time: 2 hours on days 1 and 2; 30 minutes for pump refill day 3. Repeat cycle every 21–28 days until remission (usually two to three cycles). May require hospitalization.

Single-Agent Regimens

Cladribine (Leustatin)[1,222]

Prechemo: CBC, Chem, LFTs, and RFTs (dose reduce with impaired functions). Bone marrow biopsy. Central line placement. 5-HT$_3$ and dexamethasone 10–20 mg. Mildly emetogenic.

Cladribine 0.1 mg/kg/day: Continuous infusion on days 1–7. One course. Use a 22-mm filter when preparing the solution.

Side effects: Myelosuppression. Increased risk for opportunistic infections, including fungal, herpes, and *Pneumocystis carinii*. Teach self-care measures to minimize risk of infection and bleeding. Tumor fever associated with fatigue, malaise, arthralgias, and chills. Nausea and vomiting, anorexia usually mild. Constipation and abdominal pain. Headache, insomnia, and dizziness. Tumor lysis syndrome rare even with high tumor burden.

Chair time: 1 hour days 1 and 7. One course only.

High-Dose Cytarabine (HiDAC)[1,223]

Prechemo: CBC, Chem, LFTs, and renal function tests (dose reduce with impaired functions). Bone marrow biopsy, repeat 7–14 days post-treatment. Central line placement. Saline, methylcellulose, or steroid eye drops, OU q6h, with cytarabine and continuing 48–72 hours after the last cytarabine dose is completed. 5-HT3 and dexamethasone 10–20 mg. Highly emetogenic.

Cytarabine 3000 mg/m^2/day: IV in 1000 cc NS over 1–2 hours every 12 hours on days 1, 2, and 3. IV hydration at 150 mL per hour with/without alkalinization, oral allopurinol; strict I and O, daily weights.

Side effects: Myelosuppression. Daily CBC during chemotherapy and then every other day until WBCs >500 per mcl, platelet transfusions as indicated. Tumor lysis syndrome occurs 1–5 days after initiation of treatment. Pretreat with hydration and allopurinol. With rapidly rising creatinine due to tumor lysis syndrome or neurotoxicity should discontinue cytarabine. Evaluate electrolytes, creatinine, BUN, uric acid, and PO$_4$ daily during treatment. At high doses cerebellar toxicity, including seizures, nystagmus, dysarthria, ataxia, slurred speech, difficulty with fine-motor coordination, lethargy, or somnolence. Assess baseline neurologic status and cerebellar function (coordinated movements such as handwriting and gait) before and during therapy. If cerebellar toxicity develops, treatment must be discontinued. Nausea and vomiting, anorexia. Conjunctivitis, pretreat with corticosteroid eye drops. Maculopapular rash, 6–12 hours after infusion, stomatitis. Total alopecia.

Chair time: 4 hours on infusion days. Repeat cycle every 28 days or 1 week after marrow recovery. Usually requires hospitalization.

Gemtuzumab (Mylotarg)[1,224]

Prechemo: CBC, Chem, LFTs, and renal function tests, (dose reduce with impaired functions). Bone marrow biopsy. Central line placement. 5-HT_3 and dexamethasone 10–20 mg. Diphenhydramine 25–50 mg and H_2 antagonist. Acetaminophen 650–1000 mg PO, repeat at 4 hours for two doses, then as needed. Mildly to moderately emetogenic.

Post-treatment: CBC at least weekly or BID. Bone marrow biopsy.

Gemtuzumab 9 mg/m^2: IV in 100 cc NS as a 2-hour infusion day 1. Place the bag in an ultraviolet-protected bag. Use immediately once diluted for infusion. Use a 1.2-micron filter. Do not administer by IVP or bolus.

Side effects: Infusion reaction: flushing, facial swelling, headache, dyspnea, and/or hypotension. Can be related to rate of infusion. Myelosuppression, dose-limiting toxicity. Post-infusion related syndrome: fever, chills, nausea and vomiting, urticaria, skin rash, fatigue, headache, diarrhea, dyspnea, and/or hypotension. Usually observed in the first 2 hours after infusion. Transient hypotension can be observed up to 6 hours after the infusion. Nausea and vomiting. Mucositis and stomatitis mild. Transient increases in LFTs. Diarrhea seen.

Chair time: 6 hours on day 1. Repeat with a second dose 14 days after administration of the first dose.

RELAPSE AML

Mitoxantrone + Etoposide (MV)[1,225]

Prechemo: CBC, Chem, LFTs, and renal function tests. Dose reduce with impaired renal or hepatic functions. Bone marrow biopsy, central line placement, EKG, and MUGA. 5-HT_3 and dexamethasone 10–20 mg. Moderately to highly emetogenic.

Mitoxantrone 10 mg/m^2/day: IV days 1–5, IV push over 3 minutes.
OR
IV infusion over 30 minutes. Vesicant. Diluted in 50 mL with either NS or D5W.

Etoposide 100 mg/m^2/day: IV in 2500 cc NS over 1 hour on days 1–5.

Side effects: Myelosuppression dose-limiting. Hypersensitivity reaction with etoposide. Nausea and vomiting, anorexia; mucositis, diarrhea. CHF with decreased LVEF. Increased cardiotoxicity with cumulative dose>180 mg/m^2 mitoxantrone. Urine will be green blue for 24 hours. Blue discoloration of fingernails and sclera for 1–2 days after treatment. Radiation recall. Tumor lysis syndrome, consider treating with hydration and allopurinol. Alopecia.

Chair time: 2 hours on days 1–5; second cycle given if remission is not achieved.

FLAG: Fludarabine + Cytarabine + G-CSF[1,226]

Prechemo: CBC, Chem, LFTs, and renal function tests. Dose reduce with impaired functions. Bone marrow biopsy, central line placement, EKG, and MUGA. 5-HT_3 and dexamethasone 10–20 mg. Highly emetogenic.

Fludarabine 30 mg/m²: IV in 100 cc NS over 30 minutes on days 1–5.

Cytarabine 2000 mg/m²: IV in 1000 cc NS over 4 hours, 3.5 hours after the end of the fludarabine infusion days 1–5. IV hydration at 150 mL per hour with or without alkalinization, oral allopurinol, strict I and O, daily weights.

G-CSF 5 mcg/kg/day: SQ on day 0 and then 300-mcg SQ QD until ANC recovery.

Side effects: Myelosuppression dose-limiting toxicity. Weakness, agitation, confusion, progressive encephalopathy, cortical blindness, seizures, and/or coma with high doses cytarabine. Pneumonia pulmonary hypersensitivity reaction characterized by dyspnea, cough, and interstitial pulmonary infiltrates. Immunosuppression: decrease in CD4+ and CD8+, increasing risk for opportunistic infections (fungus, herpes, and *Pneumocystis carinii*). Tumor lysis syndrome: occurs 1–5 days after initiation of treatment. Pretreat with hydration and allopurinol. Patients with rapidly rising creatinine discontinue the high-dose cytarabine. Nausea and vomiting, anorexia; mucositis, diarrhea. Maculopapular rash, erythema, and pruritus. Alopecia.

Chair time: 8 hours on days 1–5. A second cycle if remission is not achieved. May require hospitalization.

LEUKEMIA: ACUTE PROMYELOCYTIC LEUKEMIA (APL)

COMBINATION REGIMENS

All-Trans-Retinoic Acid + Idarubicin (AIDA)[1,227]

Prechemo: CBC, Chem, renal and liver functions. Monitor: CBC, coagulation studies, LFTs, triglyceride, and cholesterol levels frequently throughout therapy. Bone marrow biopsy baseline and every 5–6 weeks from the start of induction therapy. 5-HT$_3$ and dexamethasone 20-mg IV days 2, 4, 6, and 8. Mildly to moderately emetogenic.

All-Trans-Retinoic Acid (ATRA) 45 mg/m^2: PO daily. 10-mg tablets; protect from light.

Absorption enhanced when taken with food.

Idarubicin 12 mg/m^2: Slow IV push through side port of free-flowing IV on days 2, 4, 6, and 8. Vesicant. If patient has a central line, a slower infusion over 1 hour may cause less nausea and vomiting. Dose reduced for renal dysfunction. For hepatic dysfunction, give 50% of dose if serum bili is 2.5 mg/dL; do not give if serum bili is 5 mg/dL.

Drug interactions: Drugs that induce or inhibit CYP450 hepatic enzyme system.

Side effects: Alteration in oxygenation varies in severity, but has resulted in death. Usually seen with the first treatment. Signs and symptoms include fever, dyspnea, weight gain, pulmonary infiltrates, pleural, and/or pericardial effusions. Access VS, weight, and pulmonary exam at each visit. Give high-dose steroids to prevent (e.g., dexamethasone 10 mg IV every 12 hours for 3 days). Myelosuppression dose-limiting toxicity. Vitamin A toxicity: headache, benign intracranial hypertension with papilledema, earache or ear "fullness," fever, skin/mucous membrane dryness, pruritus, increased sweating, and visual disturbances. Dizziness, anxiety, paresthesias, depression, confusion, and agitation. Nausea and vomiting, anorexia; stomatitis, diarrhea. Gastrointestinal bleeding/hemorrhage abdominal pain, diarrhea, and constipation. Alopecia, darkening of nail beds, skin ulcer/necrosis, sensitivity to light, and radiation recall. Arrhythmia, flushing, hypotension, and phlebitis. Cardiotoxicity is similar characteristically but less severe than with daunorubicin and doxorubicin. Discoloration of urine from pink to red.

Chair time: 1 hour on days 2, 4, 6, and 8.

SINGLE-AGENT REGIMENS

Arsenic Trioxide (Trisenox)[1,19,228]

Prechemo: CBC, Chem, LFTs, and renal function tests. Doses reduce with impaired functions. Bone marrow biopsy, EKG. 5-HT$_3$, and dexamethasone 10 mg. Mildly emetogenic.

Induction

Arsenic Trioxide 0.15 mg/kg: IV in 100–250 cc NS or D5W daily until bone marrow remission, not to exceed 60 doses.

Consolidation

Arsenic Trioxide 0.15 mg/kg: IV in 100–250 cc NS or D5W daily for 25 doses over a period of up to 5 weeks. Give IV over 1–2 hours (or up to 4 hours if acute vasomotor reactions occur).

Side effects: Vasomotor reactions: symptoms include flushing, tachycardia, dizziness, and lightheadedness. Increasing the infusion time to 4 hours usually resolves these symptoms. Stop infusion for tachycardia and/or hypotension. Resume at decreased rate after resolution. Headaches can also occur; treat with acetaminophen as needed. APL differentiation syndrome: characterized by fever, dyspnea, weight gain, pulmonary infiltrates, and pleural or pericardial effusions, with or without leukocytosis. Can be fatal. At the first suggestion, high-dose steroids should be instituted (e.g., dexamethasone 10 mg IV bid) for at least 3 days or longer until signs and symptoms abate. Drug can cause QT interval prolongation and complete atrioventricular block. Prolonged QT interval can progress to a torsade de pointes-type fatal ventricular arrhythmia. Patients with history of QT prolongation, concomitant administration of drugs that prolong the QT interval, CHF, administration of potassium-wasting diuretics, and conditions resulting in hypokalemia or hypomagnesemia such as concurrent administration of amphotericin B have increased risk of developing this arrhythmia. EKGs should be done weekly, more often if abnormal. Hypokalemia, hypomagnesemia, and hyperglycemia. Edema. Less commonly, hyperkalemia, hypocalcemia, hypoglycemia, and acidosis. Potassium levels should be kept at > 4.0 mEq/dL and magnesium > 1.8 mg/dL. Myelosuppression usually resolves spontaneously. Disseminated intravascular coagulation (DIC).

Nausea, abdominal pain, diarrhea, constipation, anorexia, dyspepsia, abdominal tenderness or distention, and dry mouth. Increased hepatic transaminases ALT and AST. Use with caution in patients with renal impairment. Kidney is the main route of elimination of arsenic. Cough is common, dyspnea, epistaxis, hypoxia, pleural effusion, postnasal drip, wheezing, decreased breath sounds, crepitations, rales/crackles, hemoptysis, tachypnea, and rhonchi. Arthralgias, myalgias, bone, back, neck limb pain. Fatigue. Headache, insomnia, and paresthesias common. Dizziness, tremors, seizures, somnolence, and (rarely) coma. Dermatitispruritus, ecchymosis, dry skin, erythema, hyperpigmentation, and urticaria.

Chair time: 2–5 hours daily until bone marrow remission and then 2 hours daily for 25 doses.

All-Trans-Retinoic Acid (Vesanoid, Tretinoin, ATRA)[1,229]

Prechemo: CBC, Chem, LFTs, and renal function tests. Dose reduce with impaired functions. Bone marrow biopsy baseline and 5–6 weeks from the start of therapy. Oral phenothiazine or 5-HT$_3$. Mildly to moderately emetogenic.

ATRA (Tretinoin) 45 mg/m^2: PO daily in one to two divided doses. 10-mg tablets. Absorption enhanced when taken with food.

Drug interactions: Drugs that inhibit or induce CYP450 hepatic enzyme system.

Side effects: Alteration in oxygenation varies in severity but has resulted in death. Usually seen with the first treatment. Signs and symptoms include fever, dyspnea, weight gain, pulmonary infiltrates, pleural, and/or pericardial effusions. Access VS, weight, and pulmonary exam at each visit. Give high-dose steroids to prevent (e.g., dexamethasone 10-mg IV every 12 hours for 3 days). Myelosuppression dose-limiting toxicity. Vitamin A toxicity: headache, benign intracranial hypertension with papilledema, earache or ear "fullness," fever, skin/mucous membrane dryness, pruritus, increased sweating, and visual disturbances. Dizziness, anxiety, paresthesias, depression, confusion, and agitation. Nausea and vomiting, anorexia; stomatitis, diarrhea. Gastrointestinal bleeding/hemorrhage abdominal pain, diarrhea, and constipation. Alopecia, darkening of nail beds, skin ulcer/necrosis, sensitivity to light, and radiation recall. Arrhythmia, flushing, hypotension, and phlebitis. Cardiotoxicity is similar characteristically but less severe than with daunorubicin and doxorubicin.

Chair time: No chair time. Monitor CBC, coagulation studies, liver functions, triglyceride, and cholesterol levels frequently throughout therapy.

LEUKEMIA: CHRONIC LYMPHOCYTIC LEUKEMIA (CLL)

COMBINATION REGIMENS

Cyclophosphamide + Vincristine + Prednisone (CVP)[1,230]

Prechemo: CBC, Chem, renal and liver functions. Bone marrow biopsy baseline and post-treatment (stop G-CSF 7 days before bone marrow biopsy). 5-HT$_3$ and dexamethasone 20 mg. Moderately emetogenic.

Cyclophosphamide 400 mg/m^2: PO on days 1–5
OR
Cyclophosphamide 800 mg/m^2: IV in 1000 cc NS over 1 hour on day 1.
Vincristine 1.4 mg/m^2: (maximum dose 2 mg): IV push on day 1. Vesicant.
Prednisone 100 mg/m^2: PO or IV on days 1–5 (taper prednisone dose).

Side effects: Myelosuppression dose-limiting toxicity. Nausea and vomiting, anorexia, stomatitis, and gastric irritation. Hemorrhagic cystitis, preventable with hydration. Peripheral neuropathy including numbness, weakness, myalgias, and cramping. Jaw pain and paralytic ileus may require discontinuation of vincristine. Impotency. Alopecia. Tumor lysis syndrome can occur if WBC is elevated. Prevent with allopurinol and hydration. Steroid toxicities: sodium and water retention, Cushingoid changes, behavioral changes, including emotional lability, insomnia, mood swings, and euphoria. Muscle weakness and loss with prolonged use. May increase glucose and sodium and decrease potassium and affect warfarin dose.

Chair time: 2 hours on day 1. Repeat cycle every 21 days.

Cyclophosphamide + Fludarabine (CF)[1,231]

Prechemo: CBC, Chem, renal and liver functions. Bone marrow biopsy baseline and post-treatment (stop G-CSF 7 days before bone marrow biopsy). 5-HT$_3$ and dexamethasone 20 mg IVPB. Moderately emetogenic.

Cyclophosphamide 1000 mg/m^2: IV in 1000 cc NS over 1 hour on day 1.

Fludarabine 20 mg/m^2: IV in 100 cc NS over 30 minutes on days 1–5.

Bactrim DS: One tablet PO BID.

Side effects: Myelosuppression dose-limiting toxicity. Agitation, confusion, and visual disturbances. Immunosuppression: decrease in CD4$^+$ and CD8$^+$, increasing risk for opportunistic infections (fungus, herpes, and *Pneumocystis carinii*). Nausea and vomiting, anorexia; mucositis, diarrhea. Hemorrhagic cystitis preventable with hydration. Tumor lysis syndrome. Prevent with allopurinol and hydration. Maculopapular skin rash, erythema, and pruritus. Alopecia.

Chair time: 2 hours on day 1 and 1 hour on days 2–5. Repeat cycle every 21–28 days.

Fludarabine + Prednisone (FP)[1,232]

Prechemo: CBC, Chem, renal and liver functions. Bone marrow biopsy. 5-HT$_3$ IV. Mildly emetogenic.

Fludarabine 30 mg/m^2: IV in 100 cc NS over 30 minutes on days 1–5.

Prednisone 30 mg/m^2: PO on days 1–5.

Side effects: Myelosuppression dose-limiting toxicity. Agitation, confusion, and visual disturbances. Immunosuppression: decrease in CD4$^+$ and CD8$^+$, increasing risk for opportunistic infections (fungus, herpes, and *Pneumocystis carinii*). Pneumonia. Pulmonary hypersensitivity reaction characterized by dyspnea, cough, and interstitial pulmonary infiltrates. Steroid toxicities: sodium and water retention, cushingoid changes, and behavioral changes, including emotional lability, insomnia, mood swings, and euphoria. Muscle weakness and loss with prolonged use. May increase glucose and sodium and decrease potassium and affect warfarin dose. Nausea and vomiting, anorexia; mucositis, diarrhea. Maculopapular skin rash, erythema, and pruritus. Alopecia.

Chair time: 1 hour on days 1–5. Repeat the schedule every 28 days.

Chlorambucil + Prednisone (CP)[1,230]

Prechemo: CBC, Chem, renal and liver functions. Bone marrow biopsy. 5-HT$_3$ or phenothiazine PO. Mildly emetogenic.

Chlorambucil 30 mg/m^2: PO on day 1 every 2 weeks. 2-mg tablets.

Prednisone 80 mg: PO on days 1–5 every 2 weeks.

Side effects: Myelosuppression dose-limiting toxicity. Nausea and vomiting are rare. Anorexia and weight loss may occur. Pulmonary fibrosis and pneumonitis dose related and potentially life-threatening. Tumor lysis syndrome can occur if WBCs are elevated. Steroid toxicities: sodium and water retention, cushingoid changes, and behavioral changes, including emotional lability, insomnia, mood swings, and euphoria. Muscle weakness and loss with prolonged use. May increase glucose and sodium and decrease potassium and affect warfarin dose. Skin rash on face, scalp, and trunk seen in early stage of therapy.

Chair time: No chair time. Repeat cycle every 2 weeks.

Fludarabine + Rituxan (FR)[1,233]

Prechemo: CBC, Chem, renal and liver functions. Bone marrow biopsy baseline and 2 months after the completion of cycle 6. 5-HT$_3$ and dexamethasone IV. Diphenhydramine 25–50 mg and H$_2$ antagonist. Acetaminophen 650–100 mg PO. Mildly emetogenic.

Fludarabine 25 mg/m²: IV in 100 cc NS over 20–30 minutes on days 1–5.

Rituximab 50 mg/m²: IV over 4 hours without rate escalation, day 1 (first cycle only).

Rituximab 325 mg/m²: IV on day 3 (first cycle only). Start at 50-mg/hr, increasing by 50 mg/hr every 30 minutes to maximum rate of 400 mg/hr as tolerated.

Rituximab 375 mg/m²: IV over 1 hour on day 5 cycle 1. Then **day 1 only** cycles 2–6. Administer at 100mg/hr for the first 15 minutes of the infusion, and then increase rate to infuse the entire dose over the next 45 minutes. Dilute to a final concentration of 1–4 mg/mL.

Restage patient 2 months after cycle 6. Those patients demonstrating stable disease or better should be treated with:

Rituximab 375 mg/m²: IV over 3–4 hours escalating dose from 100 mg/hr in 100mg/hr increments every 30 minutes to a maximum rate of 400 mg/hr weekly for 4 weeks.

Side effects: Myelosuppression: severe and cumulative. Hypersensitivity reactions with rituxan and with high tumor burden. Premedicate. Decrease in CD4+ and CD8+, increasing risk for opportunistic infections (fungus, herpes, and *Pneumocystis carinii*). Tumor lysis syndrome can occur if WBC is elevated or large tumor burden. Prevent with allopurinol and hydration 150 mL/hr with or without alkalinization. Fatigue, agitation, confusion, and visual disturbances. Pneumonia. Pulmonary hypersensitivity reaction characterized by dyspnea, cough, and interstitial pulmonary infiltrates. Nausea and vomiting, anorexia; mucositis and, diarrhea.

Chair time: 5 hours days 1 and 3; 2 hours on day 5; and1 hour on days 2 and 4 of cycle 1. Then, 5 hours day 1 and 1 hour days 2–5 cycles 2–6. Repeat cycle every 28 days for six cycles.

Fludarabine + Cyclophosphamide + Rituxan (FCR)[1,234]

Prechemo: CBC, Chem, renal and liver functions. Bone marrow biopsy, central line placement. Diphenhydramine 25–50 mg and H_2 blocker plus acetaminophen 650–1000mg PO day 1 only. 5-HT_3 and dexamethasone IV. Mildly to moderately emetogenic.

Fludarabine 25 mg/m²: IV in 100 cc NS over 30 minutes on days 2–4 of cycle 1 only.

Fludarabine 25 mg/m²: IV on days 1–3 of cycles 2–6.

Cyclophosphamide 250 mg/m²: IV in 500 cc NS on days 2–4 of cycle 1 only.

Cyclophosphamide 250 mg/m²: IV in 500 cc NS on days 1–3 of cycles 2–6.

Rituximab 375 mg/m²: IV, day 1 of cycle 1 only. Start at 50 mg/hr with rate escalation every 30 minutes by 50 mg/hr up to a maximum of 400 mg/hr.

Rituximab 500 mg/m²: IV on day 1 on cycles 2–6. Start rate at 100 mg/hr up and increase every 30 minutes by 100 mg/hr to a maximum rate of 400 mg/hr. Dilute to a final concentration of 1–4 mg/mL

Side effects: Myelosuppression: severe and cumulative. Hypersensitivity reactions with rituxan and patients with high tumor burden. Premedicate with acetaminophen, diphenhydramine, and corticosteroids. Decrease in CD4+ and CD8+, increasing risk for opportunistic infections (fungus, herpes, and *Pneumocystis carinii*). Tumor lysis syndrome can occur if WBC is elevated or large tumor burden. Prevent with allopurinol and hydration 150 mL/hr with or without alkalinization. Fatigue. Hemorrhagic cystitis, preventable with hydration. Agitation, confusion, and visual disturbances. Pneumonia, pulmonary hypersensitivity reaction characterized by dyspnea, cough, and interstitial pulmonary infiltrates. Nausea and vomiting, anorexia; mucositis, diarrhea.

Chair time: 5–8 hours on day 1; 2 hours days 2 and 3. Repeat cycle every 4 weeks for six cycles. Delay cycle if bone marrow has not recovered.

SINGLE-AGENT REGIMENS

Alemtuzumab (Campath)[1,235]

Prechemo: CBC, Chem, renal and liver functions. Bone marrow biopsy, central line placement. 5-HT_3 and dexamethasone IV. Mildly emetogenic. Acetaminophen 650 mg and diphenhydramine 50 mg.

Alemtuzumab 30 mg: IV in 100 cc NS or D5W over 2 hours three times a week on alternate days. Administer 3 mg three times a week until tolerated (infusion-related toxicities are less than grade 2). Increase to 10 mg IV three times per week. When tolerated (infusion-related toxicities are less than grade 2), increase to the maintenance dose of 30-mg IV three times per week. Total duration of therapy, including dose escalation, is 12 weeks. Contraindications: patients with active systemic infections, HIV-positive, AIDS, or known type 1 hypersensitivity or anaphylactic reactions. Bactrim DS and Famciclovir 250 mg PO BID day 8 through 2 months after completion of therapy.

Side effects: Hypersensitivity reactions: most often seen in the first week of therapy. Fever, chills, rigors, nausea and vomiting, urticaria, skin rash, fatigue, headache, diarrhea, dyspnea, and/or hypotension. Stop the drug if reaction occurs; may treat with steroids; meperidine for rigors. Usually resolves in 20 minutes. Myelosuppression dose-limiting toxicity. Increased incidence of pancytopenia with single doses greater than 30 mg or if cumulative weekly dose exceeds 90 mg. Dramatic drop in WBCs during the first week. Opportunistic infections common, including *Pneumocystis carinii* pneumonia, pulmonary aspergillus, and herpes simplex infections. Tumor lysis with high WBCs or high tumor burden. Prevent with allopurinol and hydration. Pain, headache, asthenia, dysphasias, and dizziness.

Chair time: 2–3 hours 3 days per week for 12 weeks. Weekly CBC and CD-41.

Chlorambucil[1,236]

Prechemo: CBC, Chem, renal and liver functions. Bone marrow biopsy. Oral phenothiazine or 5-HT$_3$ PO. Mildly emetogenic.

Chlorambucil 6–14 mg/day: PO as induction therapy and then:

Chlorambucil 0.7 mg/Kg/day: PO for 2–4 days.

Side effects: Myelosuppression dose-limiting. Pulmonary fibrosis and pneumonitis, dose related; rare. Nausea and vomiting are rare. Anorexia and weight loss.

Chair time: No chair time. Repeat cycle every 21 days.

Cladribine (Leustatin, 2-CdA)[1,237]

Prechemo: CBC, Chem, renal and liver functions. Bone marrow biopsy, central line placement. Oral phenothiazine or 5-HT$_3$ PO. Mildly emetogenic.

Cladribine 0.09 mg/kg/day: IV continuous infusion on days 1–7.

Use 0.22-micron filter to add calculated dose and a sufficient amount of bacteriostatic NS to achieve a total volume of 100 mL to infusion reservoir. DO NOT use D5W.

Side effects: Myelosuppression dose-limiting toxicity. Decrease in CD4$^+$ and CD8$^+$, increasing risk for opportunistic infections (fungus, herpes, and *Pneumocystis carinii*). Tumor lysis syndrome if WBC is elevated or large tumor burden. Prevent with allopurinol and hydration 150 mL/hr with or without alkalinization. Fatigue secondary to anemia. Nausea and vomiting, anorexia; constipation, diarrhea. Headache, insomnia, and dizziness. Rash, pruritus, or injection site reactions.

Chair time: 1 hour on day 1, pump dc on day 8. Repeat cycle every 28–35 days.

Fludarabine[1,238]

Prechemo: CBC, Chem, renal and liver functions. Bone marrow biopsy. 5-HT$_3$ and dexamethasone IV. Mildly emetogenic.

Fludarabine 20–30 mg/m^2: IV in 100 cc NS on days 1–5.

Side effects: Myelosuppression: severe and cumulative. Decrease in CD4$^+$ and CD8$^+$, increasing risk for opportunistic infections (fungus, herpes, and *Pneumocystis carinii*). Fatigue secondary to anemia. Agitation, confusion, and visual disturbances. Pneumonia. Pulmonary hypersensitivity reaction characterized by dyspnea, cough, and interstitial pulmonary infiltrates. Nausea and vomiting, anorexia; mucositis, diarrhea.

Chair time: 1 hour on days 1–5. Repeat schedule every 28 days.

Prednisone[1,239]

Prechemo: CBC, Chem, renal and liver functions. Bone marrow biopsy.

Prednisone 20–30 mg/m^2/day: PO for 1–3 weeks. Take with food.

Use if patient symptomatic with autoimmune thrombocytopenia or hemolytic anemia.

Side effects: Gastric irritation, increased appetite. Steroid toxicities: sodium and water retention, cushingoid changes, behavioral changes, including emotional lability, insomnia, mood swings, and euphoria. May increase glucose and sodium and decrease potassium and affect warfarin dose. Muscle weakness, loss of muscle mass, osteoporosis, and pathologic fractures with prolonged use. Perceptual alterations: cataracts or glaucoma may develop.

Chair time: No chair time.

Bendamustine (Treanda) [1,240]

Prechemo: CBC and Chem. 5HT3 and dexamethasone 10 mg in 100 cc of NS. Diphenhydramine 25–50 mg and cimetidine 300 mg in 100 cc of NS. Mildly to moderately emetogenic.

Bendamustine (Treanda) 100 mg/m^2: IV in 500 cc NS over 30 minutes days 1 and 2.

Side effects: Infusion reactions are common. Symptoms include fever, chills, pruritus, and rash. In rare instances, severe anaphylactic and anaphylactoid reactions have occurred, particularly in the second and subsequent cycles of therapy. Myelosuppression is common. Nadirs seen in the third week of therapy and may require dose delays if marrow recovery has not occurred by day 28. Dose reduction necessary for grade 3 or 4 toxicities. Infection, including pneumonia and sepsis have been reported. Tumor lysis syndrome. Preventive measures include hydration and the use of allopurinol during the first 1–2 weeks of therapy in patients at high risk. Blood chemistries, particularly potassium and uric acid levels, should be closely monitored. Nausea and vomiting, usually mild to moderate. Diarrhea, dry mouth, mucosal inflammation, and stomatitis. Pyrexia, asthenia, fatigue, malaise, and weakness. Somnolence, cough, and headache. Rash, toxic skin reactions, and bullous exanthema have been reported. Rashes are usually mild. Can be dose related, drug should be withheld or discontinued if skin reactions are severe or progressive.

Chair time: 2 hours on days 1 and 2. Repeat cycle every 28 days up to six cycles.

LEUKEMIA: CHRONIC MYELOGENOUS LEUKEMIA (CML)

COMBINATION REGIMENS

Interferon + Cytarabine (Ara-C)[1,241]

Prechemo: CBC, Chem, renal and liver functions. Bone marrow biopsy. Oral 5-HT$_3$. Acetaminophen 650–1000 mg PO. Mildly to moderately emetogenic.

Interferon α-2b 5 X 10^6 IU/m^2: SQ daily.

Available in single-dose prefilled syringes 3, 6, and 9 million units.

Cytarabine 20-mg/m^2: SQ daily for 10 days.

Side effects: Myelosuppression. Interferon should be reduced by 50% when neutrophil count drops below 1500/mm^3, the platelet count drops below 100,000 per mm^3, or both. Both drugs should be discontinued with neutrophils less than 1000 mm^3, platelets less than 50,000 mm^3, or both. Flu-like syndrome: chills 3–6 hours after interferon. Fatigue, malaise, headache, and myalgias are cumulative and dose-limiting. Thrombophlebitis, pain at the injection site, should be treated with warm compresses. Tumor lysis syndrome occurring 1–5 days after the initiation of treatment. Nausea and vomiting, anorexia, xerostomia, and mild diarrhea. Partial alopecia.

Chair time: Administered in the office or self-administered. Repeat every 28 days.

SINGLE-AGENT REGIMENS

Imatinib (Gleevec)[1,242]

Prechemo: CBC, Chem, renal and liver functions. Bone marrow biopsy. Oral 5-HT$_3$. Mild to moderately emetogenic.

Imatinib 400–800 mg: Per day. 100- and 400-mg tablets. 400-mg/day single dose for patients in chronic-phase CML. 600-mg/day single dose for patients in accelerated phase or blast crisis. Treatment continues as long as patient derives benefit from drug. In disease progression, failure of hematologic response after 3 months, or loss of hematologic remission, increase dose to 600 mg/day (chronic CML) or to 800 mg/day given as 400 mg BID (accelerated or blast crisis).

Drug interactions: CYP3A4 inducers, inhibitors, and substrates.

Side effects: Myelosuppression, nausea, and vomiting. Diarrhea and dyspepsia. Fluid retention, especially in the older patient (primarily periorbital and lower extremity edema). May require diuretics. Pleural effusions, ascites, pulmonary edema, and weight gain. More common in accelerated phase. Muscle cramps, musculoskeletal pain, headaches, fatigue, arthralgias, and abdominal pain. Rash may occur with pruritus.

Chair time: No chair time.

Busulfan (Myleran) [1,243]

Prechemo: CBC, Chem, renal and liver functions. Bone marrow biopsy. Oral 5-HT$_3$. Mild to moderately emetogenic.

Busulfan 4–8 mg or 1.8 mg/m^2: PO daily for 2–3 weeks initially. Then: **Busulfan 1–3 mg/m^2 or 0.05 mg/m^2:** Or PO daily for maintenance. 2-mg scored tablets.

Side effects: Myelosuppression dose-limiting toxicity. Hold when leukocyte count reaches 15,000 per mL; resume when total leukocyte count is 50,000 per mL; maintenance dose of 1–3 mg qd used if remission lasts less than 3 months. Tumor lysis syndrome if WBC is elevated. Prevent with allopurinol and hydration. Nausea and vomiting mild. Mucositis dose related and may require interruption of therapy. Hyperpigmentation of skin, especially increases on the hands and nail beds. Skin rash and pruritus also observed. Cough, dyspnea, and fever after long-term therapy. Insomnia, anxiety, dizziness, and depression.

Chair time: No chair time.

Hydroxyurea[1,244]

Prechemo: CBC, Chem, renal and liver functions. Bone marrow biopsy. Oral 5-HT$_3$ or phenothizine. Mild to moderately emetogenic.

Hydroxyurea 1–5 g/day: PO, adjusted to keep WBC about 20–30 × 10^9/L. 500-mg caplets.

Side effects: Myelosuppression with leukopenia is dose-limiting. Median onset 7–10 days. Nausea and vomiting mild. Diarrhea, stomatitis, and dyspepsia. Tumor lysis syndrome if WBC count high. Muscle cramps, musculoskeletal pain, headaches, fatigue, arthralgias, abdominal pain, drowsiness and confusion. Rash, hyperpigmentation, and pruritis.

Chair time: No chair time.

Interferon α-2b[1,245]

Prechemo: CBC, Chem, renal and liver functions. Bone marrow biopsy. Oral 5-HT$_3$. Acetaminophen 650–1000 mg PO. Mildly to moderately emetogenic.

Interferon α-2b 9-million units: SQ per day 3 days per week. Available in single dose prefilled syringes 3, 6, and 9 million units.

Side effects: Myelosuppression. Flu-like syndrome: chills 3–6 hours after injection, fatigue, malaise, headache, and myalgias. Cumulative and dose-limiting. Dizziness, confusion, decreased mental status, and depression. Thrombophlebitis, pain at the injection site. Nausea, vomiting, anorexia, xerostomia, and mild diarrhea. Partial alopecia.

Chair time: Self-administered. Continue injections 3 days/week for up to 1–1.5 years.

Dasatinib (Sprycel)[1,246,247]

Prechemo: CBC, Chem, renal and liver functions. Bone marrow biopsy. Oral 5-HT$_3$. Mildly to moderately emetogenic.

Sprycel 70 mg: PO twice per day with or without food. 20-, 50-, and 70-mg tablets. Do not take within 2 hours of antacids. Do not crush or cut tablets.

Side effects: Myelosuppression, severe. Monitor CBC weekly first month, every other week for second month, and then as clinically indicated. CNS or GI bleed seen. Nausea and vomiting, anorexia, diarrhea, constipation, mucositis, and dyspepsia. Fluid retention: pleural effusion and pericardial effusion. May require diuretics. Prolongation of QT interval. Monitor potassium and magnesium levels. Rash may occur with pruritus. Headache, musculoskeletal pain, arthralgias, and myalgias. Fatigue.

Chair time: No chair time.

Nilotinib (Tasigna) [1,248]

Prechemo: CBC, Chem, Mg^{2+}, serum lipase, and LFTs. Bone marrow biopsy to determine Philadelphia chromosome-positive CML. EKG at baseline, 7 days after initiation, and periodically thereafter, as well as following dose adjustments. Oral phenothiazine or 5-HT$_3$ as needed. Mildly emetogenic protocol.

Nilotinib 400 mg: PO every 12 hours daily. 200-mg light-yellow gelatin capsules. Take whole with water. No food for at least 2 hours before and 1 hour after dosing.

Side effects: QT prolongation and sudden death. Should not be used in patients with hypokalemia, hypomagnesemia, or long QT syndrome. Hypophosphatemia, hypokalemia, hyperkalemia, hypocalcemia, and hyponatremia. Correct electrolyte abnormalities prior to initiating

Tasigna® and monitor periodically. Myelosuppression reversible by withholding dose. Dose reduction may be required. Drugs known to prolong the QT interval and strong CYP3A4 inhibitors or inducers should be avoided. Dose adjustment necessary if patient must be co-administered these drugs. Grapefruit products and other foods know to inhibit CYP3A4 should be avoided. Food increases blood levels of Tasigna®. Use with caution with hepatic impairment and/or history of pancreatitis. Check LFTs and serum lipase periodically. Hypertension, flushing, and pyrexia. Dyspnea, exertional dyspnea, cough, and dysphonia. Not recommended for patients with lactose intolerance or malabsorption. Abdominal discomfort, dyspepsia, and flatulence. Dizziness, paresthesia, and vertigo common. Musculoskeletal chest pain or pain. Exfoliative rash, ecchymosis, and facial swelling. Night sweats, eczema, urticaria, alopecia, erythema, hyperhidrosis, dry skin, and alopecia.

Chair time: No chair time. Take every 12 hours as tolerated or until progression.

LEUKEMIA: CUTANEOUS T-CELL LEUKEMIA (CTCL)

Denileukin Diftitox (ONTAK)[1, 249]

Prechemo: CBC, Chem, LFTs, renal functions, albumin baseline and weekly. 5-HT$_3$ and dexamethasone. Diphenhydramine 25-50 mg and H$_2$ antagonist to reduce hypersensitivity reactions. Mildly to moderately emetogenic.

Ontak 9-18 mcg/kg/day: IV into empty IV bag. Add up to 9 mL of sterile saline without preservative for each 1 mL of ONTK for final concentration of at least 15 mcg/mL over 15 minutes daily for 5 days. Drug comes frozen. Thaw in refrigerator in less than 24 hours or at room temp for 1 to 2 hours. DO NOT REFREEZE.

Side effects: Hypersensitivity reactions; hypotension, back pain, dyspnea, vasodilation, rash, chest pain or tightness, tachycardia. Vascular leak syndrome with hypotension, edema, and hypoalbuminemia; seen in first 2 weeks of infusion. Patients with cardiac problems at risk for myocardial infarction. Myelosuppression and cutaneous infections. Flu-like syndrome. Nausea, vomiting, anorexia, and diarrhea. Rash, pruritus, and sweating. Dyspnea, cough, SOB, pharyngitis, rhinitis. Monitor weight, blood pressure, and CBC. Nervousness, confusion, and insomnia. Hematuria, albuminuria, and pyuria. Acute renal insufficiency. Loss of visual acuity.

Chair time: 1 hour on days 1–5. Repeat every 3 weeks for six cycles.

LEUKEMIA: HAIRY CELL LEUKEMIA

Cladribine (Leustatin, 2-CdA)[1,250]

Prechemo: CBC, Chem, renal and liver functions. Bone marrow biopsy, central line placement. Oral phenothiazine or 5-HT$_3$ as needed. Mildly emetogenic.

Cladribine 0.09 mg/kg/day: IV continuous infusion on days 1–7. Use 0.22-micron filter to add calculated dose and a sufficient amount of bacteriostatic NS to achieve a total volume of 100 mL to infusion reservoir. DO NOT use D5W.

Side effects: Myelosuppression dose-limiting toxicity. Decrease in CD4$^+$ and CD8$^+$, increasing risk for opportunistic infections (fungus, herpes, and *Pneumocystis carinii*). Tumor lysis syndrome if WBC is elevated or large tumor burden. Prevent with allopurinol and hydration 150 mL/hr with or without alkalinization. Fatigue: nausea and vomiting, anorexia; constipation, diarrhea. Headache, insomnia, and dizziness. Rash and pruritus.

Chair time: 1 hour on day 1, pump d/c day 8. Administer one cycle.

Pentostatin[1,251]

Prechemo: CBC, Chem, renal and liver functions. Bone marrow biopsy. Moderately emetogenic.

Pentostatin 4mg/m^2: IV on day 1. IV push or as bolus diluted in 25–50 mL of NS or D5W over 30 minutes.

Side effects: Myelosuppression: increased risk of opportunistic infections. Dose-limiting toxicity. Nausea and vomiting, anorexia. Allergic hypersensitivity reaction: fever, chills, myalgias, and arthralgias. Headache, lethargy, and fatigue.

Immunosuppression: Decrease in CD4$^+$ and CD8$^+$, increasing risk for opportunistic infections (fungus, herpes, and *Pneumocystis carinii*).

Chair time: 1 hour on day 1; repeat cycle every 14 days for six cycles or two cycles beyond complete remission. Do not treat for more than 1 year.

Interferon α-2a[1,252]

Prechemo: CBC, Chem, renal and liver functions. Bone marrow biopsy. Oral phenothiazine or 5-HT$_3$ as needed. Mildly to moderately emetogenic.

Interferon α-2a 3-million units: SQ per day 3 days per week.

Side effects: Flu-like syndrome: fever, chills, headache, myalgias, and arthralgias. Managed with acetaminophen and increased oral fluid intake. Myelosuppression. Nausea, diarrhea, and vomiting. Anorexia cumulative and dose-limiting. Taste alteration and xerostomia. Mild proteinuria and hypocalcemia. Mild transient elevations in serum transaminases, dose-dependant. Dizziness, confusion, and decreased mental status and depression. Retinopathy with cotton-wool spots and small hemorrhages. Usually asymptomatic and resolves when drug discontinued. Dry skin, pruritus, and irritation at injection. Alopecia is partial.

Chair time: Continue SQ injections 3 days per week for up to 1–1.5 years.

Lung Cancer: Non–Small Cell Lung Cancer

ADJUVANT THERAPY

COMBINATION REGIMENS

Paclitaxel + Carboplatin[1,253]

Prechemo: CBC, Chem, LFTs, and renal function tests. 5-HT$_3$ and dexamethasone 10–20 mg. Diphenhydramine 25–50 mg and H$_2$ antagonist. Mildly to moderately etogenic.

Paclitaxel 175 mg/m²: IV in 500 cc NS over 3 hours on day 1. Use non-PVC containers and tubing with 0.22-micron inline filter.

Carboplatin AUC 6: IV in 500 cc NS on day 1. Give carboplatin after paclitaxel to decrease toxicities.

Side effects: Hypersensitivity reaction: with paclitaxel or in patients receiving more than seven courses of carboplatin therapy. Myelosuppression cumulative, dose related and dose-limiting. G-CSF recommended. Nausea and vomiting acute or delayed. Mucositis and/or diarrhea. Transient elevations in serum transaminases, bilirubin, and alkaline phosphatase. Decreases Mg^{2+}, K$^+$, Ca^{2+}, and Na$^+$. Sensory neuropathy with numbness and paresthesias; dose related and can be dose-limiting. Alopecia.

Chair time: 5 hours on day 1. Repeat every 21 days for four cycles.

Vinorelbine + Cisplatin[1,254]

Prechemo: CBC, Chem, LFTs, and renal function tests. 5-HT$_3$ and dexamethasone 10–20 mg. Moderately to highly etogenic.

Vinorelbine 25 mg/m²: IV weekly for 16 weeks. Vesicant. Dilute to a final concentration in syringe 1.5–3.0 or IV bag of 0.5–3.0 mg/mL. Infuse diluted drug IV over 6–10 minutes into sidearm port of a free-flowing

IV, either peripherally or via central line (preferred). Use port closest to the IV bag, not the patient.

Cisplatin 50 mg/m²: IV in 500–1000 cc NS on days 1 and 8. Repeat cisplatin every 28 days for four cycles.

Side effects: Myelosuppression dose related and dose-limiting. Nausea and vomiting, acute or delayed. Constipation, diarrhea, stomatitis, and anorexia. Metallic taste to foods. Severe neuropathy with numbness, tingling, and sensory loss in arms and legs. Proprioception and vibratory sense and loss of motor function. Paresthesias dose related and can be severe, requiring pain medication or Neurontin. High-frequency hearing loss. Necrosis of proximal and distal renal tubules preventing reabsorption of Mg^{2+}, Ca^{2+}, and K^+. May be avoided with adequate hydration, diuresis, as well as slower infusion time. Alopecia likely.

Chair time: 3 hours on days 1 and 8 for cisplatin; repeat every 28 days for four cycles. 1 hour weekly for vinorelbine for 16 weeks.

METASTATIC DISEASE

COMBINATION REGIMENS

Carboplatin + Paclitaxel[1,255]

Prechemo: CBC, Chem, Mg^{2+}, and renal functions. 5-HT$_3$ and dexamethasone 10–20 mg in 100 cc of NS. Diphenhydramine 25–50 mg and H$_2$ antagonist in 100 cc of NS. Mildly to moderately emetogenic.

Carboplatin AUC 6: IV in 500 cc NS on day 1. Give after paclitaxel to decrease toxicities.

Paclitaxel 175 mg/m²: IV in 500 cc NS over 3 hours on day 1. Use non-PVC containers and tubing with 0.22-micron inline filter.

Side effects: Hypersensitivity reaction: with paclitaxel or in patients receiving more than seven courses of carboplatin therapy. Myelosuppression cumulative and dose related and dose-limiting. G-CSF recommended. Nausea and vomiting, acute or delayed. Mucositis and/or diarrhea. Transient elevations in serum transaminases, bilirubin and alkaline phosphatase. Decreases Mg^{2+}, K^+, Ca^{2+}, and Na^+. Sensory neuropathy with numbness and paresthesias; dose related and can be dose-limiting. Alopecia.

Chair time: 5 hours on day 1. Repeat every 21 days until progression.

Cisplatin + Paclitaxel[1,256]

Prechemo: CBC, Chem, LFTs, and renal function tests. 5-HT$_3$ and dexamethasone 10–20 mg. Diphenhydramine 25–50 mg and H$_2$ antagonist. Moderately to highly emetogenic.

Paclitaxel 175 mg/m²: IV in 500 cc NS over 3 hours on day 1. Use non-PVC tubing and containers and a 0.22-micron inline filter.

Cisplatin 80 mg/m²: IV in 1000 cc NS on day 1. Paclitaxel administered first, followed by cisplatin.

Side effects: Hypersensitivity reaction with paclitaxel and cisplatin. Myelosuppression cumulative, dose related, dose-limiting. G-CSF recommended. Nausea and vomiting, acute or delayed. Taste alterations and anorexia. Metallic taste to food. Renal dose-limiting toxicity, may result in necrosis of proximal and distal renal tubules. Decreases Mg^{2+}, K^+, Ca^{2+}, and Na^+. May be avoided with adequate hydration, diuresis, slower infusion time. Severe neuropathy with numbness, tingling, and sensory loss in arms and legs. Proprioception and vibratory sense and loss of motor function can occur. Paresthesias dose related and can be severe, requiring pain medication or Neurontin. High-frequency hearing loss. Alopecia: total loss of body hair.

Chair time: 5 hours on day 1. Repeat cycle every 21 days until progression.

Docetaxel + Carboplatin[1,257]

Prechemo: CBC, Chem, LFTs, and renal function tests. Dexamethasone 8 mg PO bid day before, day of, and day after docetaxel. 5-HT₃ and dexamethasone 10–20 mg. Moderately to highly emetogenic.

Docetaxel 75 mg/m²: IV in 2500 cc NS on day 1. Use non-PVC container and tubing.

Carboplatin AUC 6: IV in 500 cc NS on day 1.

Side effects: Hypersensitivity reaction with cisplatin or in patients receiving more than seven courses of carboplatin. Myelosuppression, dose related and can be dose-limiting. Nausea and vomiting. Decreases Mg^{2+}, K^+, Ca^{2+}, and Na^+. Neuropathy with numbness and paresthesia. Edema, pleural effusion, and ascites. Hand-foot syndrome. Nail changes, rash, and dry, pruritic skin. Alopecia.

Chair time: 3 hours on day 1. Repeat cycle every 21 days until progression.

Docetaxel + Cisplatin[1,258]

Prechemo: CBC, Chem, LFTs, and renal function tests. 5-HT₃. Diphenhydramine 25–50 mg and H₂ antagonist. Dexamethasone 8-mg PO bid for 3 days, starting the day before treatment. Moderately emetogenic.

Docetaxel 75 mg/m²: IV in 2500 cc NS on day 1. Use non-PVC containers and tubing.

Cisplatin 75 mg/m²: IV in 500–1000 cc NS on day 1.

Side effects: Hypersensitivity reaction with docetaxel and cisplatin. Myelosuppression, dose related, and can be dose-limiting. G-CSF recommended. Nausea and vomiting, acute or delayed. Metallic taste to food. Severe neuropathy with numbness, tingling, and sensory loss in arms and legs. Proprioception and vibratory sense and loss of motor function can occur. Paresthesias dose related. Can be severe, requiring pain medication or Neurontin. High-frequency hearing loss. Renal,

dose-limiting toxicity, cumulative. May result in necrosis of proximal
and distal renal tubules. Decreases Mg^{2+}, K^+, Ca^{2+}, and Na^+. Reduce risk
with adequate hydration, diuresis, or slower infusion time. Fluid retention is a cumulative toxicity with docetaxel with peripheral edema,
pleural effusions, dyspnea at rest, cardiac tamponade, or ascites. Maculopapular, violaceous/erythematous, and pruritic rash may occur with
docetaxel. Changes in nails, onycholysis. Alopecia.

Chair time: 4 hours on day 1. Repeat cycle every 21 days until progression.

Docetaxel + Gemcitabine[1,259]

Prechemo: CBC, Chem, LFTs, and renal function tests. IV 5-HT_3.
Diphenhydramine 25–50 mg and H_2 antagonist in dexamethasone 8-mg
PO bid for 3 days, starting the before, day of, and day after treatment.
Moderately emetogenic.

Docetaxel 100 mg/m²: IV in 250 cc NS on day 8. Use non-PVC containers and tubing.

Gemcitabine 1100 mg/m²: IV in 250 cc NS over 30 minutes on days
1 and 8.

Side effects: Hypersensitivity reaction with docetaxel. Myelosuppression is dose-limiting. G-CSF recommended. Thrombocytopenia increased in older patients. Nausea, vomiting, diarrhea, and mucositis.
Neuropathy with numbness, tingling, and sensory loss in arms and legs.
High-frequency hearing loss. Flu-like syndrome with fever 6–12 hours
after gemcitabine. Dose reduce gemcitabine for elevation of serum
transaminase and bilirubin levels. Fluid retention is a cumulative toxicity with docetaxel, peripheral edema, pleural effusions, dyspnea at rest,
cardiac tamponade, or ascites. Maculopapular, violaceous/erythematous,
and pruritic rash may occur with docetaxel. Nails changes and may include onycholysis. Alopecia.

Chair time: 1 hour on day 1 and 2 hours on day 8. Repeat cycle every
21 days.

Gemcitabine + Cisplatin[1,260]

Prechemo: CBC, Chem, Mg^{2+}, and LFTs. 5-HT_3 and dexamethasone
10–20 mg in 100 cc of NS. Moderately to highly emetogenic.

Gemcitabine 1250 mg/m²: IV in 250 cc NS over 30 minutes on days
1 and 8.

Cisplatin 100 mg/m²: IV in 1000 cc NS on day 1.

Side effects: Hypersensitivity reaction with cisplatin. Myelosuppression,
with grades 3 and 4 thrombocytopenia more common in older patients.
Nausea and vomiting, acute or delayed. Diarrhea and/or mucositis.
Metallic taste. Flu-like syndrome. Nephrotoxicity with cisplatin. Decreased levels of Mg^{2+}, K^+, Ca^{2+}, Na^+, and PO_4. Elevated levels of

serum transaminases and bilirubin. Sensory neuropathy, dose related, usually reversible. Pruritic, maculopapular skin rash on trunk and extremities. Edema. High-frequency hearing loss and tinnitus. Alopecia.

Chair time: 3 hours day 1 and 1 hour on day 8. Repeat every 21 days.

Gemcitabine + Carboplatin[1,261]

Prechemo: CBC, Chem, LFTs, and renal function tests. 5-HT$_3$ and dexamethasone 10–20 mg. Mildly to moderately emetogenic.

Gemcitabine mg 1000 mg/m^2: IV in 250 cc NS over 30 minutes on days 1 and 8.

Carboplatin AUC 5: IV in 500 cc NS on day 1.

Side effects: Hypersensitivity reaction the risk increases with more than seven courses of carboplatin. Myelosuppression, cumulative and dose related. Can be dose-limiting. G-CSF recommended. Thrombocytopenia grades 3–4 more common in older patients. Nausea and vomiting, acute or delayed. Mucositis and diarrhea. Elevation of serum transaminase and bilirubin levels. Flu-like syndrome with fever in absence of infection 6–12 hours after treatment. Fluid retention cumulative toxicity with docetaxel. Peripheral edema, pleural effusions, dyspnea at rest, cardiac tamponade, or ascites. Altered renal function with decreases in Mg^{2+}, K^+, Ca^{2+}, and Na^+. Risk my be reduced with adequate hydration, diuresis, and slower infusion time. Pruritic, maculopapular skin rash, usually involving trunk and extremities. Alopecia.

Chair time: 2 hours on day 1 and 1 hour on day 8. Repeat cycle every 21 days.

Gemcitabine + Vinorelbine[1,262]

Prechemo: CBC, Chem, LFTs, and renal function tests. 5-HT$_3$ and dexamethasone 10–20 mg. Mildly to moderately emetogenic.

Gemcitabine 1200 mg/m^2: IV in 250 cc NS over 30 minutes on days 1 and 8.

Vinorelbine 30 mg/m^2: IV on days 1 and 8. Vesicant. Dilute to a final concentration in syringe 1.5–3.0 or IV bag of 0.5–3.0 mg/mL. Infuse diluted drug IV over 6–10 minutes into sidearm port of a free-flowing IV, either peripherally or via central line (preferred). Use port closest to the IV bag, not the patient. Flush vein with at least 75–125 mL of IV solution after infusion.

Side effects: Myelosuppression is dose-limiting. Prolonged infusion time (60 minutes) of gemcitabine is associated with higher toxicities. Nausea and vomiting. Constipation, diarrhea, and mucositis. Flu-like syndrome with fever in absence of infection 6–12 hours after treatment. Neuropathy, incidence increased if patient had prior vinca alkaloids. Constipation. Elevation of serum transaminase and bilirubin levels.

Edema. Pruritic, maculopapular skin rash, usually involving trunk and extremities. Alopecia is rare.

Chair time: 2 hours on days 1 and 8. Repeat cycle every 21 days until progression.

Vinorelbine + Cisplatin[1,263]

Prechemo: CBC, Chem, and Mg^{2+}. 5-HT_3 and dexamethasone 10–20 mg. Moderately to highly emetogenic.

Vinorelbine 25 mg/m²: IV push on days 1, 8, 15 and 22. Vesicant. Dilute in syringe or IV bag to concentration of 1.5–3.0 mg/mL. Infuse diluted drug IV over 6–10 minutes into sidearm port of a free-flowing IV. Flush vein with at least 75–125 mL of IV fluid after drug infusion.

Cisplatin 100 mg/m²: IV in 1000 cc NS on day 1.

Side effects: Myelosuppression, dose-limiting. Nausea and vomiting, acute or delayed. Constipation, diarrhea, stomatitis, and anorexia. Nephrotoxicity dose related. Decreases Mg^{2+}, K^+, Ca^{2+}, Na^+, and P. Jaw pain, myalgias, and arthralgias. Dyspnea. Neuropathy, incidence increased if patient had prior vinca alkaloids. High-frequency hearing loss. Alopecia.

Chair time: 3 hours on day 1 and 1 hour on days 8 and 15. Repeat cycle every 28 days.

Vinorelbine + Carboplatin[1,264]

Prechemo: CBC, Chem, LFTs, and renal function tests. 5-HT_3 and dexamethasone 10–20 mg. Moderately etogenic.

Vinorelbine 25 mg/m²: IV on days 1 and 8. Vesicant. Dilute to a final concentration in syringe 1.5–3.0 or IV bag of 0.5–3.0 mg/mL. Infuse diluted drug IV over 6–10 minutes into sidearm port of a free-flowing IV, either peripherally or via central line (preferred). Use port closest to the IV bag, not the patient. Flush vein with at least 75–125 mL of IV solution after infusion.

Carboplatin AUC 6: IV in 500 cc NS on day 1.

Side effects: Hypersensitivity reaction, risk increases when receiving more than seven courses of carboplatin. Myelosuppression dose related and can be dose-limiting. Nausea and vomiting. Constipation, diarrhea, stomatitis, and anorexia. Nephrotoxicity less common than with cisplatin and rarely symptomatic. Decreases Mg^{2+}, K^+, Ca^{2+}, and Na^+. Neuropathy, incidence increased if patient had prior vinca alkaloids. Alopecia likely.

Chair time: 3 hours on day 1 and 1 hour on day 8. Repeat cycle every 28 days.

Etoposide + Cisplatin (EP)[1,265]

Prechemo: CBC, Chem, LFTs, and renal function tests. 5-HT$_3$ and dexamethasone 10–20 mg. Mildly to moderately emetogenic.

Etoposide 120 mg/m^2: IV in 250 cc NS on days 1–3.

Cisplatin 60 mg/m^2: IV in 500–1000 cc NS on day 1.

Side effects: Hypersensitivity reaction during rapid infusion of etoposide. Myelosuppression, dose-limiting. Nausea and vomiting, acute or delayed. Mucositis and diarrhea are rare. Metallic taste to food. Neuropathy with numbness, tingling, and sensory loss in arms and legs. Proprioception and vibratory sense and loss of motor function. Paresthesias dose related, severe, requiring pain medication or Neurontin. High-frequency hearing loss and tinnitus. Nephrotoxicity, may be cumulative, can result in necrosis of proximal and distal renal tubules. Decreases Mg^{2+}, K^+, Ca^{2+}, and Na^+. May be reduced with adequate hydration, diuresis, and slower infusion time. Alopecia.

Chair time: 4 hours on day 1; 2 hours on days 2–3. Repeat cycle every 21–28 days.

Etoposide + Cisplatin + Docetaxel[1,266]

Prechemo: CBC, Chem, LFTs, and renal function tests. 5-HT$_3$ and dexamethasone 10–20 mg. Moderately to highly emetogenic.

Cisplatin 50 mg/m^2: IV in 500–1000 cc NS on days 1–8, 29, and 36.

Etoposide 50 mg/m^2: IV in 250 cc NS on days 1–5 and 29–33.

Administer concurrent thoracic radiotherapy, 4–6 weeks after the completion of combined modality therapy, followed by:

Prechemo: Dexamethasone 8-mg PO bid for 3 days, starting the day before, day of, and day after treatment. Mildly emetogenic.

Docetaxel 75 mg/m^2: IV in 250 cc NS on day 1. Use non-PVC containers and tubing. Repeat every 21 days for three cycles. Docetaxel dose can be escalated to 100 mg/m^2 IV on subsequent cycles in the absence of toxicity.

Side effects: Hypersensitivity reaction during rapid infusion of etoposide. Myelosuppression, dose-limiting. Nausea and vomiting, acute or delayed. Mucositis and diarrhea are rare. Metallic taste to food. Neuropathy with numbness, tingling, and sensory loss in arms and legs. Proprioception and vibratory sense and loss of motor function. Paresthesias dose related, severe, requiring pain medication or Neurontin. Local tissue irritation progressing to desquamation in radiation field. No oil-based lotions in radiation field. High-frequency hearing loss and tinnitus. Nephrotoxicity and may be cumulative, may result in necrosis of proximal and distal renal tubules. Decreases Mg^{2+}, K^+, Ca^{2+}, and Na^+. Risk may be reduced with adequate hydration, diuresis, and slower infusion time. Fluid retention is a cumulative toxicity with docetaxel, peripheral edema, pleural effusions, dyspnea at rest, cardiac tamponade, or ascites.

Maculopapular, violaceous/erythematous and pruritic rash may occur with docetaxel. Nails changes and may include onycholysis. Alopecia.
Chair time: 1–3 hours days 1–5, 8, 29–33, and 36 during XRT. 2 hours day 1 docetaxel, repeat cycle every 21 days for three cycles.

Bevacizumab (Avastin) + Carboplatin + Paclitaxel[1,267]

Prechemo: CBC, Chem, LFTs, and urine test for protein baseline and throughout treatment. **See carboplatin + Paclitaxel** for non-small cell lung cancer).
Bevacizumab 15 mg/kg: IV every 3 weeks. Initial infusion over 90 minutes; second dose over 60 minutes, subsequent doses over 30 minutes. DO NOT administer perioperatively—may inhibit wound healing.
Side effects: Infusion reaction with bevacizumab, escalate infusion time as above. Myelosuppression mild. Delayed wound healing: hold 28 days perioperatively. Wound dehiscence; gastrointestinal perforation, fistulas and/or intra-abdominal abscess; abdominal pain associated with constipation, vomiting, and fever. Hypertension, congestive heart failure. Arterial thromboembolic. Cerebral infarction, transient ischemic attacks, myocardial infarction, angina, and a variety of other arterial thromboembolic events. GI hemorrhage, subarachnoid hemorrhage, and hemorrhagic stroke, or thrombocytopenia may occur. Tracheoesophageal fistula. Reversible posterior leukoencephalopathy syndrome (RPLS), a rare but serious neurological disorder; headache, seizure, lethargy, confusion, blindness, and other visual and neurologic disturbances. Nephrotic syndrome and proteinuria. Dipstick or urinalysis to detect proteinuria, hold with evidence of moderate to severe proteinuria. Abdominal pain, diarrhea, nausea, vomiting, anorexia, stomatitis, and constipation common. Diarrhea can be severe. Upper respiratory infection, dyspnea. Exfoliative dermatitis.
Chair time: 90 minutes for first dose, 1 hour for second dose, 30 minutes all subsequent doses. Administer with carboplatin and paclitaxel protocol (CP) every 3 weeks for six cycles. Then continue bevacizumab alone every 3 weeks until progression or until unacceptable toxicity.

Single-Agent Regimens

Paclitaxel[1,268,269]

Prechemo: CBC, Chem, 5-HT$_3$, and dexamethasone 10–20 mg . Diphenhydramine 25–50 mg and H$_2$ antagonist. Mildly emetogenic.
Paclitaxel 225 mg/m^2: IV in 500 cc NS over 3 hours day 1. Repeat every 21 days
OR

Paclitaxel 80–100 mg/m²: IV in 250–500 cc NS weekly for 3 weeks. Repeat every 28 days. Use non-PVC containers and tubing with 0.22 micron inline filter.

Side effects: Hypersensitivity reaction. Myelosuppression dose-limiting. G-CSF recommended. Sensory neuropathy with numbness and paresthesias, dose related. Arthralgias and myalgias. Alopecia.

Chair time: 4 hours on day 1. Repeat every 21 days.

OR

2 hours weekly three times a week. Repeat every 28 days.

Docetaxel[1,270,271]

Prechemo: CBC, Chem, LFTs. Dexamethasone 8 mg PO bid day before, day of, and day after treatment. 5-HT₃ in 100 cc NS. Mildly to moderately emetogenic.

Docetaxel 75 mg/m²: IV in 250 cc NS on day 1. Repeat cycle every 21 days.

OR

Docetaxel 36 mg/m²: IV in 250 cc NS weekly for 6 weeks Repeat cycle every 8 weeks. Use non-PVC containers and tubing.

Side effects: Hypersensitivity reactions. Myelosuppression, G-CSF recommended. Nausea and vomiting. Mucositis and diarrhea. Peripheral neuropathy with paresthesias. Fluid retention with weight gain, peripheral and/or generalized edema, pleural effusion, and ascites. Hand-foot syndrome. Nail changes, rash, and dry, pruritic skin. Alopecia.

Chair time: 2 hours on day 1. Repeat every 21 days.

OR

Weekly for 6 weeks repeating every 8 weeks.

Pemetrexed (Alimta)[1,272]

Prechemo: CBC, Chem, LFTs, renal function tests. Oral phenothiazine or 5-HT₃. Mildly to moderately emetogenic.

Dexamethasone 4 mg: PO bid for 3 days, starting the day before - treatment.

Folic acid 1 mg (350–1,000 mg): PO qd, starting 5 days before the first treatment and ending 21 days after the last dose of pemetrexed.

Vitamin B12 1000 mcg: IM during the week preceding the first dose and every three cycles thereafter (may be given the same day as pemetrexed beginning with second dose).

Pemetrexed 500 mg/m²: IV in 100 cc NS over 10 minutes on day 1.

Side effects: Myelosuppression is dose-limiting toxicity. Dose reductions or treatment delay may be necessary for subsequent doses. Nausea, vomiting, and diarrhea, usually mild to moderate. Mild anorexia, stomatitis, and pharyngitis. Patients with renal or hepatic impairment may require dose adjustment. Pruritus and rash.

Chair time: 1 hour on day 1. Repeat cycle every 21 days until progression.

Gemcitabine[1,273]

Prechemo: CBC, Chem, LFTs. 5-HT$_3$ and dexamethasone 10 mg. Mildly emetogenic.

Gemcitabine 1000 mg/m^2: IV in 250 cc NS over 30 minutes on days 1, 8, and 15.

Side effects: Myelosuppression dose-limiting with grades 3 and 4 thrombocytopenia more common in older patients. Nausea and vomiting, diarrhea, mucositis. Flu-like syndrome. Mild dyspnea and drug-induced pneumonitis. Transient elevation of serum transaminases and bilirubin. Pruritic, maculopapular skin rash, usually involving trunk and extremities. Edema. Alopecia is rare.

Chair time: 1 hour days 1, 8, and 15. Repeat every 28 days.

Topotecan[1,274]

Prechemo: CBC, Chem, LFTs. 5-HT$_3$ and dexamethasone 10 mg. Mildly to moderately emetogenic.

Topotecan 1.5 mg/m^2: IV in 100 cc NS on days 1–5.

Side effects: Myelosuppression dose-limiting toxicity. If severe neutropenia occurs, reduce dose by 0.25 mg/m^2 for subsequent doses or may use G-CSF. Nausea and vomiting dose related. Diarrhea, constipation, abdominal pain. Flu-like syndrome, headache, fever malaise, arthralgias, and myalgias. Dose reduce with low protein and hepatic or renal dysfunction. Microscopic hematuria. Alopecia.

Chair time: 1 hour on days 1–5. Repeat cycle every 21 days.

Vinorelbine[1,275]

Prechemo: CBC, Chem. Oral phenothiazine or 5-HT$_3$.

Vinorelbine 25 mg/m^2: IV push on day 1. Vesicant.

Dilute to a final concentration in syringe 1.5–3.0 or IV bag of 0.5–3.0 mg/mL. Infuse diluted drug IV over 6–10 minutes into sidearm port of a free-flowing IV, either peripherally or via central line (preferred). Use port closest to the IV bag, not the patient. Flush vein with at least 75–125 mL of IV solution after infusion.

Side effects: Myelosuppression. Nausea and vomiting are mild. Stomatitis, constipation, diarrhea, and anorexia. Reduce by 50% if total bilirubin 2.1–3 mg/dL. If total bilirubin >3.0 mg/dL, reduce by 75%. Mild to moderate neuropathy with paresthesias, constipation. Alopecia.

Chair time: 1 hour on day 1. Repeat cycle every 7 days until progression.

Gefitinib (Iressa)[1,276]

Prechemo: CBC, Chem. Oral phenothiazine or 5-HT$_3$.
Gefitinib 250 mg/day: PO. (250-mg tablets.) Taken with or without food.
Available to patients:

1. Who are currently or have previously taken the drug and are benefiting.
2. Previously enrolled or new patients in non-investigational (IND) clinical trials.
3. Through the Iressa access program.

Side effects: Interstitial lung disease includes dyspnea, cough, or low-grade fever, rapidly becoming more severe. Mild to moderate diarrhea, may be interrupted for up to 14 days with severe diarrhea. Nausea and vomiting. Rash, acne, dry skin, and pruritus. May interrupt drug for 14 days until rash resolves. Elevations in blood pressure, especially in those with underlying hypertension. Amblyopia, conjunctivitis.
Chair time: No chair time. Continue treatment until disease progression.

Erlotinib (Tarceva)[1,277]

Prechemo: CBC, Chem. Oral phenothiazine or 5-HT$_3$.
Erlotinib (Tarceva) 150-mg/day: PO. (150-, 100-, and 25-mg tablets.)
Take on an empty stomach.
Side effects: Rash, from maculopapular to pustular, on the face, neck, chest, back, and arms. Most rashes are mild to moderate, begin on day 8–10, maximizing in intensity by week 2, and gradually resolving by week 2. Treat with corticosteroids, topical clindamycin, or minocycline. Diarrhea mild to moderate. Conjunctivitis and dry eyes may occur and are mild to moderate. Interstitial lung disease with dyspnea, cough, or low-grade fever, rapidly becoming more severe. Drug and food interactions with CYP3A4 inducers and inhibitors. Patients taking warfarin should have PT/INR monitored closely.
Chair time: No chair time. Continue treatment until disease progression.

LUNG CANCER: SMALL CELL LUNG CANCER

COMBINATION REGIMENS

Etoposide + Cisplatin[1,278]

Prechemo: CBC, Chem, Mg^{2+}, and renal function tests. $5-HT_3$ and dexamethasone 10–20 mg. Moderately to highly emetogenic.

Etoposide 80 mg/m²: IV in 250 cc NS over 1 hour on days 1–3.

Cisplatin 80 mg/m²: IV in 500–1000 cc NS over 1–2 hours on day 1.

Side effects: Hypersensitivity reaction to cisplatin or during rapid infusion of etoposide. Myelosuppression, dose-limiting. Nausea and vomiting, acute or delayed. Mucositis and diarrhea are rare. Metallic taste to food. Neuropathy with numbness, tingling, and sensory loss in arms and legs. Proprioception and vibratory sense and loss of motor function. Paresthesias dose related; can be severe, requiring pain medication or Neurontin. High-frequency hearing loss and tinnitus. Nephrotoxicity and may be cumulative; may result in necrosis of proximal and distal renal tubules. Decreases Mg^{2+}, K^+, Ca^{2+}. Risk may be reduced with adequate hydration, diuresis, and slower infusion time. Alopecia.

Chair time: 4 hours on day 1; 2 hours on days 2–3. Repeat every 21 days.

Etoposide + Carboplatin[1,279]

Prechemo: CBC, Chem, Mg^{2+}, renal function tests. $5-HT_3$ and 10- to 20-mg dexamethasone. Mildly to moderately emetogenic.

Etoposide 100 mg/m²: IV in 250 cc NS on days 1–3.

Carboplatin AUC 6: IV in 500 cc NS on day 1.

Side effects: Hypersensitivity reaction may occur during rapid infusion of etoposide or with more than seven courses of carboplatin therapy. Myelosuppression can be a dose-limiting toxicity. Nausea and vomiting. Mucositis and diarrhea are rare. Nephrotoxicity less common than with cisplatin and rarely symptomatic. Decreases Mg^{2+}, K^+, Ca^{2+}, and Na^+.

Peripheral sensory neuropathy. Paresthesias and numbness dose-limiting toxicity. Alopecia.

Chair time: 3 hours on day 1 and 2 hours on days 2–3. Repeat every 28 days.

Irinotecan + Cisplatin[1,280]

Prechemo: CBC, Chem, Mg^{2+}. Atropine 0.25-1.0mg IV unless contraindicated. 5-HT_3 and dexamethasone 10–20 mg. Moderately to highly emetogenic.

Irinotecan 60 mg/m²: IV in 250–500 cc D5W over 90 minutes on days 1, 8, and 15.

Cisplatin 60 mg/m²: IV in 500–1000 cc NS over 1–3 hours on day 1.

Side effects: Myelosuppression can be severe, dose-limiting toxicity. G-CSF recommended. Nausea and vomiting, acute or delayed. Early diarrhea, managed with atropine before administration of irinotecan. Late diarrhea severe and should be treated aggressively. Consider Lomotil, Imodium, tincture of opium, and hydration. Diarrhea or constipation. Abdominal pain. Dose reduce patients with low protein and hepatic and/or renal dysfunction. Decreases Mg^{2+}, K^+, Ca^{2+}. Peripheral sensory neuropathy dose-limiting. Paresthesias and numbness. High-frequency hearing loss and tinnitus. Alopecia.

Chair time: 4 hours on day 1 and 2 hours on days 2 and 3. Repeat every 28 days.

Carboplatin + Paclitaxel + Etoposide[1,281]

Prechemo: CBC, Chem, Mg^{2+}. 5-HT_3 and dexamethasone 10–20 mg. Diphenhydramine 25–50 mg and H_2 antagonist. Moderately to highly emetogenic.

Carboplatin AUC 6: IV in 500 cc NS on day 1.

Paclitaxel 200 mg/m²: IV in 500 cc NS over 3 hours on day 1. Use non-PVC tubing and containers and a 0.22-micron inline filter. Give carboplatin after paclitaxel to decrease toxicities.

Etoposide 50 mg alternating with 100 mg: PO on days 1–10. (50- and 100-mg capsules.) Store in refrigerator. Monitor patients taking warfarin; it can elevate INR (international normalized ratio).

Side effects: Hypersensitivity reaction with paclitaxel or with more than seven courses of carboplatin therapy. Myelosuppression dose-limiting. G-CSF recommended. Nausea and vomiting, acute or delayed. Mucositis and/or diarrhea. Severe neuropathy with numbness, tingling, and sensory loss in arms and legs. Proprioception and vibratory sense and loss of motor function can occur. Paresthesias are dose related and can be severe, requiring pain medication or Neurontin. High-frequency hearing loss. Nephrotoxicity, dose-limiting toxicity. Decreases Mg^{2+},

Ca^{2+}, and K^+. Risk may be reduced with adequate hydration, diuresis, and slower infusion time. Alopecia.

Chair time: 6 hours on day 1. Repeat cycle every 21 days until disease progression.

Cyclophosphamide + Doxorubicin + Vincristine (CAV)[1,282]

Prechemo: CBC, Chem, and LFTs. MUGA. 5-HT$_3$ and dexamethasone 20 mg. Moderately to highly emetogenic.

Cyclophosphamide 1000 mg/m^2: IV in 500 cc NS on day 1.

Doxorubicin 40 mg/m^2: IV push on day 1. Potent vesicant.

Vincristine 1 mg/m^2: IV push on day 1 (maximum dose 2 mg). Vesicant.

Side effects: Myelosuppression may be severe. Nausea and vomiting, acute or delayed. Stomatitis and diarrhea. Constipation, abdominal pain, or paralytic ileus as a result of nerve toxicity. Acute pericarditis-myocarditis. With high cumulative doses of doxorubicin >550 mg/m^2, cardiomyopathy may occur. Cyclophosphamide may increase the risk of doxorubicin-induced cardiotoxicity. Peripheral neuropathies. Cranial nerve dysfunction may occur (rare), as well as jaw pain, diplopia, vocal cord paresis, mental depression, and metallic taste. Use with caution in patients with abnormal liver function. Hemorrhagic cystitis, dysuria, and urinary frequency. Red-orange discoloration of urine. Provide adequate hydration. Hyperpigmentation, photosensitivity, and radiation recall. Complete alopecia.

Chair time: 2 hours on day 1. Repeat cycle every 21 days.

Cyclophosphamide + Doxorubicin + Etoposide (CAE)[1,283]

Prechemo: CBC, Chem, and LFTs. MUGA. 5-HT$_3$ and dexamethasone 20 mg. Moderately to highly emetogenic.

Cyclophosphamide 1000 mg/m^2: IV in 500 cc NS on day 1.

Doxorubicin 45 mg/m^2: IV push on day 1. Potent vesicant.

Etoposide 50 mg/m^2: IV in 250 cc NS on days 1–5.

Side effects: Allergic reaction: may occur during rapid infusion of etoposide. Myelosuppression can be severe and dose-limiting toxicity. Nausea and vomiting, acute or delayed. Stomatitis and diarrhea, not dose-limiting. Constipation, abdominal pain, or paralytic ileus. Acute pericarditis-myocarditis. With high cumulative doses >550 mg/m^2 of doxorubicin cardiomyopathy may occur. Cyclophosphamide may increase the risk of doxorubicin-induced cardiotoxicity. Use with caution in patients with abnormal liver function. Hemorrhagic cystitis, dysuria, and urinary frequency. Red-orange discoloration of urine. Provide adequate hydration. Hyperpigmentation, photosensitivity, and radiation recall. Complete alopecia.

Chair time: 3 hours on day 1; 2 hours on days 2–5. Repeat cycle every 21 days.

SINGLE-AGENT REGIMENS

Etoposide[1,284,285]

Prechemo: CBC, Chem, LFTs. Oral phenothiazine or 5-HT$_3$. Mildly to moderately emetogenic.
Etoposide 160 mg/m^2/day: PO on days 1–5
OR
Etoposide 50 mg/m^2: PO bid on days 1–21. (50- or 100-mg capsules.)
May give as a single dose up to 400 mg. With 400 mg, divide dose into two to four doses. Store in refrigerator.
Side effects: Myelosuppression may be severe. Neurotoxicities: Peripheral neuropathies may occur but are uncommon and mild. Nausea and vomiting, mild to moderate. More commonly observed with oral administration. Metallic taste to food. Alopecia.
Chair time: Repeat cycle every 28 days as tolerated or until progression.

Paclitaxel[1,286]

Prechemo: CBC, Chem, Mg^{2+}. 5-HT$_3$ and dexamethasone 10–20 mg. Diphenhydramine 25–50 mg and H$_2$ antagonist. Mildly emetogenic.
Paclitaxel 80–100 mg/m^2: IV in 250 cc NS weekly for 3 weeks.
Use non-PVC containers and tubing with 0.22-micron inline filter.
Side effects: Hypersensitivity reaction. Myelosuppression, dose-limiting G-CSF recommended. Nausea and vomiting. Stomatitis. Sensory neuropathy with numbness and paresthesias, dose related. Arthralgias and myalgias. Transient elevations in serum transaminases, bilirubin, and alkaline phosphatase. Alopecia.
Chair time: 2 hours on day 1. Repeat every 28 days until progression.

Topotecan[1,287]

Prechemo: CBC, Chem, LFTs. 5-HT$_3$ and dexamethasone 10–20 mg. Mildly to moderately emetogenic.
Topotecan 1.5 mg/m^2: IV in 100 cc NS on days 1–5.
Side effects: Myelosuppression dose-limiting toxicity. If severe neutropenia occurs, reduce dose by 0.25 mg/m^2 for subsequent doses or may use G-CSF. Nausea and vomiting dose related. Diarrhea, constipation, abdominal pain. Dose reduce with low protein and hepatic or renal dysfunction. Microscopic hematuria. Alopecia.
Chair time: 1 hour on days 1–5. Repeat every 21 days until progression.

LYMPHOMA: HODGKIN'S DISEASE

COMBINATION REGIMENS

Doxorubicin + Bleomycin + Vinblastine + Dacarbazine (ABVD)[1,288]

Prechemo: CBC, Chem, renal function tests, sedimentation rate, PFTs, and MUGA. Central line placement recommended. 5-HT$_3$, dexamethasone, and acetaminophen. Moderately to highly emetogenic.

Doxorubicin 25 mg/m^2: IV push on days 1 and 15.

Bleomycin 10 units/m^2: IV push on days 1 and 15. Test dose of 2 units before first dose to detect hypersensitivity.

Vinblastine 6 mg/m^2: IV push days 1 and 15. Vesicant.

Dacarbazine 375 mg/m^2: IV in 500–1000 cc NS over at least 1 hour on days 1 and 15. Vesicant.

Side effects: Myelosuppression may be severe. GCSF support. Nausea, vomiting, and anorexia. Mucositis and stomatitis. Constipation and paralytic ileus. Flu-like syndrome: fever, chills, malaise, myalgias, and arthralgias. Doxorubicin dose limit, >550 mg/m^2 can cause cardiomyopathies. Arrhythmias and/or EKG changes, pericarditis, or myocarditis. Discoloration of urine from pink to red. Reduce dose for increased bilirubin level or creatinine clearance. Peripheral neuropathy, including numbness, weakness, myalgias, and later, severe motor difficulties. Jaw pain. Pneumonitis with bleomycin. Radiation recall, hyperpigmentation of nail beds, and dermal crease of hands. Alopecia total.

Chair time: 2–3 hours on days 1 and 15. Repeat cycle every 28 days for 4–6 cycles.

Nitrogen Mustard + Vincristine + Procarbazine + Prednisone (MOPP)[1,289]

Prechemo: CBC, Chem, renal function tests, sedimentation rate, and MUGA. Central line placement recomended. 5-HT$_3$, dexamethasone, and acetaminophen. Moderately to highly emetogenic.

Nitrogen mustard 6 mg/m^2: IV push on day 1. Prepare immediately before administrations (within 15 minutes). Powerful vesicant. Avoid contact with skin or eyes or inhaling powder.

Vincristine 1.4 mg/m^2: IV push on days 1 and 8. Maximum dose 2 mg. Vesicant.

Procarbazine 100 mg/m^2: PO on days 1–14. (50-mg tablets.)

Prednisone 40-mg/m^2: PO on days 1–14.

Side effects: Myelosuppression, dose-limiting toxicity. Nausea, vomiting, anorexia, and taste alterations. Mucositis and stomatitis. Constipation and paralytic ileus. Procarbazine drug and food interaction: avoid tricyclic antidepressants; decreased bioavailability of digoxin; antabase-like reaction with alcohol; avoid tyramines (beer, wine, cheese, brewer's yeast, chicken liver, and bananas). Fever, chills, sweating, lethargy, myalgias, and arthralgias. Reduce dose for increased bilirubin level or creatinine clearance. Peripheral neuropathy, numbness, weakness, myalgias, and later, severe motor difficulties. Jaw pain. Tinnitus, deafness, and other signs of eighth cranial nerve damage. Paresthesias, ataxia, lethargy, headache, confusion, and/or seizures. Steroid toxicities: sodium and water retention, cushingoid changes, hyperglycemia, hypokalemia, increased sodium level, mood changes, euphoria, headache, insomnia, depression, and psychosis. Warfarin and insulin doses may need to be increased. Pneumonitis. Radiation recall, hyperpigmentation, sun sensitivity. Alopecia is total.

Chair time: 1 hour on days 1 and 15. Repeat every 28 days.

MOPP/ABVD Hybrid[1,290]

Prechemo: CBC, Chem, renal function tests, sedimentation rate, PFTs, and MUGA. Central line placement recommended. 5-HT$_3$ and dexamethasone 10–20 mg IV (hold dexamethasone day 8). Acetaminophen PO. Moderately to highly emetogenic.

Nitrogen mustard 6 mg/m^2: IV push on day 1. Powerful vesicant. Avoid contact with skin and eyes or inhaling powder. Administer within 15 minutes of reconstitution.

Vincristine 1.4 mg/m^2: IV push on day 1. Maximum dose 2 mg. Vesicant.

Procarbazine 100 mg/m^2: PO on days 1–14. (50-mg capsules.)

Prednisone 40 mg/m^2: PO on days 1–14, take with breakfast.

Doxorubicin 35 mg/m^2: IV push on day 8. Potent vesicant.

Bleomycin 10-units/m²: IV push on day 8. Test dose of 2 units before the first dose.

Hydrocortisone 100 mg: IV given before bleomycin on day 8.

Vinblastine 6 mg/m²: IV on day 8. Vesicant.

Side effects: Myelosuppression dose-limiting. Nausea, vomiting, and anorexia. Mucositis and stomatitis. Constipation and paralytic ileus. Procarbazine drug and food interaction: avoid tricyclic antidepressants; decreased bioavailability of digoxin; antabuse-like reaction with alcohol; avoid tyramines (beer, wine, cheese, brewer's yeast, chicken liver, and bananas). Acute pericarditis-myocarditis. With high cumulative doses >550 mg/m²of doxorubicin, cardiomyopathy may occur. Fever, chills, sweating, lethargy, myalgias, and arthralgias. Discoloration of urine from pink to red. Increased bilirubin level or creatinine clearance. Peripheral neuropathy, including numbness, weakness, myalgias, and late severe motor difficulties. Jaw pain. CNS toxicity with paresthesias, ataxia, lethargy, headache, confusion, and/or seizures. Steroid toxicities: sodium, water retention, cushingoid changes, hyperglycemia, hypokalemia, increased sodium levels, mood changes, euphoria, headache, insomnia, depression, and psychosis. Warfarin and insulin doses may need to be increased. Pneumonitis. Radiation recall, sun sensitivity, hyperpigmentation. Alopecia is total.

Chair time: 2 hours on days 1 and 8. Repeat cycle every 28 days.

MOPP Alternating with ABVD[1,291]

See MOPP and ABVD regimens previously outlined.
Alternate MOPP with ABVD for 12 cycles.

Stanford V[1,292]

Prechemo: CBC, Chem, renal function tests, sedimentation rate, PFTs, and MUGA. Central line placement recommended. 5-HT₃ and dexamethasone 10–20 mg IV. Acetaminophen PO. Moderately to highly emetogenic.

Nitrogen mustard 6 mg/m²: IV push on day 1. Prepare and use within 15 minutes of preparation. Powerful vesicant; avoid contact with skin and eyes or inhaling powder.

Doxorubicin 25 mg/m²: IV push on days 1 and 15. Potent vesicant.

Vinblastine 6 mg/m²: IV push on days 1 and 15. Reduce to 4 mg/m² on weeks 9 and 12 in patients >50 years of age. Vesicant.

Vincristine 1.4 mg/m²: IV push on days 8 and 22 (maximum dose 2 mg). Reduce to 1 mg/m² on weeks 9 and 12 in patients >50 years of age. Vesicant.

Bleomycin 5 units/m²: IV push on days 8 and 22. Test dose of 2 units before first dose to detect hypersensitivity.

Etoposide 60 mg/m²: IV in 250 cc NS on days 15 and 16. Enhances warfarin action by increasing INR.

Prednisone 40-mg/m²: PO every other day. Taper starting week 10. Take with breakfast.

Prophylactic: Bactrim DS PO bid, acyclovir 200-mg PO tid.

Side effects: Myelosuppression dose-limiting. Hypersensitivity reactions with bleomycin and etoposide. Nausea, vomiting, and anorexia. Mucositis and stomatitis. Constipation and paralytic ileus secondary to autonomic neuropathy. Acute pericarditis-myocarditis. With high cumulative doses >550 mg/m², doxorubicin, cardiomyopathy may occur. Fever, chills, sweating, lethargy, myalgias, and arthralgias. Discoloration of urine from pink to red. Dose reduce for increased bilirubin level or creatinine clearance. Peripheral neuropathy: numbness, weakness, myalgias, and later, severe motor difficulties. Jaw pain. Pneumonitis. Radiation recall, sun sensitivity, hyperpigmentation. Alopecia is total.

Chair time: 2 hours days 1, 8, 15, 16, and 22. Repeat every 28 days for three cycles.

Bleomycin + Etoposide + Doxorubicin + Cyclophosphamide + Vincristine + Procarbazine + Prednisone (BEACOPP)[1,293]

Prechemo: CBC, Chem, renal function tests, sed rate, PFTs, and MUGA. Central line placement recommended. 5-HT$_3$ and IV. Acetaminophen PO. Moderately to highly emetogenic.

Bleomycin 10 units/m²: IV push on day 8. Test dose of 2 units before first dose.

Etoposide 100 mg/m²: IV in 250 cc NS on days 1–3.

Doxorubicin 25 mg/m²: IV push on day 1. Vesicant.

Cyclophosphamide 650 mg/m²: IV in 500 cc NS on day 1.

Vincristine 1.4 mg/m²: IV push on day 8 (maximum dose 2 mg). Vesicant.

Procarbazine 100 mg/m²: PO on days 1–7. (50-mg tablets.)

Prednisone 40-mg/m²: PO on days 1–14. Take with breakfast.

Side effects: Myelosuppression dose-limiting toxicity. Hypersensitivity reactions with bleomycin and etoposide. Nausea, vomiting, and anorexia. Mucositis and stomatitis. Constipation and paralytic ileus secondary to autonomic neuropathy. Procarbazine drug and food interactions: avoid tricyclic antidepressants; decreased bioavailability of digoxin; antabuse-like reaction with alcohol; avoid tyramines (beer, wine, cheese, brewer's yeast, chicken liver, and bananas). Acute pericarditis-myocarditis. With high cumulative doses >550 mg/m² doxorubicin, cardiomyopathy may occur. Fever, chills, sweating, lethargy, myalgias, and arthralgias. Discoloration of urine from pink to red. Hemorrhagic cystitis, preventable with appropriate hydration. Reduce dose for increased bilirubin level or creatinine clearance. Peripheral neuropathy, including numbness, weakness, and later, severe motor difficulties. Jaw pain. Paresthesias, ataxia, lethargy, headache, confusion, and/or seizures. Steroid toxicities: sodium, water retention, cushingoid changes, hyperglycemia, hypokalemia, increased sodium levels, mood changes, euphoria, headache, insomnia, depression, and psychosis. Warfarin and insulin doses may need to be increased. Pneumonitis. Radiation recall, sun sensitivity, hyperpigmentation. Alopecia is total.

Chair time: 3 hours on day 1; 2 hours on days 2 and 3; 1 hour on day 8. Repeat every 21 days.

Bleomycin + Etoposide + Doxorubicin + Cyclophosphamide + Vincristine + Procarbazine + Prednisone (BEACOPP Escalated)[1,294]

Prechemo: CBC, Chem, renal function tests, sed rate, PFTs, and MUGA. Central line placement recommended. 5-HT$_3$ and IV. Acetaminophen PO. Moderately to highly emetogenic.

Bleomycin 10 units/m^2: IV push on day 8. Test dose of 2 units before first dose.

Etoposide 200-mg/m^2: IV in 250 cc NS infusion on days 1–3.

Doxorubicin 35 mg/m^2: IV push on day 1. Vesicant.

Cyclophosphamide 1200 mg/m^2: IV in 50–1000 cc NS on day 1.

Vincristine 1.4 mg/m^2: IV push on day 8 (maximum dose 2 mg). Vesicant.

Procarbazine 100 mg/m^2: PO on days 1–7. (50-mg tablets.)

Prednisone 40-mg/m^2: PO on days 1–14. Take with breakfast.

Side effects: Hypersensitivity reactions with bleomycin and etoposide. Myelosuppression dose-limiting toxicity. G-CSF, at 5-g/kg/day SQ, starting at day 8 and continuing until neutrophil recovery. Nausea, vomiting, and anorexia. Mucositis and stomatitis. Constipation and paralytic ileus. Procarbazine drug and food interactions: avoid tricyclic antidepressants; decreased bioavailability of digoxin; antabuse-like reaction with alcohol; avoid tyramines (beer, wine, cheese, brewer's yeast, chicken liver, and bananas). Acute pericarditis-myocarditis. With high cumulative doses >550 mg/m^2 doxorubicin, cardiomyopathy may occur. Fever, chills, sweating, lethargy, myalgias, and arthralgias. Discoloration of urine from pink to red. Hemorrhagic cystitis, preventable with appropriate hydration. Reduce dose for increased bilirubin level or creatinine clearance. Peripheral neuropathy, jaw pain. Paresthesias, ataxia, lethargy, headache, confusion, and/or seizures. Steroid toxicities: sodium, water retention, cushingoid changes, hyperglycemia, hypokalemia, increased sodium levels, mood changes, euphoria, headache, insomnia, depression, and psychosis. Warfarin and insulin doses may need to be increased. Pneumonitis. Radiation recall, sun sensitivity, hyperpigmentation. Alopecia is total.

Chair time: 3 hours on day 1; 2 hours on days 2 and 3; 1 hour on day 8. Repeat every 21 days.

Etoposide + Vincristine + Doxorubicin (EVA)[1,295]

Prechemo: CBC, Chem, renal function tests, sed rate, and MUGA. 5-HT$_3$ and dexamethasone 10–20-mg IV. Moderately to highly emetogenic.

Etoposide 200 mg/m^2: IV in 250 cc NS on days 1–5.

Vincristine 2 mg: IV push on day 1 (maximum dose, 2 mg). Vesicant.

Doxorubicin 50 mg/m^2: IV push on day 2. Vesicant.

Side effects: Hypersensitivity reactions with etoposide. Myelosuppression, may be severe. Nausea, vomiting, and anorexia. Mucositis and stomatitis. Constipation and paralytic ileus. Acute pericarditis-myocarditis. With high cumulative doses >550 mg/m^2 doxorubicin, cardiomyopathy may occur. Discoloration of urine from pink to red. Peripheral neuropathy, including numbness, weakness, myalgias, jaw pain, and later, severe motor difficulties. Radiation recall, sun sensitivity, hyperpigmentation. Alopecia is total.

Chair time: 2 hours on days 1–5. Repeat cycle every 28 days.

Etoposide + Vinblastine + Cytarabine + Cisplatin (EVAP)[1,296]

Prechemo: CBC, Chem, Mg^{2+}, renal function tests, sed rate, and MUGA. 5-HT$_3$ and dexamethasone 10–20 mg IV. Moderately to highly emetogenic.

Etoposide 120 mg/m^2: IV in 250 cc NS over 1 hour on days 1, 8, and 15.

Vinblastine 4 mg^2: IV push on day 1, 8, and 15. Vesicant.

Cytarabine 30 mg/m^2: IV in 100 cc NS over 1 hour on days 1, 8, and 15. Irritant.

Cisplatin 40 mg/m^2: IV in 500 cc NS over 1–2 hours on days 1, 8, and 15.

Side effects: Hypersensitivity reactions with etoposide and cisplatin. Myelosuppression may be severe. Nausea, vomiting, and anorexia. Mucositis and stomatitis. Metallic taste to food. Constipation and paralytic ileus secondary to autonomic neuropathy. Peripheral neuropathy, including numbness, weakness, myalgias, jaw pain, and later, severe motor difficulties. High-frequency hearing loss and tinnitus. Nephrotoxicity, dose-limiting toxicity with cisplatin. Can be prevented by adequate hydration and diuresis. Decreases in Mg^{2+}, Ca^{2+}, and K$^+$. Enhanced warfarin action by increasing PT. Dose modification for increased bilirubin level or creatinine clearance. Total alopecia.

Chair time: 4–5 hours on days 1, 8, and 15. Repeat cycle every 28 days.

Carmustine + Etoposide + Cytarabine + Melphalan (Mini-BEAM)[1,297]

Prechemo: CBC, Chem, renal function tests, sed rate, PFTs, and MUGA. Central line placement recommended. 5-HT$_3$ and dexamethasone 10–20 mg IV. Moderately to highly emetogenic.

Carmustine (BCNU) 60 mg/m^2: IV in 500 cc D5W over 1–2 hours on day 1.

Etoposide 75 mg/m^2: IV in 250 cc NS over 1 hour on days 2–5.

Cytarabine 100 mg/m^2: IV in 250 cc NS over 1 hour every 12 hours on days 2–5. Irritant.

Melphalan 30 mg/m^2: IV in 100 cc NS over 30–45 minutes on day 6. Use 0.45-filter and administer within 1 hour of reconstituting.

Side effects: Hypersensitivity reactions with etoposide and melphalan. Myelosuppression may be severe. Nausea, vomiting, and anorexia. Mucositis and stomatitis. Metallic taste to food. Constipation and paralytic ileus. Peripheral neuropathy, jaw pain. At high doses of cytarabine cerebellar toxicity, including nystagmus, dysarthria, ataxia, slurred speech, difficulty with fine motor coordination, lethargy, or somnolence. Decreases in Mg^{2+}, Ca^{2+}, and K$^+$. When on warfarin increasing INR. Reduce dose for increased bilirubin level or creatinine clearance. Pulmonary toxicity with cough and dyspnea, pulmonary infiltrates. High-frequency hearing loss and tinnitus. Intense pain and/or burning at site of injection with BCNU. Infuse over 1–2 hours and ice above IV site. Radiation recall, sun sensitivity, hyperpigmentation. Alopecia is total.

Chair time: 5 hours on day 1, 3 hours on days 2–5; 1 hour on day 6. Repeat cycle every 28 days. May require hospitalization.

SINGLE-AGENT REGIMENS

Gemcitabine (Gemzar)[1,298]

Prechemo: CBC, Chem, and LFTs. Oral phenothiazine.
OR
5-HT$_3$ and dexamethasone 10-mg IV. Mildly to moderately emetogenic.

Gemcitabine 1250 mg/m^2: IV in 250 cc NS over 30 minutes on days 1, 8, and 15.

Side effects: Myelosuppression dose-limiting, with grades 3 and 4 thrombocytopenia more common in older patients. Nausea and vomiting, diarrhea, mucositis. Flu-like syndrome. Mild dyspnea and drug-induced pneumonitis. Transient elevation of serum transaminases and bilirubin. Pruritic, maculopapular skin rash, usually involving trunk and extremities. Edema. Alopecia is rare.

Chair time: 1 hour on days 1, 8, and 15. Repeat cycle every 28 days.

LYMPHOMA: NON-HODGKIN'S LYMPHOMA

LOW-GRADE

COMBINATION REGIMENS

Cyclophosphamide + Vincristine + Prednisone (CVP)[1,299]

Prechemo: CBC, Chem, sedimentation rate. 5-HT$_3$ and dexamethasone 10–20-mg IV. Moderately emetogenic.

Cyclophosphamide 400 mg/m²: PO on days 1–5.

OR

800 mg/m²: IV in 500 cc NS on day 1. Take pills with breakfast. 25- and 50-mg tablets.

Vincristine 1.4 mg/m²: IV push on day 1 (maximum dose 2 mg). Vesicant.

Prednisone 100 mg/m²: PO on days 1–5. Take with breakfast.

Side effects: Myelosuppression dose-limiting toxicity. Cyclophosphamide cardiotoxicity with cumulative dose 140 mg/m² with no prior anthracycline exposure; 120 mg/m² with prior exposure, at greater risk. Nausea, vomiting, anorexia; mucositis, diarrhea, paralytic ileus. Hemorrhagic cystitis preventable with appropriate hydration. Peripheral neuropathy, jaw pain. Steroid toxicities: sodium, water retention, cushingoid changes, hyperglycemia, hypokalemia, increased sodium levels, mood changes, euphoria, headache, insomnia, depression, and psychosis. Warfarin and insulin doses may need to be increased. Alopecia, hyperpigmentation of nails and skin, and transverse ridging of nails may occur.

Chair time: 2 hours on day 1. Repeat cycle every 21 days for four cycles.

Cyclophosphamide + Vincristine + Prednisone (CVP) + Rituxan[1,300]

Prechemo: Use above CVP protocol and single-agent rituxan protocol.
Rituxan 375 mg/m²: On day 1 prior to **CVP**. Repeat every 21 days for 8 cycles.

Cyclophosphamide + Vincristine + Prednisone (CVP) followed by Rituxan[1,301]

Prechemo: Use above CVP protocol and single-agent rituxan protocol.
CVP: Given first every 21 days for 6-8 cycles, followed by:
Rituxan 375 mg/m²: IV weekly for 4 doses every 6 months for up to 16 doses.

Cyclophosphamide + Mitoxantrone (Novantrone) + Vincristine (Oncovin) + Prednisone (CNOP)[1,301]

Prechemo: CBC, Chem, sedimentation rate. 5-HT₃ and dexamethasone 10–20 mg IV. Moderately to highly emetogenic protocol.
Cyclophosphamide 750 mg/m²: IV in 500 cc NS on day 1.
Mitoxantrone 10 mg/m²: IV push or infusion over 5–30 minutes on day 1.
Vincristine 1.4 mg/m²: IV push on day 1 (maximum dose 2 mg). Vesicant.
Prednisone 50-mg/m²: PO on days 1–5. Take with breakfast.
Side effects: Myelosuppression dose-limiting toxicity. Patients with cumulative mitoxantrone dose 140 mg/m² with no prior anthracycline exposure; 120 mg/m² with prior exposure, at greater risk for congestive cardiomyopathy. Nausea, vomiting, anorexia; mucositis, diarrhea, paralytic ileus. Hemorrhagic cystitis preventable with appropriate hydration. Urine will be green-blue for 24 hours. Peripheral neuropathy, jaw pain. Steroid toxicities: sodium, water retention, cushingoid changes, hyperglycemia, hypokalemia, increased sodium levels, mood changes, euphoria, headache, insomnia, depression, and psychosis. Warfarin and insulin doses may need to be increased. Hyperpigmentation of nails and skin, and transverse ridging of nails may occur. Sclera may become discolored blue. Alopecia.
Chair time: 2 hours. Repeat cycle every 21 days.

Fludarabine + Mitoxantrone (Novantrone) + Dexamethasone (FND)[1,302]

Prechemo: CBC, Chem, sedimentation rate. 5-HT₃ and dexamethasone 10–20 mg IV. Moderately emetogenic.
Fludarabine 25 mg/m²: IV in 100 cc NS over 30 minutes on days 1–3.

Mitoxantrone 10 mg/m²: IV push or IV infusion over 5–30 minutes on day 1.

Dexamethasone 20 mg: PO on days 1–5. Take with breakfast.

Bactrim DS: One tablet PO bid, 3 times per week.

Side effects: Myelosuppression dose-limiting toxicity. Nausea, vomiting, anorexia; mucositis, diarrhea, paralytic ileus. Hemorrhagic cystitis, preventable with appropriate hydration. Urine will be green-blue for 24 hours. Peripheral neuropathy, jaw pain. Patients with cumulative mitoxantrone dose 140 mg/m² with no prior anthracycline exposure; 120 mg/m² with prior exposure, at greater risk for congestive cardiomyopathy. Steroid toxicities: sodium, water retention, cushingoid changes, hyperglycemia, hypokalemia, increased sodium levels, mood changes, euphoria, headache, insomnia, depression, and psychosis. Warfarin and insulin doses may need to be increased. Tumor lysis syndrome, treat with hydration and allopurinol. Metallic taste, pneumonia and pulmonary hypersensitivity reactions characterized by cough, dyspnea, and interstitial infiltrate with fludarabine. Hyperpigmentation of nails and skin, and transverse ridging of nails may occur. Sclera may become discolored blue. Alopecia.

Chair time: 1 hour days 1–3. Repeat cycle every 21 days.

Fludarabine + Cyclophosphamide (FC)[1,303]

Prechemo: CBC, Chem, sedimentation rate. 5-HT_3 and dexamethasone 10–20 mg IV. Moderately emetogenic.

Fludarabine 20 mg/m²: IV in 100 cc NS over 30 minutes on days 1–5.

Cyclophosphamide 1000 mg/m²: IV in 500 cc NS on day 1.

Bactrim DS: 1 tablet PO bid.

Side effects: Myelosuppression dose-limiting toxicity. Severe and cumulative. Fatigue: secondary to anemia. Nausea, vomiting, anorexia; mucositis, and diarrhea. Tumor lysis syndrome, treat with hydration and allopurinol. Hemorrhagic cystitis, preventable with appropriate hydration. Weakness and paresthesias as well as agitation, confusion, and visual disturbances. Pneumonia and pulmonary hypersensitivity reactions with cough, dyspnea, and interstitial infiltrate. Hyperpigmentation of nails and skin, and transverse ridging of nails may occur. Alopecia.

Chair time: 2 hours day 1 and 1 hour days 2–5. Repeat cycle every 21–28 days.

Cyclophosphamide + Doxorubicin + Vincristine + Prednisone (CHOP)[1,304]

Prechemo: CBC, Chem, sedimentation rate. MUGA. 5-HT_3 and dexamethasone 10–20 mg IV. Moderately to highly emetogenic.

Cyclophosphamide 750 mg/m²: IV in 500 cc NS on day 1.

Doxorubicin 50 mg/m²: IV push on day 1. Vesicant.

Vincristine 1.4 mg/m²: IV push on day 1 (maximum dose 2 mg). Vesicant.

Prednisone 100 mg/m²: PO on days 1 through 5. Take with breakfast.

Side effects: Myelosuppression, moderate to severe. GCSF recommended. Nausea, vomiting, anorexia; mucositis, diarrhea, and paralytic ileus. Discoloration of urine from pink to red. Hemorrhagic, cystitis preventable with appropriate hydration. Cardiotoxicity, increased risk when doxorubicin dose > 450 mg/m². Peripheral neuropathy, jaw pain. Steroid toxicities: sodium, water retention, cushingoid changes, hyperglycemia, hypokalemia, increased sodium levels, mood changes, headache, insomnia, depression, and psychosis. Hyperpigmentation of nails, radiation recall, sun sensitivity. Alopecia.

Chair time: 2 hours on day 1. Repeat cycle every 21 days for six cycles.

INTERMEDIATE-GRADE

Cyclophosphamide + Doxorubicin + Vincristine + Prednisone (CHOP)[1,304]

Prechemo: CBC, Chem, sedimentation rate. MUGA. 5-HT₃ and dexamethasone 10–20 mg IV. Moderately to highly emetogenic.

Cyclophosphamide 750 mg/m²: IV in 500 cc NS on day 1.

Doxorubicin 50 mg/m²: IV push on day 1. Vesicant.

Vincristine 1.4 mg/m²: IV push on day 1 (maximum dose 2 mg). Vesicant.

Prednisone 100 mg/m²: PO on days 1 through 5. Take with breakfast.

Side effects: Myelosuppression, moderate to severe. GCSF recommended. Nausea, vomiting, anorexia; mucositis, diarrhea, and paralytic ileus. Discoloration of urine from pink to red. Hemorrhagic cystitis, preventable with appropriate hydration. Cardiotoxicity, increased risk when doxorubicin dose > 450 mg/m². Peripheral neuropathy, jaw pain. Steroid toxicities: sodium, water retention, cushingoid changes, hyperglycemia, hypokalemia, increased sodium levels, mood changes, headache, insomnia, depression, and psychosis. Hyperpigmentation of nails, radiation recall, sun sensitivity. Alopecia.

Chair time: 2 hours on day 1. Repeat cycle every 21 days for six cycles.

Cyclophosphamide + Mitoxantrone + Oncovin + Prednisone (CNOP)[1,305]

Prechemo: CBC, Chem, sedimentation rate. 5-HT₃ and dexamethasone 10–20 mg IV. Moderately to highly emetogenic protocol.

Cyclophosphamide 750 mg/m²: IV in 500 cc NS on day 1.

Mitoxantrone 10 mg/m²: IV push or infusion over 5–30 minutes on day 1.

Vincristine 1.4 mg/m²: IV push on day 1 (maximum dose 2 mg). Vesicant.

Prednisone 100 mg/m²: PO on days 1–5. Take with breakfast.

Side effects: Myelosuppression dose-limiting toxicity. Cardiotoxicity, less than that of doxorubicin or daunorubicin. Patients with cumulative dose mitoxantrone 140 mg/m² with no prior anthracycline exposure; 120 mg/m² with prior exposure, at greater risk.

Nausea, vomiting, anorexia; mucositis, diarrhea, paralytic ileus. Hemorrhagic cystitis preventable with appropriate hydration. Urine will be green-blue for 24 hours. Sclera may become discolored blue. Peripheral neuropathy, jaw pain. Steroid toxicities: sodium, water retention, cushingoid changes, hyperglycemia, hypokalemia, increased sodium levels, mood changes, headache, insomnia, depression, and psychosis. Warfarin and insulin doses may need to be increased. Hyperpigmentation of nails and skin, and transverse ridging of nails may occur. Alopecia.

Chair time: 2 hours on day 1. Repeat cycle every 21 days.

Etoposide + Prednisone + Vincristine + Cyclophosphamide + Doxorubicin (EPOCH)[1,306]

Prechemo: CBC, Chem, LFTs, renal function tests, and MUGA. Central line placement. 5-HT₃ and dexamethasone 10–20 mg IV. Moderately to highly emetogenic.

Etoposide 50 mg/m²/day: IV continuous infusion on days 1–4.

Prednisone 60 mg/m²/day: PO on days 1–5. Take with breakfast.

Vincristine 0.4 mg/m²/day: IV continuous infusion on days 1–4. Vesicant.

Cyclophosphamide 750 mg/m²: IV in 500 cc NS on day 5. Begin after infusion.

Doxorubicin 10 mg/m²/day: Continuous infusion on days 1–4. Vesicant.

Etoposide, Viscristine, and Doxorubicin: Compatible in same solution for continuous infusion.

Bactrim DS: 1 tablet PO bid, three times per week.

Side effects: Myelosuppression dose-limiting toxicity. Nausea, vomiting, and anorexia. Mucositis, stomatitis, and diarrhea. Constipation and paralytic ileus. Cardiotoxicity with doxorubicin, increased risk with cumulative doses >450 mg/m². Arrhythmias and/or EKG changes, pericarditis, or myocarditis. Steroid toxicities: sodium, water retention, cushingoid changes, hyperglycemia, hypokalemia, increased sodium levels, mood changes, headache, insomnia, depression, and psychosis. Warfarin and insulin doses may need to be increased. Discoloration of urine from pink to red. Hemorrhagic cystitis, give appropriate hydration. Peripheral neuropathy, jaw pain. Hyperpigmentation of nails, radiation recall. Alopecia.

Chair time: 1 hour on days 1–4; 2 hours on day 5. Repeat cycle every 21 days.

Etoposide + Prednisone + Oncovin + Cyclophosphamide + Doxorubicin + Rituximab (EPOCH + Rituximab) [1,307]

Prechemo: CBC, Chem, LFTs, renal function tests, and MUGA. Central line placement. 5-HT$_3$ and dexamethasone 10–20 mg IV. Diphenhydramine and H$_2$ antagonist prior to Rituximab. Moderately to highly emetogenic.

Rituximab 375 mg/m^2: IV on day 1. Administered day 1 before continuous infusion (see Rituximab protocol for administration).

Etoposide 50 mg/m^2/day: IV continuous infusion on days 1–4.

Prednisone 60 mg/m^2/day: PO on days 1–5. Take with breakfast.

Vincristine 0.4 mg/m^2/day: IV continuous infusion on days 1–4. Vesicant.

Cyclophosphamide 750 mg/m^2: IV in 500 cc NS on day 5.

Doxorubicin 10 mg/m^2/day: Continuous infusion on days 1–4.

Etoposide, Viscristine, and Doxorubicin: Compatible in same solution for continuous infusion.

Bactrim DS: 1 tablet PO bid, three times per week.

Side effects: Myelosuppression dose-limiting toxicity. Nausea, vomiting, and anorexia; moderately to highly emetogenic. Mucositis, stomatitis, and diarrhea. Cardiotoxicity with doxorubicin, increased risk with cumulative doses >450 mg/m^2. Arrhythmias and/or EKG changes, pericarditis, or myocarditis. Steroid toxicities: sodium, water retention, cushingoid changes, hyperglycemia, hypokalemia, increased sodium levels, mood changes, headache, insomnia, depression, and psychosis. Warfarin and insulin doses may need to be increased. Discoloration of urine from pink to red. Hemorrhagic cystitis preventable with appropriate hydration. Peripheral neuropathy jaw pain. Hyperpigmentation of nails, radiation recall, sun sensitivity. Alopecia.

Chair time: 4–6 hours on day 1; 1–2 hours on days 2–5. Repeat cycle every 21 days.

Methotrexate + Doxorubicin + Cyclophosphamide + Oncovin + Prednisone + Bleomycin (MACOP-B) [1,308]

Prechemo: CBC, Chem, LFTs, renal function tests, and MUGA. 5-HT$_3$ and dexamethasone, acetaminophen. Moderately to highly emetogenic.

Methotrexate 400 mg/m^2: IV in 500–1000 cc NS on day 1 weeks 2, 6, and 10. Drug interactions include aspirin, penicillins, nonsteroidal anti-inflammatory drugs (NSAIDs), cephalosporins, phenytoin, warfarin, 5-fluorouracil, thymidine, folic acid, and omeprazole. Vigorously hydrate; moderate dose of MTX.

Leucovorin 15 mg/m²: PO every 6 hours for six doses; begin 24 hours after methotrexate.

Doxorubicin 50 mg/m²: IV push on day 1 weeks 1, 3, 5, 7, 9, and 11. Vesicant.

Cyclophosphamide 350 mg/m²: IV in 500 cc NS on day 1 weeks 1, 3, 5, 7, 9, and 11.

Vincristine 1.4 mg/m²: IV push on day 1 weeks 2, 4, 6, 8, 10, and 12. Vesicant.

Prednisone 75 mg/day: PO for 12 weeks; taper weeks 11 and 12. Take with breakfast.

Bleomycin 10 units/m²: IV on day 1 weeks 4, 8, and 12. Test dose of 2 units before first dose.

Bactrim DS: 1 tablet PO bid.

Ketoconazole 200-mg: PO daily.

Side effects: Myelosuppression dose-limiting toxicity. Nausea, vomiting, and anorexia. Mucositis and stomatitis can be severe. Constipation and paralytic ileus. Cardiotoxicity with doxorubicin, increased risk with cumulative doses >450 mg/m². Arrhythmias and/or EKG changes, pericarditis, or myocarditis. Fever, chills, sweating, lethargy, myalgias, and arthralgias common. Discoloration of urine from pink to red. Hemorrhagic cystitis preventable with appropriate hydration. Dose reduce with renal dysfunction. Peripheral neuropathy, jaw pain. CNS toxicity with paresthesias, neuropathies, ataxia, lethargy, headache, confusion, and/or seizures. Steroid toxicities: sodium, water retention, cushingoid changes, hyperglycemia, hypokalemia, increased sodium levels, mood changes, headache, insomnia, depression, and psychosis. Warfarin and insulin doses may need to be increased. Pneumonitis. Hyperpigmentation of nails, radiation recall, sun sensitivity. Alopecia.

Chair time: 2–3 hours day 1 weekly. Administer one cycle.

Methotrexate + Bleomycin + Doxorubicin + Cyclophosphamide + Vincristine + Dexamethasone (m-BACOD)[1,309]

Prechemo: CBC, Chem, LFTs, renal function tests, and MUGA. Central line placement. 5-HT$_3$ and dexamethasone acetaminophen. Moderately to highly emetogenic.

Methotrexate 200 mg/m²: IV in 500–1000 cc NS on days 8 and 15. Drug interactions include aspirin, penicillins, nonsteroidal anti-inflammatory drugs (NSAIDs), cephalosporins, phenytoin warfarin, 5-fluorouracil, thymidine, folic acid, and omeprazole. Vigorously hydrate; moderate dose of MTX.

Leucovorin 10 mg/m²: PO every 6 hours for eight doses, begin 24 hours after methotrexate.

Bleomycin 4 units/m^2: IV on day 1. Test dose of 2 units recommended before first dose.

Doxorubicin 45 mg/m^2: IV push on day 1. Vesicant.

Cyclophosphamide 600 mg/m^2: IV in 500 cc NS on day 1.

Vincristine 1 mg/m^2: IV push on day 1. Maximum dose 2 mg. Vesicant.

Dexamethasone 6 mg/m^2: PO on days 1-5. Take with breakfast.

Side effects: Myelosuppression dose-limiting toxicity. Nausea, vomiting, and anorexia. Mucositis and stomatitis can be severe. Constipation and paralytic ileus. Cardiotoxicity with doxorubicin, increased risk with cumulative doses >450 mg/m^2. Arrhythmias and/or EKG changes, pericarditis, or myocarditis. Fever, chills, sweating, lethargy, myalgias, and arthralgias common. Discoloration of urine from pink to red. Hemorrhagic cystitis, preventable with appropriate hydration. Dose reduce with renal dysfunction. Peripheral neuropathy, jaw pain. CNS toxicity with paresthesias, neuropathies, ataxia, lethargy, headache, confusion, and/or seizures. Steroid toxicities: sodium, water retention, cushingoid changes, hyperglycemia, hypokalemia, increased sodium levels, mood changes, headache, insomnia, depression, and psychosis. Warfarin and insulin doses may need to be increased. Pneumonitis. Hyperpigmentation of nails, radiation recall, sun sensitivity. Alopecia.

Chair time: Chair time 2–3 hours days 1, 8, and 15. Repeat cycle every 21 days.

ProMACE/CytaBOM[1,310]

Prechemo: CBC, Chem, LFTs, renal function tests, and MUGA. Central line placement recommended. 5-HT$_3$ and dexamethasone. Moderately to highly emetogenic.

Prednisone 60 mg/m^2/day: PO on days 1–14. Take with breakfast.

Doxorubicin 25 mg/m^2: IV push on day 1.

Cyclophosphamide 650 mg/m^2: IV in 500 cc NS on day 1.

Etoposide 120 mg/m^2: IV in 250 cc NS on day 1.

Cytarabine 300 mg/m^2: IV in 250 cc NS on day 8.

Bleomycin 5 units/m^2: IV push day 8. Test dose of 2 units before first dose.

Vincristine 1.4 mg/m^2: IV push day 8. Vesicant.

Methotrexate 120 mg/m^2: IV in 500 cc NS on day 8. Drug interactions include aspirin, penicillins, NSAIDs, cephalosporins, phenytoin, warfarin, thymidine, folic acid, and omeprazole.

Leucovorin 25 mg/m^2: PO every 6 hours for six doses, begin 24 hours after methotrexate.

Bactrim DS: 1 tablet PO bid days 1–21.

Side effects: Hypersensitivity reactions with etoposide. Myelosuppression dose-limiting toxicity. Nausea, vomiting, and anorexia. Mucositis, stomatitis, and diarrhea. Constipation and paralytic ileus. Cardiotoxicity with doxorubicin, increased risk with cumulative doses >450 mg/m^2. Arrhythmias and/or EKG changes, pericarditis, or myocarditis. Steroid toxicities: sodium, water retention, cushingoid changes, hyperglycemia, hypokalemia, increased sodium levels, mood changes, headache, insomnia, depression, and psychosis. Warfarin and insulin doses may need to be increased. Discoloration of urine from pink to red. Hemorrhagic cystitis, preventable with appropriate hydration. Peripheral neuropathy, jaw pain. Tumor lysis, syndrome, treat with hydration and allopurinol. Total alopecia, hyperpigmentation of nail beds and dermal crease of hands. Radiation recall. Sun sensitivity.

Chair time: 3 hours on days 1 and 8. Repeat cycle every 21 days.

HIGH-GRADE

Magrath Protocol (Burkitt's lymphoma)[1,311]

Prechemo: CBC, Chem, renal function tests, LFTs, sedimentation rate, MUGA. Central line placement. Ommaya reservoir placement versus lumbar puncture every cycle. 5-HT$_3$, dexamethasone. Moderately emetogenic.

Cyclophosphamide 1200-mg/m^2: IV in 500–1000 cc NS on day 1.

Doxorubicin 40-mg/m^2: IV push on day 1. Vesicant.

Vincristine 1.4 mg/m^2: IV push on day 1 (maximum dose 2 mg). Vesicant.

Prednisone 40 mg/m^2: PO on days 1–5. Take with breakfast.

Methotrexate 300 mg/m^2: IV in 500 cc NS on day 10 for 1 hour, and then:

Methotrexate 60 mg/m^2: IV continuous infusion, days 10 and 11, over 41 hours.

Drug interactions include aspirin, penicillins, NSAIDs, cephalosporins, phenytoin, warfarin, 5-fluorouracil, thymidine, folic acid, and omeprazole.

Leucovorin rescue 15 mg/m^2: IV in 100 cc NS over 15 minutes every 6 hours for eight doses starting 24 hours after methotrexate on day 12.

Intrathecal cytarabine 30 mg/m^2: IT on day 7, cycle 1 only; 45 mg/m^2 IT on day 7 for all subsequent cycles. Use preservative-free solution only.

Intrathecal preservative-free methotrexate 12.5-mg: IT on day 10, all cycles.

Side effects: Myelosuppression dose-limiting. Nausea, vomiting, and anorexia, mucositis, and stomatitis. Diarrhea is common and an indication to interrupt therapy of methotrexate. Transient increases in LFTs with methotrexate. Cardiotoxicity with doxorubicin, increased risk with cumulative doses >450 mg/m^2. Arrhythmias and/or EKG changes, pericarditis, or myocarditis. Discoloration of urine from pink to red. Hemorrhagic cystitis, preventable with appropriate hydration. Monitor BUN and creatinine levels; methotrexate can precipitate in renal tubules, resulting in acute tubular necrosis. Peripheral neuropathy jaw pain, paralytic ileus with vincristine. CNS toxicity with paresthesias, neuropathies, dizziness, blurred vision, ataxia, lethargy, headache, confusion, and/or seizures. Intrathecal chemotherapy can increase cerebrospinal fluid pressure. Steroid toxicities: sodium, water retention, cushingoid changes, hyperglycemia, hypokalemia, increased sodium levels, mood changes, headache, insomnia, depression, and psychosis. Warfarin and insulin doses may need to be increased. Tumor lysis syndrome; treat with hydration and allopurinol. SIADH with high-dose cyclophosphamide. Monitor serum Na^+, intake and output, and daily weights. Hyperpigmentation of nails, radiation recall, sun sensitivity. Alopecia.

Chair time: 2 hours days 1 and 10; 1 hour days 7 and 12. Repeat cycle every 28 days.

OR

Regimen A-CODOX-M (alternate with regimen B-IVAC)[1,312]

Prechemo: CBC, Chem, renal function tests, LFTs, sedimentation rate, and MUGA. Central line placement. Ommaya reservoir placement vs. lumbar puncture each cycle. 5-HT$_3$ and dexamethasone IV. Moderately to highly emetogenic.

Cyclophosphamide 800 mg/m^2: IV in 500–1000 cc NS on day 1.

Cyclophosphamide 200 mg/m^2: IV in 500 cc NS on days 2–5.

Doxorubicin 40 mg/m^2: IV push on day 1. Vesicant.

Vincristine 1.5 mg/m^2: IV push through free-flowing IV on days 1 and 8 in cycle 1; days 1, 8, and 15 in cycle 3. Maximum dose 2 mg. Vesicant.

Methotrexate 1200 mg/m^2: IV in 500–1000 cc NS over 1 hour on day 10, followed by:

Methotrexate 240 mg/m^2/hour: IV continuous infusion for the next 23 hours on day 10. Requires leucovorin rescue and adequate hydration. Drug interactions include aspirin, penicillins, NSAIDs, cephalosporins, phenytoin; warfarin, 5-fluorouracil, thymidine, folic acid, and omeprazole.

Leucovorin rescue 192 mg/m^2: IV in 1000 cc NS over 15 minutes starting 36 hours after the start of the methotrexate infusion, and then:

Leucovorin 12 mg/m^2: IV in 100 cc NS over 15 minutes every 6 hours until serum MTX levels < 50 nM.

CNS PROPHYLAXIS

Intrathecal cytarabine 70 mg/m^2: IT on days 1 and 3. Use preservative-free solution only.

Intrathecal methotrexate 12 mg: IT on day 15. Patients with CNS disease at presentation require additional intrathecal therapy. Use preservative-free solution only.

Side effects: Myelosuppression dose-limiting toxicity. Nausea, vomiting, and anorexia; moderately to highly emetogenic. Mucositis and stomatitis. Constipation and paralytic ileus. Diarrhea is common and an indication to interrupt therapy of methotrexate. Transient increases in LFTs can be seen with methotrexate. Cardiotoxicity with doxorubicin, increased risk with cumulative doses >450 mg/m². Arrhythmias and/or EKG changes, pericarditis, or myocarditis. Discoloration of urine from pink to red. Methotrexate, can precipitate in renal tubules, resulting in acute tubular necrosis. Hemorrhagic cystitis, hematuria, frequency preventable with uroprotection and hydration. Monitor BUN and serum creatinine levels. Tumor lysis syndrome treat with hydration and allopurinol. SIADH with high-dose cyclophosphamide. Monitor serum Na⁺, intake and output, and daily weights. Peripheral neuropathy and jaw pain with vincristine. CNS toxicity with paresthesias, neuropathies, dizziness, blurred vision, ataxia, lethargy, headache, confusion, and/or seizures. Intrathecal chemotherapy can increase cerebrospinal fluid pressure. Hyperpigmentation of nails, radiation recall, sun sensitivity. Alopecia.

Chair time: 2 hours days 1–5, 1 hour all other treatment days. Alternate regimen A (CODOX-M) with regimen B (IVAC) for four cycles.

Regimen B-IVAC[312]

Prechemo: CBC, Chem, renal function tests, LFTs, sedimentation rate, and MUGA. Central line placement. Ommaya reservoir placement vs. lumbar puncture each cycle. 5-HT₃ and dexamethasone IV. Moderately to highly emetogenic.

Ifosfamide 1500 mg/m²: IV in 500–1000 cc NS over 1 hour on days 1–5. Phenobarbital, phenytoin, cimetidine, and allopurinol increase toxicity. May enhance anticoagulant effects of warfarin.

Mesna 360 mg/m²: IV over 1 hour (dose mixed with ifosfamide), then:
Mesna 360 mg/m²: IV in 100 cc NS over 15 minutes every 3 hours days 1–5

Etoposide 60 mg/m²: IV in 250 cc NS over 1–2 hours on days 1–5.

Cytarabine 2 g/m²/day: IV in 500–1000 cc NS over 2 hours every 12 hours on days 1 and 2 for a total of four doses. IV hydration at 150/mL per hour with or without alkalinization, oral allopurinol, strict intake and output, and daily weights.

Methotrexate 12 mg: IT on day 5. Use preservative-free solution. Patients with CNS disease at presentation require additional intrathecal therapy.

Side effects: Myelosuppression dose-limiting toxicity. Nausea, vomiting, and anorexia, mucositis, and stomatitis. Constipation and paralytic ileus. High doses of cytarabine can result in cerebellar toxicity, including nystagmus, dysarthria, ataxia, slurred speech, difficulty with fine motor coordination, lethargy, or somnolence. Assess baseline neurologic status and cerebellar function (coordinated movements, such as handwriting and gait) before and during therapy. If cerebellar toxicity develops, treatment must be discontinued. Sensory/perceptual alterations: lethargy and confusion at high doses of ifosfamide, lasting 1–8 hours; reversible. Sterile phlebitis may occur at injection site. Hyperpigmentation, dermatitis, and nail ridging may occur. Total alopecia.

Chair time: 3 hours on days 1 and 2; 2 hours on days 3–5. May require hospitalization for every 12-hour treatment.

Stanford Regimen (small non-cleaved cell and Burkitt's lymphoma) [1,313]

Prechemo: CBC, Chem, renal function tests, and LFTs before each treatment. 5-HT$_3$, dexamethasone. Moderately to highly emetogenic.

Cyclophosphamide 1200 mg/m²: IV in 500–1000 cc NS on day 1.

Doxorubicin 40 mg/m²: IV push on day 1. Vesicant.

Vincristine 1.4 mg/m²: IV push on day 1 (maximum dose 2 mg). Vesicant.

Prednisone 40 mg/m²: PO on days 1–5. Take with breakfast.

Methotrexate 3000 mg/m²: IV in 1000 cc NS over 6 hours on day 10. Requires leucovorin rescue and adequate hydration. Drug interactions include aspirin, penicillins, NSAIDs, cephalosporins, phenytoin, warfarin, thymidine, folic acid, and omeprazole.

Leucovorin 25 mg/m²: IV in 100 cc NS over 15 minutes or PO every 6 hours for 12 doses beginning 24 hours after methotrexate.

Intrathecal preservative-free methotrexate 12-mg: IT on days 1 and 10 of cycles 2–4.

Side effects: Myelosuppression, may be severe. Nausea, vomiting, and anorexia, mucositis, and stomatitis. Constipation and paralytic ileus. Adequate hydration and leucovorin rescue for high-dose methotrexate to prevent acute renal tubular necrosis. Chemical arachnoiditis: Severe headaches, mochal rigidity, seizures, vomiting, fever, and an inflammatory cell infiltrate in the CSF. Cerebral dysfunction: paresis, aphasia, behavioral abnormality, and seizures with high-dose methotrexate. Occurs within 6 days of treatment. Resolves within 48–72 hours. Cardiotoxicity with doxorubicin, increased risk with cumulative doses >450 mg/m². Arrhythmias and/or EKG changes, pericarditis, or myocarditis. Peripheral neuropathy and jaw pain with vincristine. Discoloration of urine from pink to red. Total alopecia, hyperpigmentation of nail beds and dermal crease of hands. Radiation recall. Sun sensitivity.

Chair time: 2 hours day 1; 7 hours day 10. Repeat cycle every 21 days for three cycles.

MANTLE CELL LYMPHOMA

Bortezomib (Velcade) [1,314]

Prechemo: CBC, Chem, renal function tests, and LFTs. Bone marrow biopsy. 5-HT$_3$ and dexamethasone. Moderately emetogenic.

Bortezomib 1.3 mg/m^2: IV push, followed by saline flush on days 1, 4, 8, and 11, followed by a 10-day rest period.

Side effects: Myelosuppression, neutropenia, and thrombocytopenia. Nausea and vomiting, anorexia, constipation, and dehydration. Orthostatic hypotension. Fatigue, malaise, and generalized weakness. Peripheral neuropathy: mix of sensorimotor neuropathy. May improve and/or return to baseline with discontinuation of drug.

Chair time: 1 hour days 1, 4, 8, and 11. Repeat cycle every 21 days.

CD20+ B-CELL LYMPHOMAS

CHOP + Rituximab (GELA study) [1,315]

Prechemo: CBC, Chem, sedimentation rate. 5-HT$_3$ and dexamethasone. Tylenol 1000-mg PO. Diphenhydramine 50 mg and H$_2$ agonist.

Cyclophosphamide 750 mg/m^2: IV in 500 cc NS over 1 hour on day 1.

Doxorubicin 50 mg/m^2: IV push on day 1. Vesicant.

Vincristine 1.4 mg/m^2: IV push on day 1 (maximum dose 2 mg). Vesicant.

Prednisone 40 mg: PO on days 1 through 5. Take with breakfast.

Rituxan 375 mg/m^2: IV infusion on day 1. Administer first. Dilute to make final concentration of 1 or 4 mg/mL. Use infusion pump and blood pressure monitor. Initial infusion: beginning rate 50 mg/hr. Increase infusion rate by 50-mg/hr increments every 30 minutes to a maximum rate of 400 mg/hr. Subsequent infusions: initial rate of 100 mg/hr. Increase rate by 100 mg/hr every 30 minutes to a maximum rate of 400 mg/hr.

Side effects: Infusion-related reactions occur within 30 minutes to 2 hours after the beginning of the first infusion of rituximab. Myelosuppression. Potential for infection with B-lymphocytes reduced, resulting in bacterial infections not related to neutropenia. Nausea, vomiting, anorexia; mucositis, diarrhea. Cardiotoxicity with doxorubicin, increased risk with cumulative doses >450 mg/m^2. Arrhythmias and/or EKG changes, pericarditis, or myocarditis. Discoloration of urine from pink to red. Hemorrhagic cystitis; preventable with appropriate hydration. Peripheral neuropathy, jaw pain. Steroid toxicities: sodium, water retention, cushingoid changes, hyperglycemia, hypokalemia, increased sodium levels, mood changes, headache, insomnia, depression, and psychosis. Warfarin and insulin doses may need to be increased. Tumor lysis syndrome with high tumor burden or high white blood cell count. Treat/prevent with hydration and allopurinol. Skin reactions: rare and include paraneoplastic pemphigus, Stevens-Johnson syndrome, lichenoid dermatitis, vesiculobullous dermatitis, and toxic epidermal necrolysis. Rituxan should be discontinued and skin biopsy obtained to determine cause.

Chair time: First cycle 6–8 hours, second cycle 4–6 hours. Repeat cycle every 21 days.

CHOP + Rituximab (vose or Nebraska regimen)[1,316]

Prechemo: CBC, Chem, sedimentation rate. 5-HT$_3$ and dexamethasone. Tylenol 1000 mg PO Diphenhydramine 50 mg and H$_2$ agonist.

Rituxan 375 mg/m^2: IV infusion on day 1. Dilute to make final concentration of 1 or 4 mg/1 mL. Use infusion pump and blood pressure monitor. Initial infusion: beginning rate 50 mg/hr. Increase infusion rate by 50-mg/hr increments every 30 minutes to a maximum rate of 400 mg/hr. Subsequent infusions: initial rate of 100 mg/hr. Increase rate by 100 mg/hr every 30 minutes to a maximum rate of 400 mg/hr as tolerated.

Cyclophosphamide 750 mg/m^2: IV in 500 cc NS over 1 hour on day 3.

Doxorubicin 50 mg/m^2: IV push on day 3. Vesicant.

Vincristine 1.4 mg/m^2: IV push on day 3 (maximum dose 2 mg). Vesicant.

Prednisone 100 mg: PO on days 3 through 7. Take with breakfast.

Side effects: Infusion-related reactions occur within 30 minutes to 2 hours after the beginning of the first infusion of Rituximab. Myelosuppression. Potential for infection with B-lymphocytes reduced, resulting in bacterial infections not related to neutropenia. Nausea, vomiting, anorexia; mucositis, diarrhea. Cardiotoxicity with doxorubicin, increased risk with cumulative doses >450 mg/m^2. Arrhythmias and/or EKG changes, pericarditis, or myocarditis. Discoloration of urine from pink to red. Hemorrhagic cystitis; preventable with appropriate hydration. Peripheral neuropathy, jaw pain. Steroid toxicities: sodium, water retention, cushingoid changes, hyperglycemia, hypokalemia, increased sodium levels, mood changes, headache, insomnia, depression, and psychosis. Warfarin and insulin doses may need to be increased. Tumor lysis syndrome with high tumor burden or high white blood cell count. Treat/prevent with hydration and allopurinol. Skin reactions: rare and include paraneoplastic pemphigus, Stevens-Johnson syndrome, lichenoid dermatitis, vesiculobullous dermatitis, and toxic epidermal necrolysis. Rituxan should be discontinued and skin biopsy obtained to determine cause.

Chair time: 4–6 hours on day 1; 2 hours on days 2–3.

SALVAGE REGIMENS

Etoposide + Cytarabine + Cisplatin (ESHAP)[1,317]

Prechemo: CBC, Chem, Mg^{2+}. Central line placement. 5-HT$_3$ and dexamethasone. Moderately to highly emetogenic.

Etoposide 40 mg/m²: IV in 250 cc NS on days 1–4.

Methylprednisolone (Solu-Medrol) 500 mg: IV on days 1–4.

Cisplatin 25 mg/m²/day: Continuous infusion on days 1–4. May add Mg²⁺.

Cytarabine 2000 mg/m²: IV in 500–1000 cc NS on day 5 over 2 hours after cisplatin and etoposide.

Side effects: Hypersensitivity reaction when etoposide infused too quickly. Myelosuppression. Nausea and vomiting, acute or delayed. Anorexia; mucositis, diarrhea. Steroid toxicities: sodium, water retention, cushingoid changes, hyperglycemia, hypokalemia, increased sodium levels, mood changes, headache, insomnia, depression, and psychosis. Warfarin and insulin doses may need to be increased. Tumor lysis syndrome: patients with high tumor burden or high white blood cell count at risk. Treat/prevent with hydration and allopurinol. Dose reduce for renal dysfunction. Peripheral neuropathy, cerebellar toxicity, and ototoxicity.

Chair time: 2–3 hours days 1–5. Repeat every 21 days.

Dexamethasone + High-Dose Cytarabine + Cisplatin (DHAP)[1,318]

Prechemo: CBC, Chem, LFTs, renal function tests, Mg²⁺. 5-HT₃ and dexamethasone. Moderately to highly emetogenic.

Cytarabine 2000 mg/m²/day: IV in 500 cc NS over 2 hours every 12 hours, two doses on day 1. IV hydration at 150/mL per hour with or without alkalinization.

Cisplatin 100 mg/m²: IV in 1000 cc NS on day 1.

Dexamethasone 40 mg: PO or IV on days 1–4.

Side effects: Myelosuppression. Nausea and vomiting acute and delayed; anorexia and taste alterations. High doses of cytarabine can result in cerebellar toxicity, including nystagmus, dysarthria, ataxia, slurred speech, difficulty with fine motor coordination, lethargy, or somnolence. Assess baseline neurologic status and cerebellar function (coordinated movements, such as handwriting and gait) before and during therapy. If cerebellar toxicity develops, treatment must be discontinued. Cisplatin causes peripheral neuropathy and ototoxicity. Saline or steroid eye drops for 24 hours after completion of high dose cytarabine. Tumor lysis syndrome treat with hydration and allopurinol. Daily weights and intake and output recording. Discontinue therapy for rapidly increasing creatinine. Steroid toxicities: sodium, water retention, cushingoid changes, hyperglycemia, hypokalemia, increased sodium levels, mood changes, headache, insomnia, depression, and psychosis. Warfarin and insulin doses may need to be increased. Total alopecia, impaired skin/mucosal changes, including maculopapular rash.

Chair time: 5 hours day 1. Repeat cycle every 3–4 weeks. May require hospitalization.

Ifosfamide + Etoposide + Carboplatin (ICE)[1,319]

Prechemo: CBC, Chem, LFTs, renal function tests, Mg^{2+}. Bone marrow biopsy and central line placement. $5-HT_3$ and dexamethasone. Moderately to highly emetogenic.

Ifosfamide 5000 mg/m²: IV continuous infusion for 24 hours on day 2. May enhance anticoagulant effects of warfarin.

Etoposide 100 mg/m²: IV in 250 cc NS over 1–2 hours on days 1–3.

Carboplatin AUC of 5.0: IV in 500 cc NS infusion over 1 hour on day 2. Reduce dose creatinine clearance <60 cc/min or if other values are abnormal.

Mesna 5000-mg/m²: Continuous IV infusion in combination with ifosfamide on day 2.

GCSF is administered at 5 mg/kg on days 5–12.

Side effects: Myelosuppression is dose-limiting toxicity. Nausea and vomiting, anorexia. Hypersensitivity reactions after seventh dose of carboplatin. Hemorrhagic cystitis, preventable with uroprotection and hydration of 2–3 L per day. Monitor BUN and serum creatinine levels. Sensory/perceptual alterations: lethargy and confusion at high doses of ifosfamide, usually lasting 1–8 hours; reversible. Hyperpigmentation, dermatitis, and nail ridging may occur. Total alopecia.

Chair time: 2 hours on days 1 and 3; 3 hours on day 2. Repeat cycle every 14 days.

Mesna + Ifosfamide + Mitoxantrone + Etoposide (MINE)[1,320]

Prechemo: CBC, Chem, LFTs, renal function tests, Mg^{2+}. Bone marrow biopsy and central line placement. $5-HT_3$ and dexamethasone. Moderately to highly emetogenic.

Mesna 1330 mg/m²: IV in 500–1000 cc NS infused at the same time as ifosfamide on days 1–3, and then: 500 mg/day PO or IV 4 hours after ifosfamide on days 1–3.

Ifosfamide 1330 mg/m²: IV infusion on days 1–3. Phenobarbital, phenytoin, cimetidine, and allopurinol increase toxicity. May enhance anticoagulant effects of warfarin.

Mitoxantrone 8 mg/m²: IV infusion on day 1 only. IV push over 3 minutes or IV infusion over 5–30 minutes.

Etoposide 65 mg/m²: IV in 250 cc NS on days 1–3. Give over 30–60 minutes to minimize risk of hypotension. Enhances warfarin action by increasing INR. Reduce dose for increased bilirubin level or creatinine clearance.

Side effects: Hypersensitivity reaction with etoposide. Myelosuppression. Nausea, vomiting, and anorexia. Cardiotoxicity: CHF, increased risk of cardiotoxicity with cumulative dose of mitoxantrone >180 mg/m². Hemorrhagic cystitis, preventable with uroprotection and hydration of 2–3 L per day. Monitor BUN and serum creatinine levels. Urine will be green-blue; sclera may become temporarily discolored blue. Lethargy and confusion at high doses of ifosfamide, usually lasting 1–8 hours; reversible. Sterile phlebitis may occur at injection site. Hyperpigmentation, dermatitis, and nail ridging may occur. Radiation recall with etoposide. Total alopecia.

Chair time: 6 hours on days 1–3. Repeat cycle every 21 days.

PRIMARY CNS LYMPHOMA

Methotrexate + IT Methotrexate + Leucovorin + Vincristine + Procarbazine followed by Whole Brain Irradiation[1,321]

Prechemo: CBC, Chem, creatinine clearance, diagnostic lumbar puncture, Ommaya reservoir. 5-HT$_3$, dexamethasone.

Methotrexate 3.5 g/m²: IV in 1000 cc NS over 2 hours every other week for five doses.

High-dose methotrexate requires leucovorin rescue. Drug interactions include aspirin, penicillins, nonsteroidal anti-inflammatory drugs (NSAIDs), cephalosporins, phenytoin warfarin, 5-fluorouracil, thymidine, folic acid, and omeprazole.

Leucovorin 10 mg: IV in 100 cc over 15 minutes every 6 hours for 12 doses, starting 24 hours after IV methotrexate.

Vincristine 1.4 mg/m²: IV push every other week with IV methotrexate. Maximum dose 2 mg. Vesicant.

Procarbazine 100 mg/m²/day: PO for 7 days on first, third, and fifth cycle of IV methotrexate. (50-mg tablets.)

Intrathecal preservative-free methotrexate 12 mg: IT weekly on alternate weeks after systemic IV methotrexate.

Leucovorin 10 mg: IV in 100 cc over 15 minutes every 12 hours for eight doses starting 24 hours after IT methotrexate. **After chemotherapy is completed, whole brain radiation therapy to a total dose of 45 cGy.**

Side effects: Myelosuppression dose-limiting toxicity. Nausea, vomiting, and anorexia. Mucositis and stomatitis can be severe and dose-limiting. Constipation and paralytic ileus. Acute renal failure, azotemia, urinary retention, and uric acid nephropathy. Provide adequate hydration. Pneumonitis with cough and interstitial infiltrates. Fever, chills, sweating, lethargy, myalgias, and arthralgias. Hemorrhagic cystitis preventable with appropriate hydration. Peripheral neuropathy, jaw pain. CNS toxicity with paresthesias, neuropathies, ataxia, lethargy, headache, confusion, and/or seizures. Usually occurs within 6 days of high-dose methotrexate and resolves within 48–72 hours. Procarbazine drug and food interactions: avoid tricyclic antidepressants; decreased bioavailability of digoxin; antabuse-like reaction with alcohol; avoid tyramines (beer, wine, cheese, brewer's yeast, chicken liver, and bananas). Total alopecia, hyper pigmentation of nail beds and dermal crease of hands. Radiation recall, sun sensitivity.

Chair time: 2–3 hours every other week for IV methotrexate and 1 hour alternate weeks for IT methotrexate. Administer one cycle.

SINGLE-AGENT REGIMENS

Rituxan (Rituximab)[1,322]

Pretreatment: CBC, Chem. Diphenhydramine 50 mg, H_2 antagonist, and dexamethasone. Acetaminophen 1000-mg PO 30 minutes before infusion.

Rituxan 375 mg/m²: IV days 1, 8, 15, and 22. Use infusion pump and blood pressure monitor. First infusion: initial rate of 50 mg/hr. Increase infusion rate in 50-mg/hr increments every 30 minutes to a maximum rate of 400 mg/hr. If a hypersensitivity-related event develops, the infusion should be slowed or interrupted. Resume infusion at 50% of previous rate after symptoms subside. Subsequent infusions: initial rate of 100 mg/hr. Increase rate by 100 mg/hr every 30 minutes to a maximum rate of 400 mg/hr.

Side effects: Infusion-related reactions. Potential for infection: B-lymphocytes reduced, resulting in bacterial infections not related to neutropenia. Skin reactions: rare and include paraneoplastic pemphigus, Stevens-Johnson syndrome, lichenoid dermatitis, vesiculobullous dermatitis, and toxic epidermal necrolysis. Drug therapy should be discontinued and skin biopsy should be obtained to determine cause. Tumor lysis with high tumor burden or high white blood cell count at risk. Treat/prevent with hydration and allopurinol.

Chair time: 6–8 hours first dose. 4–6 hours weeks 2–4. May be repeated for one additional cycle.

Ibritumomab Tiuxetan (Zevalin) Regimen[1,323]

Pretreatment: CBC, Chem, renal function tests, and LFTs. Bone marrow biopsy, central line placement. Diphenhydramine, acetaminophen, dexamethasone.

Rituximab 250 mg/m²: IV on days 1 and 8.

Given in Radiation Oncology Department:

¹¹¹In-ibritumomab tiuxetan 5 mCi of ¹¹¹In,1.6 mg of ibritumomab tiuxetan: IV day 1.

⁹⁰Y-ibritumomab tiuxetan 0.4-mCi/kg: IV over 10 minutes on day 8 after the day 8 rituximab dose.

Dose of ⁹⁰Y-ibritumomab tiuxetan is capped at 32 mCi.

See package insert for drug preparation.

Day 1: [111]In IV over 10 minutes using 0.22-micron filter, followed by: rituximab IV within 4 hours, initially at 50 mg/hr and gradually increasing the rate in 50-mg increments if no infusion reaction occurs to a maximum of 400 mg/hr.

Biodistribution imaging 1: 2–24 hours after ^{111}In injection; image 2: 48–72 hours later; optional image 3; at 90–120 hours.

If biodistribution acceptable, on day 7–9, rituximab 250-mg/m^2 IV, and within 4 hours, ^{90}Y-ibritumomab tiuxetan IV over 10 minutes.

Side effects: Myelosuppression: severe and prolonged. Hypersensitivity reactions. Tumor lysis syndrome when white blood cell count is elevated or large tumor burden present. Prevent with allopurinol and hydration 150 mL/hr with or without alkalinization. Severe mucocutaneous reactions are rare but require discontinuation of rituximab. Asthenia, headache, pruritus, myalgias, dizziness, and fatigue. Agitation, confusion, visual disturbances. Nausea and vomiting, anorexia; mucositis, diarrhea. Radiation exposure: [90]Y is a beta-emitter, and thus, patients should protect others from exposure to their body secretions (saliva, stool, blood, and urine).

Chair time: One cycle only, 6–8 hours on days 1 and 8 for rituximab.

Fludarabine[1,324]

Prechemo: CBC and Chem. Oral phenothiazine or 5-HT$_3$. Mildly emetogenic.

Fludarabine 25 mg/m^2: IV in 100 cc NS on days 1–5.

Side effects: Myelosuppression: severe and cumulative decrease in CD4$^+$ and CD8$^+$, increasing risk for opportunistic infections (fungus, herpes, and *Pneumocystis carinii*). Fatigue. Agitation, confusion, and visual disturbances. Pneumonia pulmonary hypersensitivity reaction characterized by dyspnea, cough, and interstitial pulmonary infiltrates. Nausea and vomiting, anorexia; mucositis, diarrhea.

Chair time: 1 hour on days 1–5. Repeat cycle every 28 days.

Cladribine (Leustatin)[1,325]

Prechemo: CBC and Chem. Oral phenothiazine or 5-HT$_3$. Mildly emetogenic.

Cladribine 0.5 mg/kg: Sub Q on days 1–5.
OR
Cladribine 0.1 mg/kg/day: IV continuous infusion on days 1–7. Use .22-micron filter when preparing solution. Dilute in minimum of 100 mL NS, DO NOT use D5W.

Side effects: Myelosuppression dose-limiting toxicity. Decrease in CD4$^+$ and CD8$^+$, increasing risk for opportunistic infections (fungus,

herpes, and *Pneumocystis carinii*). Tumor lysis syndrome if WBC is elevated or large tumor burden. Prevent with allopurinol and hydration
150 mL/hr with or without alkalinization. Fatigue. Nausea and vomiting, anorexia; constipation, diarrhea. Headache, insomnia, and dizziness. Rash, pruritus, or injection site reactions.

Chair time: 1 hour on day 1, pump dc day 8. Repeat cycle every 28 days.

I 131-Tositumomab (Bexxar) [1,326]

Pretreatment: TSH, CBC, platelets >100,000/mm³; neutrophil count
>1500; chemistry, renal function tests, pregnancy test, (if applicable),
HAMA (human antimurine antibodies) if patient has had previous exposure to murine antibodies. Bone marrow biopsy >25% lymphoma of the
intratrabecular space; referral to Nuclear Medicine/Radiation Oncology
Department.

The BEXXAR therapeutic regimen consists of four components administered in two discrete steps: the dosimetric step, followed 7–14 days
later by a therapeutic step.

Premedication: Day 1

Thyroid protection initiated 24 hours prior to administration of iodine I
131-Tositumomab dosimetric dose and continued until 2 weeks after iodine I 131-Tositumomab therapeutic dose. **SSKI**—saturated solution of
potassium iodide 4 drops orally t.i.d.; or potassium iodide tablets 130
mg orally.

Premedication: Day 0

Acetaminophen 1000 mg and diphenhydramine 50 mg PO 30 minutes
prior to dosimetric and therapeutic steps.

Dosimetric Step:

Tositumomab 450 mg: intravenously in 50 ml 0.9% sodium chloride
over 60 minutes. Reduce the rate of infusion by 50% for mild to moderate infusional toxicity; interrupt infusion for severe infusional toxicity.
After complete resolution of severe infusional toxicity, infusion may be
resumed with a 50% reduction in the rate of infusion. 0.22-micron inline filter. The same IV tubing set and filter must be used throughout the
entire dosimetric or therapeutic step. A change in filter can result in loss
of drug, followed by:

Iodine I-131 Tositumomab (containing 5.0-mCi iodine-131 and 35-mg
Tositumomab) intravenously in 30 mL 0.9% sodium chloride over 20
minutes. Reduce the rate of infusion by 50% for mild to moderate infusional toxicity; interrupt infusion for severe infusional toxicity. After
complete resolution of severe infusional toxicity, infusion may be resumed with a 50% reduction in the rate of infusion.

Day 0: Whole Body Dosimetry and Biodistribution

Days 2, 3, or 4: Whole Body Dosimetry and Biodistribution

Days 6 or 7: Whole Body Dosimetry and Biodistribution

If biodistribution is acceptable begin therapeutic step. *Note:* Do not administer the therapeutic step if biodistribution is altered (see Assessment of Biodistribution of iodine I-131 Tositumomab).

Premedication: Tylenol 1000 mg and Benadryl 50 mg PO 30 minutes before treatment.

Therapeutic Step:

Tositumomab 450 mg: intravenously in 50 ml 0.9% sodium chloride over 1 hour. Reduce the rate of infusion by 50% for mild to moderate infusional toxicity; interrupt infusion for severe infusional toxicity. After complete resolution of severe infusional toxicity, infusion may be resumed with a 50% reduction in the rate of infusion, followed by:

Iodine I-131 Tositumomab (see Calculation of iodine-131 Activity for the therapeutic dose). Reduce the rate of infusion by 50% for mild to moderate infusional toxicity; interrupt infusion for severe infusional toxicity. After complete resolution of severe infusional toxicity, infusion may be resumed with a 50% reduction in the rate of infusion. Patients with $>150,000$ platelets/mm^3: The recommended dose is the activity of iodine-131 calculated to deliver 75 cGy total body irradiation and 35 mg Tositumomab, administered intravenously over 20 minutes.

Patients with NCI grade 1 thrombocytopenia (platelet counts $>100,000$ but $<150,000$ platelets/mm^3): The recommended dose is the activity of iodine-131 calculated to deliver 65 cGy total body irradiation and 35 mg Tositumomab, administered intravenously over 20 minutes. Administration is done by a nuclear medicine physician/radiation oncologist. See package insert for directions for complete preparation and administration.

Side effects: Hypersensitivity reactions. Myelosuppression prolonged and severe. Intervention with G-CSF and epoetin alfa is recommended. Transfusions of RBCs and platelets were not uncommon. Nausea, anorexia, and diarrhea. Dehydration and hypokalemia were also seen. Central neurotoxicity may occur, as well as neuropathy and optic neuritis. Radiation precautions: patients may receive outpatient treatment as long as total dose to an individual at 1 meter is 500 millirem. Remain at distance of 3 feet from other people for at least 2 days. Infants and pregnant women should not visit the patient and if necessary visits should be brief and at a distance of at least 9 feet. Do not travel by commercial transportation or go on a prolonged automobile trip with others for at least the first 2 days. Have sole use of the bathroom for at least 2 days and drink up to 3 quarts water per day for at least 2 days to prevent dehydration.

Chair time: 2 hours on day 0, body scans on day 0 (2, 3, or 4) and days 6 or 7. Therapeutic step days 7–14 (one dose within that time frame), chair time 2 hours.

Lymphoma: Cutaneous T-Cell Lymphoma (CTCL)

Single-Agent Regimens

Vorinostat (Zolinza) [327]

Prechemo: CBC, Chem, Mg^{2+}, LFTs. ECG at baseline and periodically thereafter. Oral phenothiazine or 5-HT$_3$. Mildly to moderately emetogenic.

Vorinostat 400 mg: PO daily (100-mg white gelatin capsules). Take whole with food. Dose may be reduced to 300 mg PO daily or, if necessary, 300 mg PO daily for 5 consecutive days each week if patient intolerant to therapy.

Side effects: Myelosuppression dose-related thrombocytopenia and anemia have occurred and may require dose modification or discontinuation. Nausea, vomiting, diarrhea, anorexia, dry mouth, and dysgeusia common. Anorexia, weight loss, and constipation also seen. May require antiemetics, antidiarrheals, and fluid and electrolyte replacement to prevent dehydration. Instruct patients to drink at least 2 L/day to prevent dehydration. Pulmonary embolism and deep vein thrombosis have been reported. QTc prolongation has been observed. Hyperglycemia. Monitor serum glucose, especially in diabetic or potentially diabetic patients. Severe thrombocytopenia and gastrointestinal bleeding have been reported with concomitant use of Zolinza® and other HDAC inhibitors (e.g., valproic acid). Prolongation of international normalized ratio (INR) observed with use of coumarin-derivative anticoagulants. Monitor PT/INR carefully. Fevers and chills. Use with caution in patients with hepatic impairment.

Treatment schedule: Take daily as tolerated or until progression.

MALIGNANT MELANOMA

ADJUVANT THERAPY

Interferon α-2b[1,328]

Prechemo: CBC, Chem, LFTs. Central line placement recommended. 5-HT$_3$ for IV therapy. Acetaminophen 650 mg 30 minutes before treatment and every 4 hours, may alternate with Ibuprofen 400-mg PO every 4 hours. Mild to moderately emetogenic.

Interferon α-2b 20 × 10^6 IU/m^2: IV on days 1–5 for 4 weeks. Use only Intron A powder. Do not dilute with D5W.

Then maintenance therapy:

Interferon α-2b 10 × 10^6 IU/m^2: SQ three times weekly for 48 weeks.

Side effects: Fever, chills, headache, myalgias, and arthralgias. Increase PO fluid intake. Myelosuppression, cumulative effect, dose-limiting. Nausea and diarrhea. Anorexia, cumulative and dose-limiting. Taste alteration and xerostomia. Dizziness, confusion, decreased mental status, and depression. Somnolence, irritability and poor concentration. Alopecia is partial. Dry skin, pruritus, and irritation at injection site occur.

Chair time: 1 hour on days 1–5 for 4 weeks. Treat for a total of 1 year.

METASTATIC DISEASE

COMBINATION REGIMENS

Dacarbazine (DTIC) + Carmustine (BCNU) + Cisplatin[1,329]

Prechemo: CBC, Chem, Mg^{2+}, and LFTs. Pulmonary function tests, central line placement. 5-HT$_3$ and dexamethasone. Moderately to highly emetogenic.

Dacarbazine 220 mg/m^2: IV in 500 cc NS over 1 hour on days 1–3. Vesicant.

Carmustine 150 mg/m^2: IV in 500–1000 cc of NS over 1–2 hours on day 1.

Cisplatin 25 mg/m²: IV in 500–1000 cc of NS over 1–2 hours on days 1–3.

Side effects: Fever, chills, headache, myalgias, and arthralgias. Myelosuppression with delayed nadir. Nausea and vomiting; anorexia, cumulative and dose-limiting. Taste alteration and xerostomia. Nephrotoxicity preventive with hydration. Pulmonary fibrosis. Peripheral neuropathy (sensory/motor). Paresthesias and numbness. Ototoxicity. Dry skin, flushing, pruritus, photosensitivity, and pain, irritation, and phlebitis at injection site. Alopecia.

Chair time: 4 hours on day 1; 3 hours on days 2–3. Repeat dacarbazine and cisplatin every 21 days. Repeat carmustine every 42 days.

DTIC + Cisplatin + BCNU + Tamoxifen[1,330]

Prechemo: CBC, Chem, Mg^{2+}, and LFTs. Pulmonary function tests, central line placement. 5-HT_3 and dexamethasone. Moderately to highly emetogenic.

Dacarbazine 220 mg/m²: IV in 500 cc NS over 1 hour on days 1–3 and 22–24. Vesicant.

Cisplatin 25 mg/m²: IV in 500–1000 cc of NS over 1–2 hours on days 1–3 and 22–24.

Carmustine 150 mg/m²: IV in 500 D5W on day 1.

Tamoxifen 10-mg: PO bid starting on day 4.

Side effects: Fever, chills, headache, myalgias, and arthralgias. Myelosuppression with delayed nadir. Nausea and vomiting, Anorexia cumulative and dose-limiting. Taste alteration and xerostomia. Nephrotoxicity preventive with hydration. Pulmonary fibrosis. Peripheral neuropathy (sensory/motor). Paresthesias and numbness ototoxicity. Hot flashes. Alopecia, dry skin, flushing, pruritus, photosensitivity, and pain, irritation, and phlebitis at injection site.

Chair time: 3–4 hours on days 1–3 and 22–24. Repeat cycle every 6 weeks.

Cisplatin + Vinblastine + Dacarbazine (CVD)[1,331]

Prechemo: CBC, Chem, Mg^{2+}, and LFTs. Pulmonary function tests, central line placement. 5-HT_3 and dexamethasone. Moderately to highly emetogenic.

Cisplatin 20 mg/m²: IV in 500 cc of NS over 1–2 hours on days 1–5.

Vinblastine 1.6 mg/m²: IV push on days 1–5. Vesicant.

Dacarbazine 800 mg/m²: IV in 500–1000 cc NSon day 1. Vesicant.

Side effects: Fever, chills, headache, myalgias, and arthralgias. Myelosuppression dose-limiting toxicity, delayed nadir. Nausea and vomiting. Anorexia, cumulative, and dose-limiting. Taste alteration and xerostomia. Nephrotoxicity, prevented with vigorous hydration. Peripheral neuropathy, sensory/motor. Paresthesias and numbness paralytic ileus.

Ototoxicity. Alopecia. Dry skin, flushing, pruritus, photosensitivity, and pain, irritation, and phlebitis at injection site. Pulmonary fibrosis.

Chair time: 4–5 hours on days 1–5. Repeat cycle every 21–28 days.

Interferon (IFN) + DTIC[1,332]

Prechemo: CBC, Chem, LFTs. Central line placement. 5-HT$_3$, dexamethasone. Acetaminophen 650 mg 30 minutes before treatment and every 4 hours, may alternate with Ibuprofen 400 mg PO every 4 hours. Mild to moderately emetogenic.

Induction:

Interferon α-2b 15 × 10^6 IU/m^2: IV on days 1–5, 8–12, and 15–19. DO NOT USE D5W. Use only Intron A powder (interferon α-2b).

Maintenance Therapy:

Interferon α-2b 10 × 10^6 IU/m^2: SC 3 times per week.

Dacarbazine 200 mg/m^2: IV in 500–1000 cc NS on days 22–26. Vesicant.

Side effects: Fever, chills, headache, myalgias, and arthralgias. Myelosuppression, cumulative effect, dose-limiting. Nausea and diarrhea. Anorexia, cumulative, and dose-limiting. Taste alteration and xerostomia. Dizziness, confusion, decreased mental status, and depression. Somnolence, irritability, and poor concentration. Pulmonary fibrosis. Dry skin, pruritus, and pain, irritation, and phlebitis at injection site. Alopecia is partial.

Chair time: 1–2 hours on days 1–5, 8–12, 15–19, and 22–26. Repeat every 28 days.

Cisplatin + Vinblastine + Dacarbazine + IL-2 + Interferon[1,333]

Prechemo: CBC, Chem, Mg^{2+}, LFTs. Central line placement. 5-HT$_3$ and dexamethasone. Acetaminophen 650 mg 30 minutes before treatment and every 4 hours, may alternate with Ibuprofen 400-mg PO every 4 hours. Mildly to moderately emetogenic.

Cisplatin 20 mg/m^2: IV in 500–1000 cc of NS over 1–2 hours on days 1–4 and 22–25.

Vinblastine 1.5 mg/m^2: IV push on days 1–4 and 22–25. Vesicant.

Dacarbazine 800 mg/m^2: IV in 500 mL of NS over 1–2 hours days 1 and 22. Vesicant.

Interleukin-2 9 × 10^6 IU/m^2: IV as a 24-hour continuous infusion on days 5–8 and 17–20. IL-2 administered in the hospital—high dose.

Interferon α-2b 5 × 10^6 IU/m^2: SC on days 5–9, 17–21, and 26–30.

Side effects: Chills, rigor, fever, and headache. Myalgia and arthralgias. Myelosuppression dose-limiting toxicity. Nausea and vomiting, acute or delayed. Peripheral neuropathy sensory/motor. Nephrotoxicity with vigorous hydration. Oliguria, proteinuria, elevated creatinine, tubular cell injury, and decreased renal blood flow with IL-2. Hepatomegaly, hypoalbuminemia, and elevated LFT. Hold for signs of hepatic failure including encephalopathy, increasing ascites, liver pain, or hypoglycemia. Capillary leak syndrome: peripheral edema, CHF, pleural effusions, and pericardial effusions. Strict I and O, vital signs every 2–4 hours. Ototoxicity. Diffuse erythematous rash, desquamation. Pruritus and alopecia.

Chair time: 5 hours on days 1 and 22; 3 hours on days 2–4 and 23–25. Repeat cycle every 6 weeks. May require hospitalization for IL-2.

Temozolomide + Thalidomide[1,334]

Prechemo: CBC, Chem, and LFTs. Oral phenothiazine or 5-HT$_3$. Mildly to moderately emetogenic.

Temozolomide 75 mg/m^2/day: PO for 6 weeks. (5-, 20-,100-, 250-mg capsules.)

Thalidomide 200–400 mg/m^2/day: PO for 6 weeks. (50-, 100-, 200-mg capsules.) Requires registration with STEPS program and authorization every 28 days.

Side effects: Teratogenic effect: most serious toxicity of thalidomide. Severe birth defects or death to an unborn fetus. Myelosuppression dose-limiting toxicity. Nausea and vomiting. Diarrhea, constipation, and/or anorexia. Constipation is primary GI toxicity with thalidomide. Deep vein thrombosis and pulmonary embolism, consider prophylactic warfarin. Fatigue, orthostatic hypotension, and dizziness. Peripheral neuropathy. Daytime sedation. Maculopapular skin rash, urticaria, and dry skin. Stevens-Johnson syndrome reported. Discontinue thalidomide if skin rash develops.

Chair time: No chair time. Repeat cycle every 10 weeks until disease progression.

SINGLE-AGENT REGIMENS

Dacarbazine (DTIC)[1,335,336]

Prechemo: CBC, Chem, and LFTs. Central line placement recommended. 5-HT$_3$ and dexamethasone. Moderately to highly emetogenic.

Dacarbazine 250 mg/m^2: IV in 500 cc NS on days 1–5. Repeat cycle every 21 days.

OR

Dacarbazine 850 mg/m^2: IV in 500–1000 cc NS on day 1. Repeat cycle every 3–6 weeks. Vesicant.

Side effects: Myelosuppression is a dose-limiting toxicity with delayed nadir. Nausea and vomiting. Paresthesias, neuropathies, ataxia, lethargy, headache, confusion, and seizures have all been observed. Malaise, headache, myalgia, hypotension. Pain at injection site during infusion, erythema and urticaria, phlebitis. Photosensitization. Alopecia.

Chair time: 2 hours on days 1–5. Repeat cycle every 21 days.

OR

3 hours on day 1. Repeat cycle every 3–6 weeks.

Interferon[1,337]

Prechemo: CBC, Chem, LFTs. Central line placement. Oral phenothiazide or 5-HT$_3$. Acetaminophen 650 mg 30 minutes before treatment and every 4 hours, may alternate with Ibuprofen 400 mg PO every 4 hours. Mildly emetogenic.

Interferon α-2b 20 $\times$ 10^6 IU/m^2: IM/ Sub Q 3 times per week for 12 weeks.

Side effects: Fever, chills, headache, myalgias, and arthralgias. Increase patient's PO fluid intake. Myelosuppression, cumulative effect, dose-limiting. Nausea and diarrhea. Anorexia cumulative and dose-limiting. Taste alteration and xerostomia. Dizziness, confusion, decreased mental status, and depression. Somnolence, irritability, and poor concentration. Alopecia is partial. Dry skin, pruritus, and irritation at injection site occur.

Chair time: 1 hour for self-injection teaching.

Aldesleukin (IL-2) [1,338]

Prechemo: CBC, Chem, LFTs, renal function tests. Pulmonary function tests. Central line placement. 5-HT$_3$ and dexamethasone. Acetaminophen 650 mg 30 minutes before treatment and every 4 hours, may alternate with Ibuprofen 400 mg PO every 4 hours. Mildly to moderately emetogenic.

Aldesleukin 100,000 IU/kg: IV in 500 cc D5W over 15 minutes on days 1–5 and 15–19.

Side effects: Chills, rigors, high fevers, and headache. Myalgia and arthralgias. Confusion, irritability, disorientation, impaired memory, expressive aphasia, sleep disturbances, depression, hallucinations, and psychoses may occur, resolving within 24–48 hours after last dose. Capillary leak syndrome. Strict I and O, vital signs 2–4 hours. Nausea and vomiting; diarrhea common, can be severe; stomatitis common but mild. Oliguria, proteinuria, increased creatinine, and LFTs. Anuria. Hepatomegaly and hypoalbuminemia. Myelosuppression. Diffuse erythematous rash with desquamation. Pruritus. Usually administered in hospital setting.

Chair time: 1 hour on days 1–5 and 15–19. Repeat cycle every 28 days.

Temozolomide[1,339]

Prechemo: CBC, Chem, and LFTs. Oral 5-HT$_3$. Mildly to moderately emetogenic.

Temozolomide 150 mg/m^2: PO days 1–5. (5-, 20-,100-, 250-mg capsules.) If well tolerated, can increase dose to 200 mg/m^2 PO on days 1–5.

Side effects: Myelosuppression dose-limiting toxicity with delayed nadir. Nausea and vomiting. Diarrhea, stomatitis, and/or anorexia. Fatigue, orthostatic hypotension, and dizziness. Peripheral neuropathy. Lethargy, fatigue, headache, ataxia, dizziness. Rash, itching, and mild alopecia may occur.

Chair time: No chair time. Repeat cycle every 28 days until progression.

MALIGNANT MESOTHELIOMA

COMBINATION REGIMENS

Doxorubicin + Cisplatin[1,340]

Prechemo: CBC, Chem, Mg^{2+}. Multigated angiogram (MUGA) scan. HT_3 and dexamethasone. Moderately to highly emetogenic.

Doxorubicin 60 mg/m²: IV push on day 1. Potent vesicant.

Cisplatin 60 mg/m²: IV in 500–1000 cc NS on day 1.

Side effects: Myelosuppression may be severe. Nausea and vomiting acute or delayed. Stomatitis. Cardiac: Acutely, pericarditis-myocarditis syndrome may occur. With high cumulative doses of doxorubicin >550 mg/m², cardiomyopathy may occur. Red-orange discoloration of urine. Nephrotoxicity is dose related with cisplatin, provide with adequate hydration. Decreased Mg^{2+}, K^+, Ca^{2+}, Na^+, and P. Peripheral sensory neuropathy. Paresthesias and numbness. Risk increases with cumulative doses. High-frequency hearing loss and tinnitus with cisplatin. Hyperpigmentation, photosensitivity, and radiation recall. Complete alopecia.

Chair time: 3 hours on day 1. Repeat cycle every 21–28 days.

Cyclophosphamide + Doxorubicin + Cisplatin (CAP)[1,341]

Prechemo: CBC, Chem, Mg^{2+}. Multigated angiogram (MUGA) scan. HT_3 and dexamethasone. Moderately to highly emetogenic.

Cyclophosphamide 500 mg/m²: IV in 500 cc NS on day 1.

Doxorubicin 50 mg/m²: IV push on day 1. Potent vesicant.

Cisplatin 80 mg/m²: IV in 500–1000 cc NS on day 1.

Side effects: Myelosuppression may be severe. Nausea and vomiting acute or delayed. Stomatitis. Cardiac: acutely, pericarditis-myocarditis syndrome may occur. With high cumulative doses doxorubicin >550 mg/m², cardiomyopathy may occur. Hemorrhagic cystitis, dysuria, and increased urinary frequency. Provide adequate hydration. Red-orange discoloration of urine. Nephrotoxicity dose related with cisplatin, provide adequate hydration. Decreased Mg^{2+}, K^+, Ca^{2+}, Na^+, and P. Peripheral sensory neuropathy. Paresthesias and numbness, increases with cumulative doses. High-frequency hearing loss and tinnitus with cisplatin. Hyperpigmentation, photosensitivity, and radiation recall. Complete alopecia.

Chair time: 3 hours on day 1. Repeat cycle every 21 days.

Gemcitabine + Cisplatin[1,342]

Prechemo: CBC, Chem, Mg^{2+}, and LFTs. 5-HT$_3$ and dexamethasone. Moderately to highly emetogenic.

Gemcitabine 1000 mg/m^2: IV in 250 cc NS over 30 minutes on days 1, 8, and 15.

Cisplatin 100 mg/m^2: IV in 500–1000 cc NS on day 1.

Side effects: Myelosuppression dose-limiting. Thrombocytopenia more common in older patients. Prolonged infusion time of gemcitabine (>60 minutes) leads to higher toxicities. Nausea and vomiting, acute or delayed. Diarrhea and/or mucositis. Asymptomatic fever. Nephrotoxicity with cisplatin; provide adequate hydration, diuresis, slower infusion time. Neuropathy with numbness, tingling, and sensory loss. Ototoxicity. Decreased Mg^{2+}, K^+, Ca^{2+}, Na^+, and P. Elevation of serum transaminase and bilirubin levels. Pruritic, maculopapular skin rash, usually involving trunk and extremities. Edema. Alopecia.

Chair time: 3 hours on day 1 and 1 hour on days 8 and 15. Repeat cycle every 28 days.

Gemcitabine + Carboplatin [1,343]

Prechemo: CBC, Chem, Mg^{2+}, and LFTs. 5-HT$_3$ and dexamethasone. Diphenhydramine 25–50 mg and H_2 antagonist for hypersensitivity reactions.

Gemcitabine 1000 mg/m^2: IV in 250 cc NS over 30 minutes on days 1, 8, and 15.

Carboplatin AUC 5: IV in 500 cc NS on day 1.

Side effects: Hypersensitivity reaction risk increases with more than seven courses of carboplatin. Myelosuppression dose-limiting, grades 3 and 4 thrombocytopenia more common in older patients. G-CSF recommended. Prolonged infusion time of gemcitabine (>60 minutes) leads to higher toxicities. Nausea and vomiting acute or delayed. Diarrhea and/or mucositis. Asymptomatic fever. Nephrotoxicity with carboplatin, provide adequate hydration. Elevation of serum transaminase and bilirubin levels. Pruritic, maculopapular skin rash, usually involving trunk and extremities. Edema. Alopecia.

Chair time: 2 hours on day 1 and 1 hour on days 8 and 15. Repeat cycle every 28 days.

Pemetrexed + Cisplatin[1,344]

Prechemo: CBC, Chem, Mg^{2+}. 5-HT$_3$. Dexamethasone 4 mg PO bid for 3 days, starting the day before treatment. Folic acid 1 mg PO qd, starting 5 days before the first treatment ending 21 days after the last dose of pemetrexed. Vitamin B12 1000 mcg IM during the week preceding the first dose and every three cycles thereafter (may be given the same day as pemetrexed from second dose on for convenience). 5-HT$_3$ and dexamethasone. Moderately to highly emetogenic.

Pemetrexed 500 mg/m^2: IV in 100 cc of NS over 10 minutes on day 1.

Cisplatin 75 mg/m^2: IV in 500–1000 cc NS over 2 hours on day 1, 30 minutes after pemetrexed.

Side effects: Myelosuppression is dose-limiting toxicity. Administer vitamin B12 and folic acid supplements to minimize hematologic toxicities. Nausea and vomiting acute or delayed. Anorexia, stomatitis, and pharyngitis. Nephrotoxicity with cisplatin; may require dose adjustments, provide adequate hydration, diuresis, as well as slower infusion time. Decreased Mg^{2+}, K^+, Ca^{2+}, Na^+, and P. Neuropathy with numbness, tingling, and sensory loss, cumulative effect. Ototoxicity. Pruritus and rash with pemetrexed. Alopecia.

Chair time: 3 hours on day 1. Repeat cycle every 21 days.

MULTIPLE MYELOMA

COMBINATION REGIMENS

Melphalan + Prednisone[1,345]

Prechemo: CBC, Chem, renal function tests, and LFTs. Bone marrow biopsy. Oral 5-HT$_3$. Mildly to moderately emetogenic.

Melphalan 8–10 mg/m²: PO on days 1–4. (2-mg tablets.) Take on empty stomach.

Prednisone 60-mg/m²: PO on days 1–4. Take with food. Repeat every 42 days.

Side effects: Myelosuppression dose-limiting, prolonged and cumulative. Nadir 4–6 weeks. Gastric irritation, increased appetite. Nausea and vomiting. Steroid toxicities: sodium and water retention, cushingoid changes, behavioral changes, including emotional lability, insomnia, mood swings, and euphoria. Increase glucose and sodium levels, decrease potassium levels. Insulin and warfarin doses may need to be adjusted. Muscle weakness, loss of muscle mass, osteoporosis, and pathological fractures with prolonged use of steroids. Cataracts or glaucoma.

Chair time: No chair time.

Vincristine + Doxorubicin + Dexamethasone (VAD)[1,346]

Prechemo: CBC, Chem, renal function tests, and LFTs. Bone marrow biopsy, MUGA, central line placement. 5-HT$_3$ and dexamethasone. Mildly to moderately emetogenic.

Vincristine 0.4 mg/day: IV continuous infusion on days 1–4. Vesicant.

Doxorubicin 9 mg/m²/day: IV continuous infusion on days 1–4. Potent vesicant.

Dexamethasone 40 mg: PO on days 1–4, 9–12, and 17–20.

Mix vincristine and doxorubicin together in 50–100 mL to run over 4 days.

Side effects: Myelosuppression dose-limiting toxicity. Nausea and vomiting. Constipation and paralytic ileus. Gastric irritation, increased appetite. Cardiotoxicity: doxorubicin doses >550 mg/m^2 may result in cardiomyopathy. Acutely, pericarditic-myocarditis syndrome may occur and can be acute or delayed. Discoloration of urine from pink to red. Peripheral neuropathy with numbness, weakness, myalgias, and late severe motor difficulties. Jaw pain. Steroid toxicities: sodium, water retention, cushingoid changes, hyperglycemia, hypokalemia, increased sodium levels, mood changes, headache, insomnia, depression, and psychosis. Muscle weakness, loss of muscle mass, osteoporosis, and pathological fractures with prolonged use. Warfarin and insulin doses may need to be increased. Cataracts or glaucoma. Alopecia.

Chair time: 30 minutes on day 1 and 5. Repeat every 28 days.

Thalidomide + Dexamethasone [1,347]

Prechemo: CBC, Chem, renal function tests, and LFTs. Bone marrow biopsy.

Thalidomide 200 mg: PO daily. (50- and 100-mg tablets.) Take at bedtime.

Dexamethasone 40 mg: PO on days 1–4, 9–12, and 17–20 (odd cycles).

Dexamethasone 40 mg: PO on days 1–4 (even cycles). Should be taken with food.

Side effects: Thalidomide is teratogenic. Must complete registration with Celgene STEPS program and authorization every 28 days. Drowsiness, fatigue, peripheral neuropathy. Increased sedation with barbiturates, alcohol, chlorampromazine, and reserpine. Constipation can be severe. Initiate prophylactic bowel program. Gastric irritation, increased appetite. Maculopapular skin rash, urticaria, and dry skin. Stevens-Johnson syndrome has been reported. Steroid toxicities: sodium and water retention, cushingoid changes, hyperglycemia, hypokalemia, increased sodium level. Warfarin and insulin doses may need to be increased. Muscle weakness, loss of muscle mass, osteoporosis, and pathological fractures with prolonged use. Mood changes, euphoria, headache, insomnia, depression, and psychosis. Cataracts or glaucoma may develop.

Chair time: No chair time. Repeat cycles every 28 days.

M2 Protocol [1,348]

Prechemo: CBC, Chem, renal function tests, and LFTs. Bone marrow biopsy, pulmonary function tests. 5-HT$_3$ and dexamethasone. Moderately to highly emetogenic.

Vincristine 0.03 mg/kg: IV push through side port of free-flowing IV day 1. Vesicant.

Carmustine (BCNU) 0.5 mg/kg: IV in 500 cc D5W on day 1.

Melphalan 0.25 mg/kg: PO on days 1–4. (2-mg tablets.)

Cyclophosphamide 10 mg/kg: IV in 500 cc NS on day 1.

Prednisone 1 mg/kg: PO on days 1–7; taper after first week; discontinue on day 21.

Side effects: Myelosuppression dose-limiting, delayed and cumulative. Double nadir on days 7–14 and 4–6 weeks after treatment. Nausea and vomiting. Constipation and paralytic ileus. Gastric irritation, increased appetite with prednisone. Hemorrhagic cystitis: preventable with appropriate hydration. Pulmonary toxicity with carmustine doses >1400 mg. Peripheral neuropathy, including numbness, weakness, myalgias, and late severe motor difficulties. Jaw pain. Alopecia. Steroid toxicities: sodium and water retention, cushingoid changes, hyperglycemia, hypokalemia, increased sodium level. Warfarin and insulin doses may need to be increased. Muscle weakness, loss of muscle mass, osteoporosis, and pathological fractures with prolonged use; mood changes, euphoria, headache, insomnia, depression, and psychosis; cataracts or glaucoma.

Chair time: 3 hours on day 1. Repeat cycle every 35 days.

Vincristine + Carmustine + Melphalan + Cyclophosphamide + Prednisone (VBMCP)[1,349]

Prechemo: CBC, Chem, renal function tests, and LFTs. Bone marrow biopsy, pulmonary function tests. 5-HT$_3$ and dexamethasone. Moderately to highly emetogenic.

Vincristine 1.2-mg/m²: IV push through side port of free-flowing IV on day 1.

Carmustine 20 mg/m²: IV in 500 cc D5W on day 1.

Melphalan 8-mg/m²: PO on days 1–4.

Cyclophosphamide 400-mg/m²: IV in 500 cc NS on day 1.

Prednisone 40-mg/m²/day: PO on days 1–7 (all cycles) and

Prednisone 20 mg/m²/day: PO on days 8–14 (first three cycles only).

Side effects: Myelosuppression. Nausea and vomiting. Constipation and paralytic ileus. Gastric irritation, increased appetite with prednisone. Hemorrhagic cystitis: provide appropriate hydration. Pulmonary toxicity with carmustine doses >1400 mg. Peripheral neuropathy including numbness, weakness, myalgias, and late severe motor difficulties. Jaw pain. Alopecia. Steroid toxicities: sodium and water retention, cushingoid changes, hyperglycemia, hypokalemia, increased sodium. Warfarin and insulin doses may need to be increased; muscle weakness, loss of muscle mass, osteoporosis, and pathological fractures with prolonged use; mood changes, euphoria, headache, insomnia, depression and psychosis; cataracts or glaucoma.

Chair time: 2–3 hours day 1. Repeat cycle every 35 days for 10 cycles (induction) and then every 42 days for 3 cycles and then every 56 days until relapse.

Liposomal Doxorubicin (Doxil) + Bortezomib (Velcade)[1,350]

Prechemo: CBC, Chem, LFTs, and renal function tests. Bone marrow biopsy and MUGA. 5-HT$_3$ and dexamethasone. Mildly to moderately emetogenic.

Bortezomib 1.3 mg/m^2: IV push followed by saline flush on days 1, 4, 8, and 11.

Liposomal Doxorubicin 30 mg/m^2: IV in 250 cc D5W on day 4 after bortezomib. Initial rate 1 mg/min to help minimize the risk of infusion reactions.

Side effects: Infusion reactions. Myelosuppression, particularly thrombocytopenia, can be severe. Nausea, vomiting, and diarrhea. Mucositis/stomatitis is mild to moderate. Anorexia, constipation, and dehydration also seen. Cardiac: acutely, pericarditis, and/or myocarditis, electrocardiographic changes, or arrhythmias. Not dose related. With high cumulative doses of Doxil >550 mg/m^2, cardiomyopathy may occur. Fatigue, malaise, and generalized weakness. Peripheral neuropathy. Red-orange discoloration of urine. Hand-foot syndrome on hands and in areas under tight clothing with skin rash, swelling, erythema, pain, and /or desquamation. Hyperpigmentation of nails, urticaria, and radiation recall.

Chair time: 1 hour on days 1, 8, and 11. 2 hours, day 4. Repeat every 21 days.

Lenalidomide (Revlimid) + Dexamethasone[1,351]

Prechemo: CBC, Chem, LFTs. Pregnancy test for women of childbearing age. Bone marrow biopsy. Oral 5-HT$_3$ if nausea occurs. Mildly emetogenic.

Lenalidomide 25 mg: By mouth daily on days 1–21. (5-, 10-, 15-, and 25-mg capsules.) Take with water. Do not break, chew, or open capsules.

Dexamethasone 40 mg: Pulse dose. Days 1–4, 9–12, and 17–20 for the first four cycles and then dexamethasone 40 mg PO on days 1–4 of each subsequent cycle.

Side effects: Lenalidomide is teratogenic; it is an analogue of thalidomide. Register with RevAssist® program. Myelosuppression severe, dose delay/reductions. Deep venous thrombosis (DVT) and pulmonary embolism. Use with care with impaired renal function. Diarrhea common, constipation, nausea with vomiting, and stomach pain. Dry mouth. Anorexia. Nasopharyngitis, cough dyspnea, pharyngitis, epistaxis, dyspnea on exertion, rhinitis, and bronchitis. Arthralgia, back pain, muscle cramps, and myalgias. Fatigue, dizziness, vertigo, headache, hypoesthesia, insomnia, depression, and peripheral neuropathy. Pruritus, rash, and dry skin. Edema in extremities with or without pain. Steroid toxicities: sodium, water retention, cushingoid changes, hyperglycemia, hypokalemia, increased sodium levels, mood changes, headache, insomnia, depression, and psychosis. Warfarin and insulin doses may need to be increased.

Chair time: No chair time. Repeat cycle every 28 days.

SINGLE-AGENT REGIMENS

Dexamethasone[1,350]

Pretreatments: CBC, Chem, renal function tests, and LFTs. Bone marrow biopsy. Oral H_2 antagonist or PPI to prevent gastritis. Mildly emetogenic.

Dexamethasone 40 mg: IV or PO on days 1–4, 9–12, and 17–20. Take with food.

Side effects: Elevated white blood cell count secondary to demargination. Gastric irritation, increased appetite. Steroid toxicities: sodium and water retention, cushingoid changes, hyperglycemia, hypokalemia, increased sodium level. Warfarin and insulin doses may need to be increased. Muscle weakness, loss of muscle mass, osteoporosis, and pathological fractures with prolonged use. Mood changes, euphoria, headache, insomnia, depression, and psychosis. Cataracts or glaucoma.

Chair time: No chair time. Repeat cycle every 21 days.

Melphalan[1,351]

Prechemo: CBC, Chem, RFTs, and LFTs. Bone marrow biopsy. 5-HT_3 and dexamethasone. Moderately to severly emetogenic.

Melphalan 90–140 mg/m²: IV in 100 cc NS over minimum of 15 minutes on day 1.

Side effects: Hypersensitivity reactions, can be severe. Symptoms include diaphoresis, hypotension, and cardiac arrest. Myelosuppression dose-limiting, prolonged, and cumulative. Nadir 4–6 weeks. Nausea and vomiting. Alopecia rare.

Chair time: 1 hour on day 1. Repeat every 28–42 days.

Thalidomide[1,352]

Pretreatment: CBC, Chem, renal function tests, and LFTs. Pregnancy test in women of child bearing age. Bone marrow biopsy.

Thalidomide 200–800 mg/m²: PO daily. (50-, 100- and 200-mg tablets.) Take at bedtime.

Side effects: Teratogenic. Patients must be using birth control. Registration with Celgene STEPS program to dispense. Drowsiness, fatigue, peripheral neuropathy. Increased sedation with barbiturates, alcohol, chlorampromazine, and reserpine. Constipation; can be severe. Initiate prophylactic bowel program. Maculopapular skin rash, urticaria, and dry skin. Stevens-Johnson syndrome, reported.

Chair time: No chair time. Continue treatment until progression or undue toxicity.

Bortezomib (Velcade)[1,353]

Prechemo: CBC, Chem, renal function tests, and LFTs. Bone marrow biopsy. 5-HT_3 and dexamethasone. Mildly to moderately emetogenic.

Bortezomib 1.3 mg/m^2: IV push followed by saline flush on days 1, 4, 8, and 11. If disease is progressive after two cycles or stable after four cycles, may add:

Dexamethasone 20 mg: PO daily on the day of and the day after bortezomib.

Side effects: Myelosuppression, expecially neutropenia and thrombocytopenia. Nausea and vomiting, anorexia, constipation, and dehydration. Orthostatic hypotension. Fatigue, malaise, and generalized weakness. Mix of sensorimotor neuropathy. Steroid toxicities: sodium and water retention, cushingoid changes, behavioral changes, including emotional lability, insomnia, mood swings, and euphoria. May increase glucose and sodium levels, decrease potassium level, and affect warfarin dose. Muscle weakness, loss of muscle mass, osteoporosis, and pathological fractures with prolonged use. Cataracts or glaucoma.

Chair time: 1 hour on days 1, 4, 8, and 11. Repeat cycle every 21 days.

Interferon α-2b[1,354]

Prechemo: CBC, Chem, LFTs. Central line placement. Acetaminophen 650 mg 30 minutes before treatment and every 4 hours, may alternate with Ibuprofen 400 mg PO every 4 hours. Oral 5-HT_3. Mildly to moderately emetogenic.

Interferon α-2b: 2 million units Sub Q or IM 3 times per week.

Side effects: Fever, chills, headache, myalgias, and arthralgias. Increase PO fluid intake. Myelosuppression, cumulative effect, dose-limiting. Nausea and diarrhea. Anorexia cumulative and dose-limiting. Taste alteration and xerostomia. Dizziness, confusion, decreased mental status, and depression. Somnolence, irritability, and poor concentration. Dry skin, pruritus, and irritation at injection site occur. Alopecia is partial.

Chair time: 1 hour for self-injection teaching. Use as maintenance therapy in patients with significant response to induction chemotherapy.

MYELODYSPLASTIC SYNDROME

SINGLE-AGENT REGIMENS

Azacitidine (Vidaza)[1,357]

Prechemo: CBC, Chem, renal function tests, and LFTs. Bone marrow biopsy. Oral 5-HT$_3$ or phenothiazine 30 minutes prior to daily dosing. Mildly to moderately emetogenic.

Azacitidine 75 mg/m^2: SC days 1–7. Minimum of four cycles, therapeutic effects may not be seen until five or more cycles completed. Dose may be increased to 100 mg/m^2 if no beneficial effect is seen after two treatment cycles and if no toxicity other than nausea and vomiting.

Side effects: Myelosuppression may require dose reductions. Baseline WBC >3.0 X 10^9/L, ANC >1.5 X 10^9/L, and platelets > 75 X 10^9/L. Dose adjustments should then be based on nadir counts and bone marrow biopsy cellularity at the time of the nadir. Anemia may occur or be exacerbated. Nausea and vomiting, diarrhea, constipation, stomatitis, and tongue ulceration. Dysphagia, dyspepsia, and abdominal distention. Elevated serum creatinine, renal failure, renal tubular acidosis seen. If unexplained reductions in serum bicarbonate levels (<20 mEq/L) or elevations in BUN or serum creatinine occur, delay treatment until values return to normal or baseline, then reduce dose by 50%. Decreased breath sounds, pleural effusion, rhonchi atelectasis, exacerbation of dyspnea, postnasal drip, and chest wall pain. Hypotension, syncope. Lethargy, increased fatigue, malaise, and hypoesthesia. Erythema, pruritus, swelling, pain, bruising, injection site granuloma, and injection site pigmentation changes. Rotate injection sites. Peripheral edema, urticaria, and dry skin reported.

Chair time: 30 minutes on days 1–7. Repeat cycle every 28 days as tolerated.

Arsenic Trioxide (Trisenox)[1,358]

Prechemo: CBC, Chem, renal function tests, and LFTs. 12-lead EKG and weekly throughout treatment. Oral 5-HT$_3$ or phenothiazine if nausea occurs. Mildly emetogenic.

Arsenic trioxide 0.3 mg/kg: IV in 100–250 cc NS over 1–4 hours on days 1–5 and then twice weekly for 11 weeks.

Side effects: Vasomotor reactions, flushing, tachycardia, dizziness, headaches, and lightheadedness. Increase infusion time to 4 hours to resolve. APL differentiation syndrome: characterized by fever, dyspnea, weight gain, pulmonary infiltrates, and pleural or pericardial effusions, with or without leukocytosis. Can be fatal. Treat with dexamethasone 10 mg IV bid for at least 3 days or longer until signs and symptoms abate. QT interval prolongation and complete atrioventricular block, can progress to a torsade de pointes-type fatal ventricular arrhythmia. Hypokalemia, hypomagnesemia, and hyperglycemia. Less commonly, hyperkalemia, hypocalcemia, hypoglycemia, and acidosis occur. Keep potassium level >4.0 mEq/dL and magnesium >1.8 mg/dL. Myelosuppression. Edema. Disseminated intravascular coagulation (DIC). Nausea and vomiting, abdominal pain, diarrhea, constipation, anorexia, dyspepsia, abdominal tenderness or distention, and dry mouth. Increased hepatic transaminases ALT and AST seen. Use with caution in patients with renal impairment. Cough, dyspnea, epistaxis, hypoxia, pleural effusion, postnasal drip, wheezing, decreased breath sounds, crepitations, rales/crackles, hemoptysis, tachypnea, and rhonchi. Arthralgias, myalgias, generalized pain. Fatigue, insomnia, and paresthesias. Dizziness, tremors, seizures, somnolence, and (rarely) coma. Pruritus, ecchymosis, dry skin, erythema, hyperpigmentation, and urticaria. Injection site reactions.

Chair time: 2 hours on days 1–5 and then twice weekly for 11 weeks. May repeat cycle if response is seen.

Lenalidomide (Revlimid)[1,359]

Prechemo: CBC, Chem, LFTs. Pregnancy test for women of childbearing age. Bone marrow biopsy to determine a deletion 5q cytogenetic abnormality with or without additional cytogenetic abnormalities. Oral 5-HT$_3$ if nausea occurs.

Lenalidomide 10 mg: PO daily until disease progression or daily for 21 days, repeat every 28 days. (5-, 10-, 15-, and 25-mg capsules.) Take with water. Do not break, chew, or open capsules.

Side effects: Teratogenic. Lenalidomide is an analogue of thalidomide. Register with RevAssist® program. Myelosuppression severe, dose delay/reductions. Blood product support and/or growth factors. Deep venous thrombosis (DVT) and pulmonary embolism. Use with care with impaired renal function. Diarrhea, constipation, nausea with vomiting, and stomach pain. Dry mouth. Anorexia. Nasopharyngitis, cough dyspnea, pharyngitis, epistaxis, dyspnea on exertion, rhinitis, and bronchitis. Arthralgia, back pain, muscle cramps, and myalgias. Fatigue, dizziness, vertigo, headache, hypoesthesia, insomnia, depression, and peripheral neuropathy. Pruritus, rash, and dry skin. Edema.

Chair time: No chair time. Weekly CBC first 8 weeks of therapy and then monthly.

Decitabine (Dacogen)[1,360,361]

Prechemo: CBC, Chem. Bone marrow biopsy.

Dacogen 15 mg/m^2: IV in 100 cc NS over 3 hours every 8 hours for 3 days.

OR

Dacogen 20 mg/m^2: IV in 100 cc NS over 1 hour daily for 5 days.

OR

Dacogen 10 mg/m^2: IV in 100 cc NS over 1 hour daily for 10 days.

OR

Dacogen 10 mg/m^2: Subcutaneously BID for 5 days.

Side effects: Myelosuppression. Growth factors and prophylactic antibiotics are recommended. Transfusions as indicated. Fatigue with pyrexia, arthralgias, myalgias, bone, and back pain. Nausea and vomiting, anorexia, stomatitis. Constipation and diarrhea. Ecchymosis, rash, and petechiae.

Chair time: 4 hours for 3-day protocol; 2 hours for 5- or 10-day protocol. 30 minutes for subcutaneous dosing. Repeat cycle every 6 weeks for a minimum of four cycles; complete or partial response may take longer than four cycles. Continue as long as the patient continues to benefit.

OVARIAN CANCER

COMBINATION REGIMENS

Carboplatin + Cyclophosphamide (CC)[1,362]

Prechemo: CBC, Chem, renal function tests, and LFTs, CA-125. 5-HT$_3$ and dexamethasone. Moderately to highly emetogenic.

Carboplatin 300 mg/m^2: IV in 500 cc NS on day 1.

Cyclophosphamide 600 mg/m^2: IV in 500 cc NS on day 1.

Side effects: Hypersensitivity reactions, risk increases with more than seven courses of carboplatin. Myelosuppression dose-limiting. Nausea and vomiting. Increased LFTs and bilirubin. Hemorrhagic cystitis, dysuria, and increased urinary frequency. Decreased Mg^{2+}, K$^+$, Ca^{2+}, Na$^+$, and P. Hyperpigmentation of skin and nails. Alopecia.

Chair time: 3 hours on day 1. Repeat cycle every 28 days.

Cisplatin + Cyclophosphamide (CP)[1,363]

Prechemo: CBC, Chem, renal function tests, LFTs, and CA-125. 5-HT$_3$ and dexamethasone. Moderately to highly emetogenic.

Cisplatin 100 mg/m^2: IV in 1000 cc NS on day 1.

Cyclophosphamide 600 mg/m^2: IV in 500 cc NS on day 1.

Side effects: Myelosuppression severe and dose-limiting. Nausea and vomiting acute or delayed. Nephrotoxicity dose related with cisplatin. Hemorrhagic cystitis, dysuria, and urinary frequency. Decreased Mg^{2+}, K$^+$, Ca^{2+}, Na$^+$, and P. Hyperpigmentation of skin and nails. Dose-limiting peripheral sensory neuropathy. Paresthesias and numbness. Ototoxicity. Complete alopecia.

Chair time: 4 hours on day 1. Repeat cycle every 28 days.

Cisplatin + Paclitaxel (CT)[1,364]

Prechemo: CBC, Chem, renal function tests, LFTs, and CA-125. Central line placement. 5-HT$_3$ and dexamethasone. Diphenhydramine 25–50 mg and H$_2$ antagonist. Moderately to highly emetogenic.

Cisplatin 75 mg/m^2: IV in 1000 cc NS on day 2.

Paclitaxel 135 mg/m^2: IV over 24 hours on day 1.

Side effects: Hypersensitivity reaction with paclitaxel. Myelosuppression cumulative and dose-limiting. G-CSF support recommended. Nausea and vomiting acute or delayed. Nephrotoxicity is dose related. Provide adequate hydration. Decreased Mg^{2+}, K$^+$, Ca^{2+}, Na$^+$, and P. Severe neuropathy with numbness, tingling, and sensory loss. Increased risk with cumulative dose. Alopecia.

Chair time: 1 hour on day 1 and 3 hours on day 2. Repeat cycle every 21 days.

Carboplatin + Paclitaxel[1,365]

Prechemo: CBC, Chem, renal function tests, LFTs, and CA-125. 5-HT$_3$ and dexamethasone. Diphenhydramine 25–50 mg and H$_2$ antagonist. Moderately to highly emetogenic.

Paclitaxel 175 mg/m^2: IV in 500 cc NS over 3 hours day 1.

Carboplatin AUC 6.0–7.5: IV in 500 cc NS on day 1. Given after paclitaxel to decrease toxicities.

Side effects: Hypersensitivity reaction with paclitaxel or with more than seven courses of carboplatin. Myelosuppression, cumulative and dose-limiting. G-CSF support recommended. Nausea and vomiting acute or delayed. Decreased Mg^{2+}, K$^+$, Ca^{2+}, Na$^+$, and P. Severe neuropathy with numbness and tingling. Proprioception, vibrating sense, and motor function loss. Increased risk with cumulative dosing. Alopecia.

Chair time: 5 hours on day 1. Repeat cycle every 21 days until disease progression.

Carboplatin + Docetaxel[1,366]

Prechemo: CBC, Chem, renal function tests, LFTs, and CA-125. 5-HT$_3$ and dexamethasone 8-mg PO bid day before, day of, and day after treatment. Moderately to highly emetogenic.

Carboplatin AUC 6: IV in 500 cc NS on day 1.

Docetaxel 60 mg/m^2: IV in 250 cc NS on day 1. Use non-PVC containers and tubings.

Side effects: Hypersensitivity reaction with docetaxel and risk increases with more than seven courses of carboplatin. Myelosuppression cumulative and dose-limiting. G-CSF support recommended. Nausea and vomiting. Decreased Mg^{2+}, K^+, Ca^{2+}, Na^+, and P. Peripheral neuropathy. Pruritic rash, nail changes, onycholysis, and alopecia.

Chair time: 4 hours on day 1. Repeat cycle every 21 days.

Gemcitabine + Liposomal Doxorubicin[1,367]

Prechemo: CBC, Chem, LFTs. Oral 5-HT_3 or IV 5-HT_3 and dexamethasone 10 mg. Mildly to moderately emetogenic.

Gemcitabine 1000 mg/m^2: IV in 250 cc NS on days 1 and 8.

Liposomal doxorubicin 30 mg/m^2: IV in 250 cc D5W over 1 hour on day 1.

Side effects: Infusion reaction with liposomal doxorubicin with first dose or cumulative doses. Less frequent with slower infusion. Myelosuppression dose-limiting especially with thrombocytopenia. Prolonged infusion time of gemcitabine (>60 minutes) associated with higher toxicities. Flu-like syndrome. Nausea, vomiting, stomatitis, and diarrhea usually mild. Early non-dose related pericarditis and/or myocarditis, electrocardiographic changes, or arrhythmias. With high cumulative doses liposomal doxorubicin >550 mg/m^2, cardiomyopathy may occur. Elevation of serum transaminase and bilirubin levels. Hand-foot syndrome dose related. Rash, erythema, and desquamation may be seen in areas under tight clothing. Edema. Hyperpigmentation of nails, urticaria, and radiation recall can occur. Alopecia is rare.

Chair time: 2 hours weekly for 3 weeks. Repeat cycle every 21 days.

Gemcitabine + Cisplatin[1,368]

Prechemo: CBC, Chem, LFTs, creatinine clearance, and CA-125. 5-HT_3 and dexamethasone 10–20 mg. Moderately to highly emetogenic.

Gemcitabine 800–1000 mg/m^2: IV in 250 cc NS over 30 minutes on days 1 and 8.

Cisplatin 30 mg/m^2: IV on days 1 and 8 in 1000 cc NS.

Side effects: Hypersensitivity reaction. Myelosuppression G-CSF recommended. Diarrhea and/or mucositis. Fever, malaise, chills, headache, and myalgias. Nephrotoxicity, neurotoxicity, electrolyte imbalance. Elevation of serum transaminase and bilirubin levels. Pruritic, maculopapular skin rash, involving trunk and extremities. Edema. Ototoxicity. Alopecia.

Chair time: 3 hours on days 1 and 8. Repeat cycle every 21 days.

Gemcitabine + Carboplatin[1,369]

Prechemo: CBC, Chem, LFTs, renal function tests, and CA-125. 5-HT_3 and dexamethasone. Diphenhydramine 25–50 mg and H_2 antagonist. Moderately emetogenic.

Gemcitabine 1000 mg/m²: IV in 250 cc NS over 30 minutes on days 1 and 8.

Carboplatin AUC 4: IV in 500 cc NS on day 1.

Side effects: Hypersensitivity reaction; risk increases with more than seven courses of carboplatin. Myelosuppression dose-limiting, grades 3 and 4 thrombocytopenia more common in older patients. G-CSF recommended. Infusion time gemcitabine >60 minutes leads to higher toxicities. Nausea and vomiting; acute or delayed. Diarrhea and/or mucositis. Flu-like syndrome with asymptomatic fever. Nephrotoxicity with carboplatin, provide adequate hydration and diuresis. Alopecia.

Chair time: 3 hours on day 1 and 1 hour on day 8. Repeat cycle every 21 days.

Intraperitoneal (IP) Cisplatin + Paclitaxel[1,370,371]

Prechemo: CBC, Chem (including Mg^{2+}) and CA125. Central line placement. IP port placement. Moderately to severely emetogenic.

Premedicate: Dexamethasone 20 mg PO 12 and 6 hours prior to chemo day 1. $5HT_3$ and dexamethasone 10–20 mg day 2 and 8. Diphenhydramine 25–50 mg and H_2 antagonist day 1 and 8. Aprepitant 125 mg PO 1 hour prior to chemo day 2. 80 mg PO days 3 and 4.

DAY 1:

Paclitaxel 135 mg/m²: IV over 24 hours. Use non-PVC containers and tubing with 0.22-micron inline filter.

DAY 2:

D5 ½ NS + 20 KCl/L + 2gms MgSo4/L IV@ 500 cc/hr × 2 hours

Cisplatin 75–100 mg/m²: IP in 1–2 L warmed normal saline by gravity wide open. Flush catheter and D/C huber when infused. Reposition patient from right side to left side Q 15 min × 1 hour.

D5 ½ NS + 20 meq KCl + 2 gms MgSO4/L IV@ 250cc/hr × 2 hours.

DAY 8:

Paclitaxel 60 mg/m²: IP in 1–2 L warmed normal saline by gravity wide open. Flush catheter and D/C huber after paclitaxel infused. Reposition patient from right side to left side Q 15 min × 1 hour.

Side effects: Hypersensitivy reaction. Paclitaxel. Premedicate as described days 1 and 8. Myelosuppression is cumulative, dose related, and can be dose-limiting. G-CSF support recommended. Monitor CBC prior to treatment days 1 and 8 of each cycle. Nausea and vomiting moderate to severe, may be acute or delayed. Nephrotoxicity is dose related with cisplatin. Ensure normal creatinine prior to treatment day 2 of each cycle. Decreases Mg^{2+}, K^+, Ca^{2+}, Na^+, and P. Sensory neuropathy with numbness and paresthesias, dose related.Total alopecia.

Chair time: 1 hour day 1, 5–6 hours day 2, and 3 hours day 8. Repeat cycle every 21 days for six cycles.

SINGLE-AGENT REGIMENS

Altretamine (Hexalen) [1,372]

Prechemo: CBC, Chem, renal function tests, CA-125. Oral phenothiazine or 5-HT$_3$.

Altretamine 260 mg/m^2/day: PO in four divided doses after meals and at bedtime. 50-mg capsules.

Side effects: Myelosuppression, dose-limiting toxicity. Nausea and vomiting is cumulative and dose-limiting. Diarrhea and cramps, dose-limiting. Peripheral sensory neuropathy. Agitation, confusion, hallucinations, depression, mood disorders, and Parkinson-like symptoms. Elevations in BUN or creatinine.

Chair time: No chair time. Repeat cycle every 14–21 days.

Liposomal Doxorubicin (Doxil) [1,373]

Prechemo: CBC, Chem, CA-125. MUGA. 5-HT$_3$ and dexamethasone 10–20mg. Moderately to highly emetogenic.

Liposomal doxorubicin 50 mg/m^2: IV over 1 hour on day 1. Dilute doses up to 90 mg in 250 cc of D5W.

Side effects: Infusion reactions with rapid infusion. Myelosuppression dose-limiting. Nausea and vomiting. Mild stomatitis and/or diarrhea. Pericarditis and/or myocarditis, electrocardiographic changes, or arrhythmias, not dose related. With cumulative doses >550 mg/m^2, cardiomyopathy. Typical hand-foot syndrome and rash, erythema, and desquamation in areas of restricted blood flow (e.g., areas where clothing is tight). Hyperpigmentation of nails, skin rash, urticaria, and radiation recall. Alopecia.

Chair time: 2 hours on day 1. Repeat cycle every 28 days.

Paclitaxel [1,374]

Prechemo: CBC, Chem, Mg^{2+}, and CA-125. 5-HT$_3$ and dexamethasone 10–20 mg. Diphenhydramine 25–50 mg and H$_2$ antagonist. Mildly emetogenic.

Paclitaxel 135 mg/m^2: IV in 500 cc NS over 3 hours on day 1. Use non-PVC containers and tubing with 0.22-micron inline filter.

Side effects: Hypersensitivity reaction. Myelosuppression dose-limiting. G-CSF recommended. Nausea and vomiting. Stomatitis. Sensory neuropathy with numbness and paresthesias, dose related. Arthralgias and myalgias. Transient elevations in serum transaminases, bilirubin, and alkaline phosphatase. Alopecia.

Chair time: 4 hours on day 1. Repeat every 21 days until progression.

Topotecan[1,375]

Prechemo: CBC, Chem, LFTs, and CA-125. 5-HT$_3$ and dexamethasone 10 mg. Mildly to moderately emetogenic.

Topotecan 1.5 mg/m^2: IV in 100 cc NS on days 1–5.

Side effects: Myelosuppression severe and dose-limiting. If severe neutropenia occurs dose reduce by 0.25 mg/m^2 or use G-CSF for future cycles. Nausea and vomiting, dose related. Diarrhea, and/or constipation, abdominal pain. Microscopic hematuria. Alopecia.

Chair time: 1 hour on days 1–5. Repeat every 21 days until progression.

Gemcitabine[1,376]

Prechemo: CBC, Chem, LFTs, and CA-125. Oral phenothiazine or 5-HT$_3$ and dexamethasone 10 mg. Mildly to moderately emetogenic.

Gemcitabine 800 mg/m^2: IV in 250 cc NS over 30 minutes on days 1, 8, and 15.

Side effects: Myelosuppression dose-limiting with grades 3 and 4 thrombocytopenia more common in older patients. Nausea, vomiting, diarrhea, and mucositis. Flu-like syndrome. Mild dyspnea and drug-induced pneumonitis. Transient elevation of serum transaminases and bilirubin. Pruritic, maculopapular skin rash, usually involving trunk and extremities. Edema. Alopecia is rare.

Chair time: 1 hour on days 1, 8, and 15. Repeat cycle every 28 days.

Etoposide[1,377]

Prechemo: CBC, Chem, LFTs, and CA-125. Oral phenothiazine or 5-HT$_3$. Mildly emetogenic protocol.

Etoposide 50 mg/m^2: PO on days 1–21. (50- or 100-mg capsules.) Give as single dose up to 400 mg; for doses >400 mg, divide into two to four doses. Refrigerate.

Side effects: Myelosuppression may be severe. Nausea and vomiting mild to moderate. More commonly observed with oral administration. Metallic taste to food. Neurotoxicities: peripheral neuropathies mild. Alopecia.

Chair time: Repeat cycle every 28 days as tolerated or until disease progression.

OVARIAN CANCER: GERM CELL

COMBINATION REGIMENS

Etoposide + Bleomycin + Cisplatin (BEP) [1,378]

Prechemo: CBC, Chem, renal function tests. Pulmonary function tests and chest x-ray baseline and before each cycle of therapy. 5-HT$_3$ and dexamethasone 10–20 mg. Acetaminophen 30 minutes before bleomycin. Moderately to severely emetogenic.

Bleomycin 30 units: IV push or infusion over 15 minutes on days 2, 9, and 16. A test dose of two units recommended before the first dose to detect hypersensitivity.

Etoposide 100 mg/m^2: IV in 250 cc NS over 1 hour on days 1–5.

Cisplatin 20 mg/m^2: IV in 500–1000 cc NS over 1–2 hours on days 1–5.

Side effects: Allergic reaction with bleomycin, infusion reaction with Etoposide during rapid infusion. Myelosuppression dose-limiting. Nausea and vomiting acute or delayed. Pulmonary toxicity with bleomycin, dose-limiting. Increased risk with dose >400 units. Nephrotoxicity dose related with cisplatin. Risk may be reduced with adequate hydration. Decreased Mg^{2+}, K, Ca^{2+}, Na$^+$, and P. Peripheral sensory neuropathy, dose-limiting. Paresthesias and numbness. Ototoxicity. Alopecia.

Chair time: 3 hours on days 1–5 and 1 hour on days 9 and 16. Repeat every 21 days.

PANCREATIC CANCER

LOCALLY ADVANCED DISEASE

5-Fluorouracil + Radiation Therapy (GITSG)[1,379]

Prechemo: CBC, Chem, and CA 19-9. Oral phenothiazine or 5-HT$_3$. Mildly emetogenic.

Fluorouracil 500 mg/m^2/day: IV push days 1–3 and 29–31, then weekly begining day 71.

Radiation therapy: Total dose, 4000 cGy. Chemotherapy and radiation started on the same day and given concurrently.

Side effects: Myelosuppression, dose-limiting. Nausea and vomiting and dehydration may worsen throughout treatment. Mucositis and diarrhea severe and dose-limiting. Local tissue irritation in radiation field progressing to desquamation. Do not use oil-based lotions or creams in radiation field. Hyperpigmentation, photosensitivity, nail changes, and hand-foot syndrome dose-limiting. Photophobia, increased lacrimation, conjunctivitis, and blurred vision.

Chair time: 1 hour on days 1–3 and 29–31, 1 hour weekly beginning on day 71.

METASTATIC DISEASE

COMBINATION REGIMENS

5-Fluorouracil + Leucovorin[1,380]

Prechemo: CBC, Chem, and CA 19-9. Oral phenothiazine or 5-HT$_3$. Mildly emetogenic.

5-FU 425 mg/m^2/day: IV push 1 hour after start of leucovorin on days 1–5.

Leucovorin 20 mg/m^2/day: IV push on days 1–5.

Side effects: Myelosuppression, dose-limiting. Nausea and vomiting. Mucositis and diarrhea severe and dose-limiting. Alopecia, diffuse thinning of hair. Hyperpigmentation, photosensitivity, and nail changes may occur. Hand-foot syndrome dose-limiting. Photophobia, increased lacrimation, conjunctivitis, and blurred vision.

Chair time: 1 hour on days 1–5. Repeat cycle every 28 days for six cycles.

Gemcitabine + Capecitabine (Xeloda)[1,381]

Prechemo: CBC, Chem, LFTs, renal function tests, CA 19-9. Oral phenothiazine or 5-HT$_3$ and dexamethasone 10 mg. Mildly to moderately emetogenic.

Gemcitabine 1000 mg/m²: IV in 250 cc NS on days 1 and 8.

Capecitabine 650 mg/m²: PO bid on days 1–14. (150- and 500-mg tablets.) Do not cut tablets. Administer within 30 minutes of a meal with plenty of water. Monitor international normalized ratios (INRs) closely in patients taking warfarin; may increase INR.

Side effects: Myelosuppression dose-limiting, grades 3 and 4 thrombocytopenia more common in older patients. Prolonged infusion time (>60 minutes) gemcitabine associated with higher toxicities. Nausea and vomiting, diarrhea, and/or mucositis. Flu-like syndrome. Xeloda contraindicated when creatinine clearance >30 mL/min. Creatinine clearance of 30–50 mL/min at baseline should be dose reduced to 75% of total Xeloda dose. Reduce dose for hyperbilirubinemia. Hand-foot syndrome. Pruritic, maculopapular skin rash, edema. Alopecia is rare.

Chair time: 1 hour days 1 and 8. Repeat cycle every 21 days until progression.

Gemcitabine + Docetaxel + Capecitabine (GTX)[1,382]

Prechemo: CBC, Chem, LFTs, renal function tests, and CA 19-9. 5-HT$_3$ IV, Dexamethasone 8-mg PO bid day before, day of, and day after docetaxel. Moderately emetogenic.

Gemcitabine 750 mg/m²: IV in 250 cc NS over 75 minutes days 4 and 11.

Docetaxel 30 mg/m²: IV in 250 cc NS on days 4 and 11. Use non-PVC containers and tubing.

Capecitabine 1000–1500 mg/m²: PO bid on days 1–14. (150- and 500-mg tablets.) Do not cut tablets. Administer within 30 minutes of a meal with plenty of water. Monitor INRs closely in patients taking warfarin; may increase INR.

Side effects: Hypersensitivity reactions with docetaxel. Myelosuppression dose-limiting. Nausea and vomiting, diarrhea, and mucositis. Peripheral neuropathy, paresthesias, and numbness. Flu-like syndrome. Xeloda contraindicated when creatinine clearance >30 mL/min. For baseline creatinine clearance 30–50 mL/min dose reduced to 75% of total Xeloda dose. Reduce dose for hyperbilirubinemia. Hand-foot syndrome. Pruritic, maculopapular skin rash, edema.

Chair time: 3 hours on days 4 and 11. Repeat cycle every 21–28 days until disease progression.

Gemcitabine + Cisplatin[1,383]

Prechemo: CBC, Chem, LFTs, creatinine clearance, and CA 19-9. 5-HT$_3$ and dexamethasone 10–20 mg. Moderately to highly emetogenic.
Gemcitabine 1000 mg/m²: IV in 250 cc NS on days 1, 8, and 15.
Cisplatin 50 mg/m²: IV in 1000 cc NS on days 1 and 15.
Side effects: Hypersensitivity reaction. Myelosuppression, G-CSF recommended. Diarrhea and/or mucositis. Fever, malaise, chills, headache, and myalgias. Nephrotoxicity, neurotoxicity, electrolyte imbalance. Elevation of serum transaminase and bilirubin levels. Pruritic, maculopapular skin rash, involving trunk and extremities. Edema. Ototoxicity. Alopecia.
Chair time: 3 hours on days 1 and 15. 1 hour on day 8. Repeat cycle every 28 days.

Gemcitabine + Cisplatin (modified)[1,384]

Prechemo: CBC, Chem, LFTs, creatinine clearance, and CA 19-9. 5-HT$_3$ and dexamethasone 10–20 mg. Moderately to highly emetogenic.
Gemcitabine 600–750 mg/m²: IV in 250 cc NS on days 1 and 15.
Cisplatin 25-30 mg/m²: IV in 1000 cc NS on days 1 and 15.
Side effects: Hypersensitivity reaction. Myelosuppression G-CSF recommended. Diarrhea and/or mucositis. Fever, malaise, chills, headache, and myalgias. Nephrotoxicity, neurotoxicity, electrolyte imbalance. Elevation of serum transaminase and bilirubin levels. Pruritic, maculopapular skin rash, involving trunk and extremities. Edema. Ototoxicity. Alopecia.
Chair time: 3 hours on days 1 and 15. Repeat cycle every 28 days.

Gemcitabine + Cisplatin (fixed dose rate)[1,385,386]

Prechemo: CBC, Chem, LFTs, creatinine clearance, and CA 19-9. 5-HT$_3$ and dexamethasone 10–20 mg. Moderately to highly emetogenic.
Gemcitabine 1000 mg/m²: IV in 250 cc NS @10 mg/m²/min on days 1 and 8.
Cisplatin 20 mg/m²: IV in 1000 cc NS on days 1 and 8.
Side effects: Hypersensitivity reaction. Myelosuppression. G-CSF recommended. Diarrhea and/or mucositis. Fever, malaise, chills, headache, and myalgias. Nephrotoxicity, neurotoxicity, electrolyte imbalance. Elevation of serum transaminase and bilirubin levels. Pruritic, maculopapular skin rash, involving trunk and extremities. Edema. Ototoxicity. Alopecia.
Chair time: 3 hours on days 1 and 8. Repeat cycle every 21 days.

Gemcitabine + Oxaliplatin (GemOx)[1,387]

Prechemo: CBC, Chem, Mg^{2+}, LFTs, and CA 19-9. 5-HT$_3$ and dexamethasone 10–20 mg. Moderately emetogenic.

Gemcitabine 1000 mg/m^2: IV over 100 minutes (10 mg/m^2/min) on day 1.

Oxaliplatin 100 mg/m^2: IV in 250 cc D5W over 2 hours on day 2.

Side effects: Myelosuppression dose-limiting with grade 3 and 4 thrombocytopenia more common in older patients. Prolonged infusion time of gemcitabine >60 minutes is associated with higher toxicities. Nausea and vomiting, diarrhea, mucositis. Peripheral sensory neuropathy with distal paresthesias dose-limiting. Acute dysesthesias in the laryngopharyngeal region can occur within hours or 1–3 days after therapy. Exposure to cold can exacerbate these symptoms. Avoid cold beverages and food as well as cold air. Flu-like syndrome. Elevation of serum transaminase and bilirubin levels. Pruritic, maculopapular skin rash. Edema. Alopecia is rare.

Chair time: 2 hours on day 1 and 3 hours on day 2. Repeat every 2 weeks until progression.

Gemcitabine + Irinotecan (Gemiri)[1,388]

Prechemo: CBC, Chem, LFTs, renal function tests, and CA 19-9. 5-HT$_3$ and dexamethasone 10 mg. Atropine 0.5–1.0 mg IV unless contraindicated. Moderately to highly emetogenic.

Gemcitabine 1000 mg/m^2: IV in 250 cc NS over 30 minutes on days 1 and 8.

Irinotecan 100 mg/m^2: IV in 500 cc D5W over 90 minutes on days 1 and 8.

Side effects: Myelosuppression dose-limiting, G-CSF recommended. Nausea and vomiting. Diarrhea, acute (cholinergic effect) or delayed, can be severe; treat aggressively, dose-limiting. Mucositis. Flu-like syndrome. Elevation of serum transaminase and bilirubin levels. Pruritic, maculopapular skin rash. Edema. Alopecia is mild.

Chair time: 3 hours on days 1 and 8. Repeat every 21 days until progression.

5-Fluorouracil + Doxorubicin + Mitomycin (FAM)[1,389]

Prechemo: CBC, Chem, LFTs, CA 19-9, and MUGA scan. 5-HT$_3$ and dexamethasone 20 mg. Moderately to highly emetogenic.

Fluorouracil 600 mg/m^2/day: IV push on days 1, 8, 29, and 36.

Doxorubicin 30 mg/m^2: IV push on days 1 and 29. Potent vesicant.

Mitomycin 10 mg/m^2: IV push on day 1. Potent vesicant.

Side effects: Myelosuppression dose-limiting and cumulative. Nausea and vomiting, mucositis, and diarrhea can be severe and dose-limiting.

Hemolytic-uremic syndrome. Red-orange discoloration of urine. Hyperpigmentation, photosensitivity, radiation recall, and nail changes. Hand-foot syndrome can be dose-limiting. Doxorubicin can cause cardiomyopathy with cumulative doses >550 mg/m². Photophobia, increased lacrimation, conjunctivitis, and blurred vision. Alopecia.

Chair time: 1 hour on days 1, 8, 29, and 36. Repeat cycle every 56 days.

Gemcitabine + Erlotinib (Tarceva)[1,390]

Prechemo: CBC, Chem, LFTs, CA19-9. Oral phenothiazine or 5-HT$_3$ (oral or IV).

Gemcitabine 1000 mg/m²: IV in 250 cc NS weekly for 7 weeks, 1 week rest, subsequent cycles: 1000 mg/m² IV weekly for 3 weeks with 1 week rest.

Erlotinib 100-mg: PO daily. (25-, 100-, and 150-mg tablets.) 1 hour prior to eating or 2 hours after eating. Dose modification: decrease in 50-mg increments.

Side effects: Myelosuppression dose-limiting with grade 3 and 4 thrombocytopenia more common in older patients. Nausea and vomiting, mucositis. Diarrhea mild to moderate. Flu-like syndrome. Elevation of serum transaminase and bilirubin levels. Rash with Tarceva, from maculopapular to pustular on the face, neck, chest, back, and arms. Treat with corticosteroids, topical clindamycin, or minocycline. Conjunctivitis and dry eyes. Interstitial lung disease with dyspnea, low-grade fever, rapidly becoming more severe. Erlotinib should be stopped immediately with worsening, unexplained pulmonary symptoms. Inducers of the CYP3A4 pathway may increase metabolism of erlotinib and decrease plasma concentrations, and inhibitors of the CYP3A4 pathway may increase the metabolism of erlotinib and increase plasma concentrations.

Chair time: 1 hour weekly for 7 weeks, 1 week rest. Then, 1 hour weekly. Repeat cycle every 28 days.

Streptozocin + Mitomycin + 5-Fluorouracil (SMF)[1,391]

Prechemo: CBC, Chem, and CA 19-9. 5-HT$_3$ and dexamethasone 10–20 mg. Moderately to highly emetogenic.

Streptozocin 1000 mg/m²: IV over 1 hour on days 1, 8, 29, and 36. Administer with 1–2 L of hydration to avoid renal toxicity.

Mitomycin 10 mg/m²: IV push on day 1. Potent vesicant.

Fluorouracil 600 mg/m²: IV push on days 1, 8, 29, and 36.

Side effects: Myelosuppression cumulative and dose-limiting. Renal dysfunction with streptozocin; transient proteinuria and azotemia, may progress to permanent renal failure. Hemolytic-uremic syndrome. Dose-limiting. Nausea and vomiting. Mucositis and diarrhea severe and dose-limiting. Hyperpigmentation, photosensitivity, and nail changes. Hand-foot syndrome dose-limiting. Hypoglycemia or hyperglycemia. Photophobia, increased lacrimation, conjunctivitis, and blurred vision.

Chair time: 3 hours on days 1, 8, 29, and 36. Repeat cycle every 72 days until progression.

SINGLE-AGENT REGIMENS

Gemcitabine [1,392,393]

Prechemo: CBC, Chem, and LFTs. Oral phenothiazine or 5-HT$_3$ and dexamethasone 10 mg. Mildly to moderately emetogenic.

Gemcitabine 1000 mg/m^2: IV in 250 cc NS over 30 minutes weekly for 7 weeks, 1-week rest. Subsequent cycles weekly for 3 weeks with 1 week break.

OR

Gemcitabine 1000 mg/m^2: IV over 100 minutes at 10 mg/m^2/min on days 1, 8, and 15. Both regimens repeated every 28 days.

Side effects: Myelosuppression dose-limiting with grades 3 and 4 thrombocytopenia more common in older patients. Toxicity increases with longer infusions. Nausea, vomiting, diarrhea, and mucositis. Flu-like syndrome. Mild dyspnea and pneumonitis. Transient elevation of serum transaminases and bilirubin. Pruritic, maculopapular skin rash, usually involving trunk and extremities. Edema. Alopecia is rare.

Chair time: 1–2 hours on days 1, 8, and 15. Repeat cycle every 28 days.

Capecitabine (Xeloda)[1,394]

Prechemo: CBC, Chem, LFTs, creatinine clearance. Oral phenothiazine or 5-HT$_3$. Mildly to moderately emetogenic.

Capecitabine 1250 mg/m^2/day: PO bid on days 1–14.[1,136]

Dose may be decreased to 850–1000 mg/m^2 PO bid on days 1–14. May reduce toxicities without compromising efficacy. 150- and 500-mg tablets. Administer within 30 minutes of a meal with plenty of water. Monitor INRs closely when taking warfarin, may increase INR.

Side effects: Nausea and vomiting. Diarrhea, stomatitis. Contraindicated with creatinine clearance >30 mL/min, dose reduce for creatinine clearance of 30–50 mL/min at baseline to 75% of dose. Hand-foot syndrome characterized by tingling, numbness, pain, erythema, dryness, rash, swelling, increased pigmentation, and/or pruritus of the hands and feet. Stop at first signs of hand-foot syndrome or diarrhea. Blepharitis, tear-duct stenosis, acute and chronic conjunctivitis. Reduce dose with elevations in serum bilirubin alkaline phosphatase and hepatic transaminase (SGOT, SGPT) levels.

Chair time: No chair time. Repeat cycle every 21 days for a total of eight cycles.

PROSTATE CANCER

COMBINATION REGIMENS

Flutamide + Leuprolide[1,395]

Pretreatment: CBC, Chem, LFTs, renal function tests, and prostate-specific antigen (PSA). Oral phenothiazine or 5-HT$_3$. Mildly emetogenic.

Flutamide 250 mg: PO TID. 125-mg capsules. Monitor INR when on warfarin increases anticoagulant effect. Start 2 weeks before leuprolide.

Leuprolide 7.5 mg: IM monthly or 22.5 mg IM every 3 months or 30 mg IM every 4 months.

Side effects: Nausea, vomiting, diarrhea, and/or constipation, mild. Decreased libido and impotence. Gynecomastia. Tumor flare within the first 2 weeks with increased bone pain. Hot flashes. Leuprolide can increase BUN and creatinine levels. Peripheral edema secondary to sodium retention. Yellow-green discoloration of urine with flutamide.

Chair time: Office visits every 4, 12, or 16 weeks for leuprolide injections

Flutamide + Goserelin[1,396]

Pretreatment: CBC, Chem, LFTs, renal function tests, and PSA. Oral phenothiazine or 5-HT$_3$. Mildly emetogenic.

Flutamide 250 mg: PO TID. 125-mg capsules. Monitor INR when on warfarin increases anticoagulant effect.

Goserelin 10.8 mg: SQ every 12 weeks. Inject into upper abdomen parallel to the abdominal wall. May use lidocaine before injection.

Side effects: Nausea, vomiting, diarrhea, and/or constipation. Decreased libido, impotence, hot flashes, and gynecomastia. Tumor flare within first 2 weeks with increased bone pain. Yellow-green discoloration of urine with flutamide.

Chair time: Office visits every 12 weeks for goserelin injections.

Estramustine + Etoposide[1,397]

Prechemo: CBC, Chem, LFTs, renal function tests, and PSA. Oral phenothiazine or 5-HT$_3$. Mildly to moderately emetogenic.

Estramustine 15 mg/kg/day: PO in four divided doses on days 1–21. (140-mg capsules.) Store in refrigerator. Take at least 1 hour before or 2 hours after meals. Milk products and calcium-rich foods may impair absorption. Contraindicated thrombophlebitis or thromboembolic disorder.

Etoposide 50 mg/m^2/day: PO in two divided doses on days 1–21. (50- or 100-mg capsules.) Store capsules in refrigerator. May prolong PT/INR when on warfarin.

Side effects: Myelosuppression dose-limiting toxicity. Nausea and vomiting within 2 hours of ingestion; intractable vomiting after prolonged therapy (6–8 weeks). Diarrhea. Gynecomastia with breast tenderness. Hot flashes. Dose reduce etoposide with abnormal renal function. Rash, pruritus, dry skin, peeling skin of fingertips, thinning hair, and night sweats.

Chair time: No chair time. Weekly CBCs; repeat cycle every 28 days.

Estramustine + Vinblastine[1,398]

Prechemo: CBC, Chem, LFTs, and PSA. Oral phenothiazine or 5-HT$_3$. Mildly to moderately emetogenic.

Estramustine 600 mg/m^2: PO daily on days 1–42. (140-mg capsules.) Store in refrigerator. Take at least 1 hour before or 2 hours after meals. Milk products and calcium-rich foods may impair absorption of drug. Contraindicated with thrombophlebitis or thromboembolic disorder.

Vinblastine 4 mg/m^2: IV push weekly for 6 weeks. Vesicant.

Side effects: Myelosuppression dose-limiting. Nausea and vomiting within 2 hours of ingestion; intractable vomiting after prolonged therapy (6–8 weeks). Diarrhea, abdominal pain, constipation, or adynamic ileus. Peripheral neuropathy, jaw pain. Stomatitis can be severe. Gynecomastia with breast tenderness. Dose reduce estramustine for hepatic dysfunction. Rash, pruritus, dry skin, peeling skin of fingertips, and night sweats. Alopecia is mild.

Chair time: 1 hour weekly for 6 weeks. Repeat cycle every 8 weeks.

Paclitaxel + Estramustine[1,399]

Prechemo: CBC, Chem, LFTs, renal function tests, and PSA. Central line placement. 5-HT$_3$ and dexamethasone 10–20 mg. Diphenhydramine 25–50 mg and H$_2$ antagonist before paclitaxel day 1. Oral phenothiazine or 5-HT$_3$ before estramustine.

Paclitaxel 120 mg/m^2: IV infuse continuously over 96 hours days 1–4. Use non-PVC containers and tubing with 0.22-micron inline filter.

Estramustine 600 mg/m²: PO daily; start 24 hours before paclitaxel. 140-mg capsules. Store in refrigerator. Take at least 1 hour before or 2 hours after meals. Milk products and calcium-rich foods may impair absorption of drug. Contraindicated with thrombophlebitis or thromboembolic disorder.

Side effects: Hypersensitivity reaction with paclitaxel. Myelosuppression, may be dose-limiting. Nausea and vomiting occur within 2 hours of ingestion; intractable vomiting after prolonged therapy. Diarrhea. Sensory neuropathy. Proprioception, vibrating sense, and motor function loss. Gynecomastia with breast tenderness. Rash, pruritus, dry skin, peeling skin of fingertips, and night sweats. Alopecia.

Chair time: 2 hours day 1. Repeat cycle every 21 days as tolerated.

Mitoxantrone + Prednisone[1,400]

Prechemo: CBC, Chem, LFTs, and PSA. MUGA scan. Oral phenothiazine or 5-HT$_3$. Mildly emetogenic.

Mitoxantrone 12 mg/m²: IV day 1. Vesicant. Dilute in at least 50 mL D5W or NS.

Prednisone 5 mg: PO bid daily. 5-mg tablet. Administer with meals or antacid.

Side effects: Myelosuppression dose-limiting toxicity. Gastric irritation. May increase appetite and cause weight gain. Nausea and vomiting. Mucositis and diarrhea not severe. Increased susceptibility to infections, may mask infections. Cardiomyopathy with cumulative doses of mitoxantrone >140 mg/m². CHF, hypertension, and edema. Hypokalemia and hypocalcemia with increased excretion of potassium and calcium. Osteoporosis, loss of muscle mass, muscle weakness with long-term, high-dose steroid therapy. Cataracts or glaucoma. Emotional lability, insomnia, mood swings, euphoria, and psychosis. Blue discoloration of fingernails, sclera, and urine for 1–2 days after treatment. Alopecia.

Chair time: 1 hour on day 1. Repeat cycle every 21 days.

Docetaxel + Estramustine[1,401]

Prechemo: CBC, Chem, renal function tests, and PSA. Oral phenothiazine or 5-HT$_3$. Mildly emetogenic.

Dexamethasone 4 mg: PO bid day before, day of, and day after treatment. Oral phenothiazine or 5-HT$_3$ on days 1–3 of weeks 1 and 2.

Docetaxel 40–80 mg/m²: IV in 250 cc NS day 2. Use non-PVC containers and tubing.

Estramustine 280 mg: PO TID on days 1–5. (140-mg capsules.) Store in refrigerator. Take at least 1 hour before or 2 hours after meals. Milk products and calcium-rich foods may impair absorption of drug. Contraindicated with thrombophlebitis or thromboembolic disorder.

Side effects: Hypersensitivity reactions with docetaxel. Myelosuppression dose-limiting. Nausea and vomiting occur within 2 hours of ingestion; intractable vomiting may occur after prolonged therapy. Diarrhea. Peripheral neuropathy. Fluid retention syndrome with weight gain, peripheral and/or generalized edema, pleural effusion, and ascites. Gynecomastia with breast tenderness. Dose reduce for hepatic dysfunction. Rash and dry, pruritic skin seen. Nail changes, discoloration of nail beds, onycholysis. Alopecia.

Chair time: 2 hours on day 2. Repeat cycle every 21 days.

Docetaxel + Prednisone[1, 402]

Prechemo: CBC, Chem, LFTs, renal function tests, and PSA. Oral or IV 5-HT$_3$.

Docetaxel 75 mg/m^2: IV in 250 cc NS on day 1. Use non-PVC containers and tubing.

Prednisone 5 mg: PO bid. 5-mg tablet. Administer with meals or an antacid.

Side effects: Hypersensitivity reactions with docetaxel. Myelosuppression dose-limiting. Peripheral neuropathy. Fluid retention syndrome with weight gain, peripheral and/or generalized edema, pleural effusion, and ascites. CHF, hypertension, and edema in susceptible patients. Dose reduce for hepatic dysfunction. Gastritis, increased appetite, and weight gain. Steroids suppress immune system. Hypokalemia and hypocalcemia with increased excretion of potassium and calcium. Cataracts, glaucoma, osteoporosis, loss of muscle mass, and muscle weakness with long-term, high-dose therapy. Emotional lability, insomnia, mood swings, euphoria, and psychosis.

Chair time: 2 hours on day 1. Repeat cycle every 21 days for up to 10 cycles.

SINGLE-AGENT REGIMENS

Paclitaxel[1, 403,404]

Prechemo: CBC, Chem, Mg^{2+}, and PSA. Central line placement. 5-HT$_3$ and dexamethasone 10–20 mg. Diphenhydramine 25–50 mg and H$_2$ antagonist. Mildly to moderately emetogenic.

Paclitaxel 135–170 mg/m^2: IV over 24 hours on day 1. Use non-PVC containers and tubing with 0.22-micron inline filter. Repeat cycle every 3 weeks.

OR

Paclitaxel 150 mg/m^2: IV in 500 cc NS over 1 hour weekly for 6 weeks. Repeat every 8 weeks.

Side effects: Hypersensitivity reaction. Myelosuppression dose-limiting G-CSF recommended. Nausea and vomiting. Stomatitis. Sensory neuropathy with numbness and paresthesias, dose related. Arthralgias and myalgias. Transient elevations in serum transaminases, bilirubin, and alkaline phosphatase. Alopecia.

Chair time: 2 hours on day 1. Repeat cycle every 3 weeks.

OR

Every 8 weeks.

Docetaxel[1,405]

Prechemo: CBC, Chem, LFTs, and PSA. Dexamethasone 8 mg bid day before, day of, and day after treatment. 5-HT$_3$ in 100 cc NS. Mildly to moderately emetogenic.

Docetaxel 75 mg/m²: IV in 250 cc NS on day 1. Repeat cycle every 21 days.

OR

Docetaxel 20–40 mg/m²: IV weekly for 3 weeks Repeat cycle every 4 weeks. Use non-PVC containers and tubing.

Side effects: Hypersensitivity reactions. Myelosuppression, G-CSF recommended. Nausea and vomiting, mild. Mucositis and diarrhea. Peripheral neuropathy with paresthesias. Fluid retention with weight gain, peripheral and/or generalized edema, pleural effusion, and ascites. Nail changes, rash, and dry, pruritic skin. Hand-foot syndrome. Alopecia.

Chair time: 2 hours on day 1. Repeat cycle every 21 days.

OR

Every 4 weeks.

Estramustine[1,406]

Pretreatment: CBC, Chem, LFTs, and PSA. Oral phenothiazine or 5-HT$_3$.

Estramustine 14 mg/kg/day: PO in three to four divided doses. 140-mg capsules. Store in refrigerator. Take at least 1 hour before or 2 hours after meals. Milk products and calcium-rich foods may impair absorption of drug. Contraindicated with thrombophlebitis or thromboembolic disorders.

Side effects: Nausea and vomiting occur within 2 hours of ingestion, are usually mild to moderate. Intractable vomiting may occur after prolonged therapy (6–8 weeks). Diarrhea. Gynecomastia with breast tenderness. Myelosuppression, rare. Abnormal calcium and phosphorus levels. Rash, pruritus, dry skin, peeling skin of fingertips, thinning hair, and night sweats.

Chair time: No chair time. Repeat daily as tolerated or until progression.

Goserelin (Zoladex)[1,407]

Pretreatment: CBC, Chem, LFTs, renal function tests, and PSA. Oral phenothiazine or 5-HT$_3$ if needed.

Goserelin 3.6 mg: SC every 28 days; 10.8 mg SQ every 12 weeks. Inject into upper abdomen parallel to the abdominal wall. Lidocaine before injection.

Side effects: Nausea and vomiting rare and mild. Constipation or diarrhea uncommon. Decreased libido and impotence, gynecomastia with breast tenderness. Tumor flare usually within the first 2 weeks with increased bone pain, urinary retention. Hot flashes.

Chair time: No chair time. Office visits every 28 days.

OR

Every 12 weeks for injections.

Leuprolide (Lupron)[1,408,409]

Pretreatment: CBC, Chem, LFTs, and PSA. Oral phenothiazine or 5-HT$_3$ if needed.

Leuprolide 7.5-mg: IM every 28 days.

OR

22.5 mg IM every 3 months.

OR

30 mg IM every 4 months.

Side effects: Nausea and vomiting rare. Decreased libido and impotence, gynecomastia with breast tenderness. Tumor flare usually within the first 2 weeks with increased bone pain, urinary retention. Hot flashes. Myelosuppression rare. Use with caution with abnormal renal function, can increase BUN and creatinine. Depression.

Chair time: No chair time. Office visits monthly.

OR

Every 3 months.

OR

Every 4 months for injections.

Bicalutamide[1,410]

Pretreatment: CBC, Chem, LFTs, and PSA. Oral phenothiazine or 5-HT$_3$ if needed.

Bicalutamide 50 mg: PO BID. Patients refractory to other antiandrogen agents may start with a higher dose of 150-mg PO daily. 50-mg tablet. May increase anticoagulant effect of warfarin.

Side effects: Nausea, vomiting, and diarrhea rare. Constipation mild. Decreased libido, impotence, gynecomastia, nipple pain, and galactorrhea. Hot flashes. Myelosuppression rare. Use with caution in patients with abnormal liver function. Monitor LFTs at baseline and throughout treatment.

Chair time: No chair time. Daily until progression.

Flutamide[1,411]

Pretreatment: CBC, Chem, LFTs, renal function tests, and PSA. Oral phenothiazine or 5-HT$_3$.

Flutamide 250 mg: PO TID. 125-mg capsules. May increase anticoagulation effect of warfarin.

Side effects: Nausea, vomiting, and diarrhea mild. Decreased libido and impotence, gynecomastia with breast tenderness. Hot flashes. Myelosuppression rare. Yellow-green discoloration of urine.

Chair time: No chair time. Daily until progression.

Nilutamide[1,412]

Pretreatment: CBC, Chem, LFTs, renal function tests, and PSA. Oral phenothiazine or 5-HT$_3$ if needed.

Nilutamide 300 mg: PO days 1–30 and then 150-mg PO daily. (50- and 150-mg tablets.) May increase anticoagulation effect with warfarin. Treatment should begin the day of or the day after surgical castration.

Side effects: Nausea and anorexia, constipation mild. Decreased libido, impotence, gynecomastia, nipple pain, and galactorrhea. Hot flashes. Abstain from alcohol while taking nilutamide because of increased risk of intolerance. Use with caution with abnormal liver function. Contraindicated with severe liver impairment or severe respiratory insufficiency. Dyspnea is rare but is related to interstitial pneumonitis, a serious side effect. Pneumonitis observed within the first 3 months; incidence may be higher in patients of Asian descent. Impaired adaptation to dark, abnormal vision, and alterations in color vision.

Chair time: No chair time. Daily until progression.

Prednisone[1,400]

Prechemo: CBC, Chem, renal and liver functions. H$_2$ antagonist to prevent gastritis.

Prednisone 5 mg: PO BID. Take with food.

Side effects: Gastric irritation, increased appetite. Steroid toxicities: sodium and water retention, cushingoid changes, behavioral changes, including emotional lability, insomnia, mood swings, and euphoria. May increase glucose and sodium and decrease potassium and affect warfarin dose. Muscle weakness, loss of muscle mass, osteoporosis, and pathologic fractures with prolonged use. Cataracts or glaucoma may develop.

Chair time: No chair time. Continue daily until progression.

Ketoconazole[1,413]

Pretreatment: CBC, Chem, LFTs, and PSA. Oral phenothiazine or 5-HT₃.

Ketoconazole 1200 mg: PO daily. Do not give antacids, cimetidine, ranitidine, famotidine, sucralfate, or other drugs that increase gastric pH for at least 2 hours after taking ketoconazole.

Side effects: Breast enlargement and tenderness may occur in some men, lasting weeks to duration of therapy. Oligospermia, azoospermia, decreased libido, and impotence. Nausea and vomiting. Anorexia. Diarrhea, abdominal pain, flatulence, and constipation. Dizziness, headache, nervousness, insomnia, lethargy, somnolence, and paresthesia. Rash, dermatitis, purpura, urticaria.

Chair time: No chair time. Treat daily as tolerated or until progression.

Aminoglutethimide (Cytadren)[1,414]

Pretreatment: CBC, Chem, LFTs, thyroid function tests, and PSA. Oral phenothiazine or 5-HT₃ if needed.

Aminoglutethimide 250 mg: PO QID. If tolerated, may increase to 500 mg PO QID (250-mg tablets.) Decreases levels of warfarin, phenytoin, phenobarbital, theophylline, medroxyprogesterone, digoxin, and dexamethasone by enhancing their metabolism.

Hydrocortisone 40 mg: PO QD to prevent adrenal insufficiency. Higher doses (100 mg) sometimes used during initial 2 weeks to reduce frequency of adverse events.

Side effects: Maculopapular skin rash, usually occurring in the first week of therapy. Self-limited with resolution in 5–7 days. May be accompanied by malaise and low-grade fever. Fatigue, lethargy, and somnolence. Onset is within the first week of therapy. Dizziness, nystagmus, and ataxia are less common. Mild nausea and vomiting. Hypothyroidism: monitor thyroid function. Adrenal insufficiency in the absence of hydrocortisone replacement. Presents as postural hypotension, hyponatremia, and hyperkalemia. Myelosuppression rarely occurs.

Chair time: No chair time. Treatment is daily as tolerated or until progression.

RENAL CELL CANCER

COMBINATION REGIMENS

Interferon α-2a + IL-2[1,415]

Prechemo: CBC, Chem, LFTs, renal function tests. Acetaminophen 650–1000 mg PO. Oral phenothiazine or 5-HT$_3$. Mildly to moderately emetogenic.

Interferon α-2a 9-million units: SQ days 1–4, weeks 1–4.

Interleukin-2 12-million units: SQ days 1–4, weeks 1–4.

Side effects: Myelosuppression. Flu-like syndrome; chills 3–6 hours after interferon. Fatigue, malaise, headache, and myalgias are cumulative and dose-limiting. Increase PO fluid intake. Continue acetaminophen every 4 hours, may alternate with Ibuprofen. Nausea and vomiting, anorexia, xerostomia, and mild diarrhea. Mild proteinuria and hypocalcemia. Vascular leak syndrome: weight gain, arrhythmias, and/or tachycentias, hypotension, edema, oliguria, and renal insufficiency, pleural effusions, and pulmonary congestion. Dizziness, confusion, and decreased mental status and depression. Somnolence, delirium, are common but usually resolve after interleukin-2 is stopped. Diffuse erythematous rash, may desquamate. Pruritus (with or without rash) and irritation at injection site. Partial alopecia.

Chair time: No chair time. Administer in the office or self-administer. Repeat cycle every 6 weeks.

5-Fluorouracil + Gemcitabine[1,416]

Prechemo: CBC, Chem, and LFTs. Central line placement. Oral phenothiazine or 5-HT$_3$. Mildly to moderately emetogenic.

5-Fluorouracil 150 mg/m²/day: IV continuous infusion on days 1–21.

Gemcitabine 600 mg/m²: IV in 250 cc NS on days 1, 8, and 15.

Side effects: Myelosuppression dose-limiting with grades 3 and 4 thrombocytopenia more common in older patients. Nausea and vomiting. Diarrhea, and/or mucositis can be severe and dose-limiting. Flu-like side effects with fever in absence of infection 6–12 hours after treatment. Elevation of serum transaminase and bilirubin levels. Pruritic, maculopapular skin rash, usually involving trunk and extremities. Hyperpigmentation, photosensitivity, and nail changes. Hand-foot syndrome dose-limiting. Photophobia, increased lacrimation, conjunctivitis, and blurred vision. Edema. Diffuse thinning of hair.

Chair time: 1 hour on days 1, 8, and 15. Repeat every 28 days until progression.

SINGLE-AGENT REGIMENS

Low-Dose IL-2 (Aldesleukin)[1,417]

Prechemo: CBC, Chem, LFTs, renal function tests. Central line placement. Oral phenothiazine or 5-HT$_3$. DO NOT USE corticosteroids. Acetaminophen 650–1000 mg PO.

Interleukin-2. 3 million units/day: IV continuous infusion on days 1–5.

Side effects: Myelosuppression with sever anemia. Nausea and vomiting; diarrhea severe, may require bicarbonate replacement. Flu-like syndrome: fever, chills, headache, malaise, myalgias, and arthralgias; managed with acetaminophen, nonsteroidal anti-inflammatory drugs, and increased oral fluid intake. Capillary leak syndrome: peripheral edema, CHF, pleural effusions, and pericardial effusions reversible once treatment is stopped. Dyspnea, tachypnea, pulmonary edema with hypoxia, as a result of fluid shifts. Oliguria, proteinuria, and increased serum creatinine and BUN levels. Elevated LFTs. Hepatomegaly and hypoalbuminemia. Diffuse erythematous rash, which may desquamate. Pruritus.

Chair time: 1 hour on day 1. Repeat cycle every 14 days for 1 month.

Interferon α-2a[1,418]

Prechemo: CBC, Chem, renal and liver functions. Acetaminophen 650–1000 mg PO. Oral phenothiazine or 5-HT$_3$. Mildly to moderately emetogenic.

Interferon α-2a. 5 to 15 million units: SQ per day 3–5 times per week.

Side effects: Flu-like syndrome: fever, chills, headache, myalgias, and arthralgias. Managed with increased oral fluid intake and acetaminophen (may alternate with Ibuprofen). Myelosuppression. Nausea, vomiting, and diarrhea. Anorexia cumulative and dose-limiting. Taste alteration and xerostomia. Mild proteinuria and hypocalcemia. Mild transient elevations in serum transaminases, dose-dependent toxicity with pre-existing liver abnormalities. Dry skin, pruritus, and irritation at injection. Dizziness, confusion, decreased mental status, and depression. Retinopathy with cotton-wool spots and small hemorrhages; usually asymptomatic and resolves when drug discontinued. Partial alopecia.

Chair time: No chair time. Teach patient to self-administer.

Sorafenib (Nexavar)[1,419]

Prechemo: CBC, Chem, LFTs. Oral phenothiazine. Mildly to moderately emetogenic.

Nexavar 400 mg: PO BID. (200-mg tablets.) Taken on empty stomach (at least 1 hour before or 2 hours after a meal).

Side effects: Rash on trunk and neck, red raised rash with pruritus; resolves after 6 weeks. Hand-foot syndrome with hardened calluses that turn into blisters with moist desquamation, ulceration with severe pain and sloughing of skin. Grade 3 hand-foot syndrome requires interruption/discontinuation of drug therapy. Resume at 50% of the dose when symptoms resolve. Diarrhea, nausea and vomiting, constipation, mucositis, stomatitis, dyspepsia, and dysphagia are common. Hypertension, monitor blood pressure weekly. May resolve after 6 weeks or treat for hypertension as necessary. Splinter hemorrhages of the nails. Multiple drug interactions: CYP3A4 inducers decrease sorafenib serum concentrations and CYP2C9 pathway (INR may increase with patients on warfarin therapy).

Chair time: No chair time. Daily as tolerated until progression.

Sunitinib Malate (Sutent)[1,420]

Prechemo: CBC, Chem, LFTs, and renal function tests. Oral phenothiazine or 5-HT$_3$. Mildly to moderately emetogenic.

Sutent 50 mg: PO per day. 4 weeks on, 2 weeks off. (12.5-, 25-, and 50-mg capsules.) May be taken with or without food. Dose modification: increase or decrease by 12.5 mg based on individual safety and tolerance.

Side effects: Diarrhea, nausea and vomiting, stomatitis, constipation, and abdominal pain. Decreases in left ventricular ejection fraction dysfunction (LVEF). Monitor for signs and symptoms of congestive heart failure (CHF). Patients with cardiac history should have a baseline LVEF. Hypertension, epistaxis. Arthralgia, back pain, and myalgias. Multiple drug interactions: CYP3A4 pathway.

Chair time: No chair time. Take daily for 4 weeks. Repeat cycle every 6 weeks.

Temsirolimus (Torisel)[1,421]

Prechemo: CBC, Chem, serum cholesterol, and triglycerides. PO or IV 5HT$_3$. Diphenhydramine 25–50 mg. Mildly emetogenic.

Temsirolimus 25 mg: IV in 100 cc NS over 30–60 minutes once a week. Use DEHP-free containers and tubing; inline filter not greater than 5 microns.

Side effects: Hypersensitivity reactions; treatment resumed at the discretion of the physician at a slower rate, up to 60 minutes. Myelosuppression; hold for absolute neutrophil count (ANC) <1000 per mm^3 or platelet count <75,000 per mm^3. Dose reduce once toxicities have resolved. Immunosuppression; opportunistic infections. Avoid live vaccines and close contact with those who have received live vaccines. Hyperglycemia/glucose intolerance likely. Mucositis, anorexia, nausea, diarrhea, abdominal pain, constipation, vomiting, and dysgeusia. Cough, hypoxia, fever, and interstitial lung disease. Increases in serum triglycerides and cholesterol. Initiate or increase the dose of lipid-lowering agents as needed. Fatal bowel perforation. Rapidly progressive and sometimes fatal acute renal failure. Elevations in alkaline phosphatase and AST. Hypertension. Venous thromboembolism, thrombophlebitis rare. Asthenia, back pain, arthralgia, and pain. Abnormal wound healing, use with caution in the perioperative period. Patients with central nervous system tumors and/or receiving anticoagulation therapy may be at an increased risk of developing intracerebral bleeding. Use of concomitant strong CYP3A4 inhibitors should be avoided. Rash common. Pruritus, nail disorders, dry skin, and acne.

Chair time: 1 hour on day 1. Repeat weekly until progression or unacceptable toxicity occurs.

SOFT TISSUE SARCOMAS

COMBINATION REGIMENS

Doxorubicin + Dacarbazine (AD)[1,422]

Prechemo: CBC, Chem. Central line placement, MUGA scan. 5-HT$_3$ and dexamethasone 20 mg. Moderately to highly emetogenic.

Doxorubicin 15 mg/m^2/day: IV continuous infusion days 1–4. Potent vesicant.

Dacarbazine 250 mg/m^2/day: IV continuous infusion on days 1–4. Potent vesicant.

Side effects: Myelosuppression dose-limiting toxicity. Nausea and vomiting. Flu-like syndrome: fever, chills malaise, myalgias, and arthralgias. Discoloration of urine from pink to red. Cardiac: acutely, pericarditis-myocarditis syndrome may occur. With high cumulative doses doxorubicin >550 mg/m^2, cardiomyopathy. Paresthesias, neuropathies, ataxia, lethargy, headache, confusion, and seizures. Hyperpigmentation, photosensitivity, and radiation recall. Complete alopecia.

Chair time: 1 hour on day 1. Repeat cycle every 21 days.

Mesna + Doxorubicin + Ifosfamide + Dacarbazine (MAID)[1,423]

Prechemo: CBC, Chem, renal function tests. Central line placement. MUGA scan. 5-HT$_3$ and dexamethasone 10–20 (days 1–4). Moderately to highly emetogenic.

Mesna 2500 mg/m^2/day: IV continuous infusion days 1–4.

Doxorubicin 20 mg/m^2/day: IV continuous infusion on days 1–3. Potent vesicant.

Ifosfamide 2500 mg/m^2/day: IV continuous infusion on days 1–3.

Dacarbazine 300 mg/m^2/day: IV continuous infusion on days 1–3. Potent vesicant.

Side effects: Myelosuppression dose-limiting. Flu-like syndrome: fever, chills, malaise, myalgias, and arthralgias. Nausea and vomiting.

Mucositis and/or diarrhea. Hemorrhagic cystitis with hematuria, dysuria, urinary frequency. Increased BUN and serum creatinine levels, decreased urine creatinine clearance, acute tubular necrosis, pyelonephritis, glomerular dysfunction, and metabolic acidosis. Risk may be reduced with adequate hydration. Lethargy, confusion, seizure, cerebellar ataxia, weakness, hallucinations, and cranial nerve dysfunction. Somnolence, depressive psychosis. Photosensitivity and radiation recall. Alopecia.

Chair time: 1 hour daily days 1–4, refill infusion daily. Repeat cycle every 21 days.

Cyclophosphamide + Vincristine + Doxorubicin + Dacarbazine (CYVADIC)[1,424]

Prechemo: CBC, Chem, MUGA scan. 5-HT$_3$ and dexamethasone 20 mg. Moderately to highly emetogenic.

Cyclophosphamide 500 mg/m^2: IV in 500 cc NS on day 1.

Vincristine 1.5 mg/m^2: IV push on day 1. Maximum dose is 2 mg. Vesicant.

Doxorubicin 50 mg/m^2: IV push on day 1. Potent vesicant.

Dacarbazine 750 mg/m^2: IV in 500–1000 cc NS on day 1. Potent vesicant.

Side effects: Myelosuppression dose-limiting toxicity. Nausea and vomiting severe. Constipation, abdominal pain, or paralytic ileus. Aggressive bowel program suggested. Flu-like syndrome: fever, chills malaise, myalgias, and arthralgias. Cardiac: Acutely, pericarditis-myocarditis syndrome may occur. With cumulative doses of doxorubicin >550 mg/m^2, cardiomyopathy may occur. Hemorrhagic cystitis, dysuria, and increased urinary frequency. Reduced risk with adequate hydration. Discoloration of urine from pink to red. Hyperpigmentation, photosensitivity, and radiation recall. Peripheral neuropathies, paralytic ileus. Bone, back, limb, jaw, and partial gland pain. Paresthesias, neuropathies, ataxia, lethargy, headache, confusion, and seizures. Alopecia.

Chair time: 4 hours on day 1. Repeat cycle every 21 days.

Cyclophosphamide + Doxorubicin + Vincristine (CAV) Alternating with Ifosfamide + Etoposide (IE)[1,425]

Prechemo: CBC, Chem, LFTs, and renal function tests. MUGA scan. 5-HT$_3$ and dexamethasone 20 mg. Moderately to highly emetogenic.

Cyclophosphamide 1200 mg/m^2: IV in 500–1000 cc NS on day 1.

Doxorubicin 75 mg/m^2: IV push on day 1. Potent vesicant.

Vincristine 2-mg: IV push on day 1. Vesicant.

Alternate every 21 days with:

Ifosfamide 1800 mg/m^2: IV in 500–1000 cc NS on days 1–5. Drug interactions phenobarbital, phenytoin, cimetidine, and allopurinol increase toxicity. Ifosfamide may enhance anticoagulant effects of warfarin. **Mesna 15 minutes** before, 4 and 8 hours after, ifosfamide dose.

OR

Mesna tablets at 40% of ifosfamide dose at 2 and 6 hours after ifosfamide.

Etoposide 100 mg/m²/day: IV in 250 cc NS over 1 hour on days 1–5.

Side effects: Myelosuppression may be severe. Nausea and vomiting, acute or delayed. Stomatitis and diarrhea not dose-limiting. Constipation, abdominal pain, or paralytic ileus. Cardiac: acutely, pericarditis-myocarditis syndrome may occur. With cumulative doses of doxorubicin >550 mg/m², cardiomyopathy may occur. Cyclophosphamide may increase the risk of doxorubicin-induced cardiotoxicity. Peripheral neuropathies. Cranial nerve dysfunction rare, jaw pain, diplopia, vocal cord paresis, mental depression, and metallic taste. Hemorrhagic cystitis, hematuria; hydration with 2–3 L per day and uroprotection with mesna 20% of ifosfamide dose. Red-orange discoloration of urine. Dose reduction in the presence of liver dysfunction. Lethargy and confusion at high doses of ifosfamide, usually lasting 1–8 hours and is reversible. Hyperpigmentation, photosensitivity, and radiation recall. Complete alopecia.

Chair time: 2 hours on day 1 with CAV, 3–4 hours days 1–5 with IE. Alternate CAV with IE every 21 days for a total of 17 cycles.

SINGLE-AGENT REGIMENS

Doxorubicin[1,424]

Prechemo: CBC, Chem, MUGA scan. 5-HT$_3$ and dexamethasone 10–20 mg. Mildly to moderately emetogenic.

Doxorubicin 75 mg/m²: IV push on day 1. Potent vesicant.

Side effects: Myelosuppression may be severe. Nausea and vomiting. Dose reduce with liver dysfunction. Pericarditis-myocarditis syndrome. With cumulative doses >550 mg/m² of doxorubicin, cardiomyopathy. Red-orange discoloration of urine. Hyperpigmentation, photosensitivity, and radiation recall occur. Complete alopecia.

Chair time: 1 hour on day 1. Repeat cycle every 21 days until progression.

Gemcitabine[1,426]

Prechemo: CBC, Chem, and LFTs. Oral phenothiazine or 5-HT$_3$ and dexamethasone 10 mg. Mildly to moderately emetogenic.

Gemcitabine 1000 mg/m²: IV in 250 cc NS over 30 minutes weekly for 7 weeks, 1 week rest.

Subsequent Cycles:

Gemcitabine 1000 mg/m²: IV in 250 cc NS over 30 minutes weekly for 3 weeks. Repeat cycle every 28 days.

Side effects: Myelosuppression dose-limiting with grades 3 and 4 thrombocytopenia more common in older patients. Nausea, vomiting, diarrhea, and mucositis. Flu-like syndrome. Mild dyspnea and drug-induced pneumonitis. Transient elevation of serum transaminases and bilirubin. Pruritic, maculopapular skin rash, usually involving trunk and extremities. Edema. Alopecia is rare.

Chair time: 1 hour weekly. Repeat cycle weekly for 7 weeks then 1 week off. Weekly for 3 weeks with 1 week off. Repeat cycle every 28 days subsequent cycles.

TESTICULAR CANCER

ADJUVANT THERAPY

Cisplatin + Etoposide + Bleomycin (PEB)[1,427]

Prechemo: CBC, Chem, renal function test, LDH, and Beta-HCG. Baseline pulmonary function tests, chest x-ray, and before each cycle of therapy. 5-HT$_3$ and dexamethasone 10–20 mg. Acetaminophen 30 minutes before bleomycin. Mildly to moderately emetogenic.

Cisplatin 20 mg/m^2: IV in 500 cc NS on days 1–5.

Etoposide 100 mg/m^2: IV in 250 cc NS on days 1–5.

Bleomycin 30 units: IV push or infused over 15 minutes on days 2, 9, and 16. Test dose of two units recommended before first dose to detect hypersensitivity.

Side effects: Hypersensitivity reaction with bleomycin and cisplatin. Myelosuppression dose-limiting. Nausea and vomiting, acute or delayed; mucositis and diarrhea are rare. Metallic taste and anorexia. Pulmonary toxicity is dose-limiting in bleomycin. Usually presents as pneumonitis with cough, dyspnea, dry inspiratory crackles, and infiltrates on CXR. Nephrotoxicity is dose related with cisplatin. Decreases Mg^{2+}, K^+, Ca, and Na^+. SIADH. Peripheral sensory neuropathy. Paresthesias and numbness. Ototoxicity. Alopecia.

Chair time: 3–4 hours on days 1–5, 1 hour on days 9 and 16. Repeat every 21 days.

ADVANCED DISEASE

Etoposide + Bleomycin + Cisplatin (BEP)[1,428]

Prechemo: CBC, Chem, renal function tests, LDH, and Beta-HCG. Pulmonary function tests and chest x-ray study at baseline and before each cycle of therapy. 5-HT$_3$ and dexamethasone 10–20 mg. Acetaminophen 30 minutes before bleomycin. Moderately to highly emetogenic.

Bleomycin 30 units: IV push or infused over 15 minutes on days 2, 9, and 16. A test dose of two units recommended before the first dose to detect hypersensitivity.

Etoposide 100 mg/m^2: IV in 250 cc NS over 1 hour on days 1–5.

Cisplatin 20 mg/m^2: IV in 500 cc NS over 1–2 hours on days 1–5.

Side effects: Allergic reaction with bleomycin, infusion reaction with etoposide during rapid infusion. Myelosuppression dose-limiting. Nausea and vomiting acute or delayed. Pulmonary toxicity dose-limiting in bleomycin. Nephrotoxicity dose related with cisplatin. Risk may be reduced with adequate hydration. Decreased Mg^{2+}, K, Ca^{2+}, Na^+, and P. Peripheral sensory neuropathy dose-limiting. Paresthesias and numbness. Ototoxicity. Alopecia.

Chair time: 3 hours on days 1–5 and 1 hour days 9 and 16. Repeat cycle every 21 days.

Etoposide + Cisplatin (EP)[1,429]

Prechemo: CBC, Chem, Mg^{2+}, LDH, and Beta-HCG. 5-HT$_3$ and dexamethasone 10–20 mg. Moderately to highly emetogenic.

Etoposide 100 mg/m^2: IV in 250 cc NS on days 1–5.

Cisplatin 20 mg/m^2: IV in 500 cc NS on day 1.

Side effects: Hypersensitivity reaction with etoposide or cisplatin. Myelosuppression dose-limiting toxicity. Nausea and vomiting, acute or delayed. Mucositis and diarrhea are rare. Metallic taste and anorexia. Nephrotoxicity dose related with cisplatin. Risk may be reduced with adequate hydration. Decreases Mg^{2+}, K^+, Ca^{2+}, and Na^+. SIADH. Peripheral sensory neuropathy with paresthesias and numbness. Ototoxicity. Alopecia.

Chair time: 3 hours on day 1 and 1 hour days 2–5. Repeat cycle every 21 days.

Cisplatin + Vinblastine + Bleomycin (PVB)[1,430]

Prechemo: CBC, Chem, renal function tests, LDH, and Beta-HCG. PFTs and chest x-ray study baseline and before each cycle of therapy. 5-HT$_3$ and dexamethasone 10–20 mg. Acetaminophen 30 minutes before bleomycin. Moderately to highly emetogenic.

Cisplatin 20 mg/m^2: IV in 500 cc NS on days 1–5.

Vinblastine 0.15 mg/kg: IV push on days 1 and 2. Vesicant.

Bleomycin 30 units: IV push or infused over 15 minutes on days 2, 9, and 16. Test dose of two units recommended before the first dose to detect hypersensitivity.

Side effects: Hypersensitivity reaction bleomycin (fever and chills) or cisplatin. Myelosuppression dose-limiting toxicity. Nausea and vomiting, acute or delayed. Mucositis and diarrhea are rare. Constipation resulting from neurotoxicity, abdominal pain, or paralytic ileus. Pulmonary toxicity dose-limiting in bleomycin. Nephrotoxicity is dose related with cisplatin. Risk reduced with adequate hydration. Decreases Mg^{2+}, K^+, Ca^{2+}, Na^+, and phosphorus. Paresthesias, peripheral neuropathy, depression, headache, malaise, jaw pain, urinary retention, tachycardia, orthostatic hypotension, and seizures. High-frequency hearing loss and tinnitus. Alopecia.

Chair time: 3 hours on days 1–5 and 1 hour on days 9 and 16. Repeat every 21 days.

Vinblastine + Dactinomycin + Bleomycin (VAB-6)[1,431]

Prechemo: CBC, Chem, LFTs, renal function tests, LDH, and Beta-HCG. PFTs and chest x-ray at baseline and before each cycle of therapy. Central line placement. 5-HT_3 and dexamethasone 20 mg. Acetaminophen 30 minutes before bleomycin. Moderately to highly emetogenic.

Vinblastine 4 mg/m²: IV push on day 1. Vesicant.

Dactinomycin 1 mg/m²: IV push on day 1. Vesicant.

Bleomycin 30 units: IV push or infused over 15 minutes on day 1, and then:

Bleomycin 20 units/m²: IV continuous infusion on days 1–3. Test dose of two units recommended before the first dose to detect hypersensitivity.

Cisplatin 20 mg/m²: IV in 500 cc NS over 1 hour on day 4.

Cyclophosphamide 600 mg/m²: IV in 500 cc NS over 1 hour on day 1.

Side effects: Hypersensitivity reaction bleomycin (fever and chills) or cisplatin. Myelosuppression dose-limiting. Nausea and vomiting, acute or delayed. Irritation and ulceration along the entire GI mucosa. Diarrhea with or without cramps. Anorexia common. Constipation, abdominal pain, or ileus. Pulmonary toxicity dose-limiting in bleomycin. Hepatotoxicity, dose reduce if occurs. Nephrotoxicity or hemorrhagic cystitis. Risk reduced with adequate hydration. Dose reduce for alterations in renal function. Decreases Mg^{2+}, K^+, Ca^{2+}, Na^+, and phosphorus. Paresthesias, peripheral neuropathy, depression, headache, jaw pain, urinary retention, tachycardia, orthostatic hypotension, and seizures. Flulike syndrome: malaise, myalgia, fever, depression. Hyperpigmentation, radiation recall, photosensitivity, rash, and nail changes. Alopecia.

Chair time: 2 hours on days 1 and 4. Repeat cycle every 21 days.

SALVAGE REGIMENS

Vinblastine + Ifosfamide + Cisplatin + Mesna (VeIP)[1,432]

Prechemo: CBC, Chem, renal function tests, LDH, and Beta-HCG. Central line placement. 5-HT_3 and dexamethasone 10–20 mg. Moderately to highly emetogenic.

Vinblastine 0.11 mg/kg: IV push on days 1 and 2. Vesicant.

Ifosfamide 1200 mg/m²: IV in 500–1000 cc NS on days 1–5.

Cisplatin 20 mg/m²: IV in 500 cc NS on days 1–5.

Mesna 400 mg/m²: IV in 100 cc NS given 15 minutes before first ifosfamide dose, and then:

Mesna 1200 mg/m²/day: IV continuous infusion for 5 days.

Side effects: Myelosuppression is cumulative dose-limiting. G-CSF support recommended. Nausea and vomiting acute or delayed. Mucositis and/or diarrhea. Constipation, abdominal pain, ileus rare. Nephrotoxicity and/or hemorrhagic cystitis. Prevented with mesna and vigorous hydration. Decreases Mg^{2+}, K^+, Ca^{2+}, Na^+, and phosphorus. Sensory neuropathy with numbness and paresthesias. Somnolence, confusion, depressive psychosis, or hallucinations with ifosfamide. Paresthesias, jaw pain, urinary retention, and tachycardia. Total alopecia.

Chair time: 3–4 hours on days 1–5. Repeat cycle every 21 days.

Etoposide + Ifosfamide + Cisplatin + Mesna (VIP)[1,433]

Prechemo: CBC, Chem, LFTs, renal function tests, LDH, and Beta-HCG. Central line placement. 5-HT_3 and dexamethasone 10–20 mg. Moderately to highly emetogenic.

Etoposide 75 mg/m²: IV in 250 cc NS over 30–60 minutes on days 1–5.

Ifosfamide 1200 mg/m²: IV in 500–1000 cc NS on days 1–5.

Cisplatin 20 mg/m²: IV over 1 hour on days 1–5.

Mesna 400 mg/m²: IV in 100 cc NS given 15 minutes before first ifosfamide dose, and then:

Mesna 1200 mg/m²/day: IV continuous infusion for 5 days.

Side effects: Myelosuppression dose-limiting. Nausea and vomiting acute or delayed. Mucositis, diarrhea, and anorexia. Metallic taste common. Use etoposide with caution with abnormal liver function. Dose reduction recommended. Hypotension if etoposide infused too rapidly. Nephrotoxicity and/or hemorrhagic cystitis possible, prevent with mesna and vigorous hydration. Decreases Mg^{2+}, K^+, Ca^{2+}, Na^+, and phosphorus. Sensory neuropathy with numbness and paresthesias. Somnolence, confusion, depressive psychosis, or hallucinations with ifosfamide. Radiation recall, skin changes. Total alopecia.

Chair time: 4–5 hours on days 1–5. Repeat cycle every 21 days.

STAGE I SEMINOMA

Carboplatin[1,434]

Prechemo: CBC, Chem, renal function tests, LDH, and Beta-HCG. 5-HT_3 and dexamethasone. Moderately to highly emetogenic.

Carboplatin AUC 7: IV in 500 cc NS on day 1.

Side effects: Hypersensitivity reactions, increased risk with more than seven courses. Myelosuppression dose related. Nausea and vomiting may be acute or delayed. Mucositis and diarrhea can be severe and dose-limiting. Use with caution with abnormal renal function. Instruct patients to maintain adequate oral hydration. Decreases Mg^{2+}, K^+, Ca^{2+}, and Na^+. Hyperpigmentation, photosensitivity, and nail changes. Hand-foot syndrome. Alopecia is uncommon.

Chair time: 2 hours on day 1. Give one cycle only.

THYMOMA

Cyclophosphamide + Doxorubicin + Cisplatin (CAP)[1,435]

Prechemo: CBC, Chem, renal function tests. MUGA scan. 5-HT$_3$ and dexamethasone. Moderately to highly emetogenic.

Cyclophosphamide 500 mg/m²: IV in 500 cc NS on day 1.

Doxorubicin 50 mg/m²: IV push on day 1. Potent vesicant.

Cisplatin 50 m²: IV in 500 cc NS over 1–3 hours on day 1.

Side effects: Hypersensitivity reaction with cisplatin. Cyclophosphamide can cause rhinitis and irritation of nose and throat. Myelosuppression dose-limiting. Nausea and vomiting, acute or delayed mucositis. Metallic taste. Nephrotoxicity dose related with cisplatin, risk may be reduced with adequate hydration. Hemorrhagic cystitis, dysuria, and increased urinary frequency. Decreases Mg^{2+}, K^+, Ca^{2+}, Na^+, and P. Acutely, pericarditis or myocarditis can occur. With cumulative doses >550 mg/m² of doxorubicin, cardiomyopathy. Peripheral sensory neuropathy dose-limiting with paresthesias and numbness. High-frequency hearing loss and tinnitus. Hyperpigmentation, photosensitivity, and radiation recall occur. Alopecia.

Chair time: 3–4 hours on day 1. Repeat cycle every 21 days.

Cisplatin + Etoposide[1,436]

Prechemo: CBC, Chem, and renal function tests. 5-HT$_3$ and dexamethasone 10–20 mg. Moderately to highly emetogenic.

Cisplatin 60 mg/m²: IV in 500–1000 cc NS over 1–3 hours day 1.

Etoposide 120 mg/m²: IV in 250 cc NS days 1–3.

Side effects: Hypersensitivity reaction with cisplatin or during rapid infusion of etoposide. Myelosuppression dose-limiting. Nausea and vomiting, acute or delayed. Nephrotoxicity dose related. Decreases Mg^{2+}, K^+, Ca^{2+}, Na^+, and P. Peripheral sensory neuropathy. High-frequency hearing loss and tinnitus. Alopecia.

Chair time: 3–4 hours days 1 and 1 hour days 2 and 3. Repeat cycle every 21 days.

Cisplatin + Doxorubicin + Vincristine + Cyclophosphamide (ADOC)[1,437]

Prechemo: CBC, Chem, and renal function tests. 5-HT$_3$, and dexamethasone 10–20 mg. Moderately to highly emetogenic.

Cisplatin 50 mg/m²: IV in 500–1000 cc NS over 1–2 hours on day 1.

Doxorubicin 40 mg/m²: IV push on day 1. Potent vesicant.

Vincristine 0.6 mg/m²: IV push on day 3. Vesicant.

Cyclophosphamide 700 mg/m²: IV in 500 cc NS over 1 hour on day 4.

Side effects: Myelosuppression dose-limiting. Severe nausea and vomiting. May be acute or delayed. Mucositis may occur. Constipation, abdominal pain, and paralytic ileus possible. Aggressive bowel protocol. Nephrotoxicity dose related with cisplatin. Hemorrhagic cystitis, dysuria, and increased urinary frequency. Risk reduced with adequate hydration. Acutely, pericarditis or myocarditis may occur. With cumulative doses >550 mg/m² of doxorubicin, cardiomyopathy. Peripheral sensory neuropathy dose-limiting. Paresthesias and numbness. Hyperpigmentation, photosensitivity, and radiation recall occur. Alopecia.

Chair time: 3 hours on day 1, 1 hour on day 3, and 2 hours on day 4. Repeat cycle every 28 days.

THYROID CANCER

COMBINATION REGIMENS

Doxorubicin + Cisplatin (AP)[1,438]

Prechemo: CBC, Chem, renal function tests. MUGA scan. 5-HT$_3$ and dexamethasone 10–20 mg. Moderately to highly emetogenic.
Doxorubicin 60 mg/m^2: IV push on day 1. Potent vesicant.
Cisplatin 40 m$^{2:}$ IV in 500 cc NS over 1–3 hours on day 1.
Side effects: Hypersensitivity reaction with cisplatin. Myelosuppression dose related. Nausea and vomiting, acute or delayed mucositis. Metallic taste. Nephrotoxicity dose related with cisplatin, hemorrhagic cystitis, dysuria, and increased urinary frequency. Risk reduced with adequate hydration. Decreases Mg^{2+}, K^+, Ca^{2+}, Na^+, and P. Acutely, pericarditis or myocarditis can occur. With cumulative doses >550 mg/m^2 of doxorubicin, cardiomyopathy. Peripheral sensory neuropathy dose-limiting with paresthesias and numbness. High-frequency hearing loss and tinnitus. Hyperpigmentation, photosensitivity, and radiation recall occur. Alopecia.
Chair time: 3–4 hours on day 1. Repeat cycle every 21 days.

SINGLE-AGENT REGIMENS

Doxorubicin[1,438]

Prechemo: CBC, Chem. MUGA scan. 5-HT$_3$ and dexamethasone 10–20 mg. Mildly to moderately emetogenic.
Doxorubicin 60 mg/m^2: IV push on day 1. Potent vesicant.
Side effects: Myelosuppression may be severe. Nausea and vomiting. Dose reduce with liver dysfunction. Pericarditis-myocarditis syndrome. Cumulative doses >550 mg/m^2 of doxorubicin, cardiomyopathy. Red-orange discoloration of urine. Hyperpigmentation, photosensitivity, and radiation recall. Complete alopecia.
Chair time: 1 hour on day 1. Repeat cycle every 21 days.

REFERENCES

1. Wilkes GM, Barton-Burke M. *Oncology Nursing Drug Handbook 2006.* Sudbury, MA: Jones and Bartlett Publishers; 2006.

2. Nigro ND, Seydel HG, Considine B, Vaitkevicius VK, Leichmanl, Kinzie JJ. Combined preoperative radiation and chemotherapy for squamous cell carcinoma of the anal canal. *Cancer.* 1983;51:1826–1829.

3. Bartelink H, et al. Concomitant radiotherapy and chemotherapy is superior to radiotherapy alone in the treatment of locally advanced anal cancer: results of a phase III randomized trial of the European Organization for Research and Treatment of Cancer Radiotherapy and Gastrointestinal Cooperative Groups. *J Clin Oncol.* 1997;15:2040–2049.

4. Hung A, et al. Cisplatin-based combined modality therapy for anal carcinoma: a wider therapeutic index. *Cancer.* 2003;97:1195–1202.

5. Flam MS, et al. Role of mitomycin in combination with fluorouracil and radiotherapy, and of salvage chemoradiation in the definitive nonsurgical treatment of epidermoid carcinoma of the anal canal: results of a phase III randomized Intergroup study. *J Clin Oncol.* 1996;16:227–253.

6. Thongprasert S, Napapan S, Charoentum C, Moonprakan S. Phase II study of gemcitabine and cisplatin as first line chemotherapy in inoperable biliary tract carcinoma. *Ann Oncol.* 2005;16:279–281.

7. Knox JJ, et al. Combining gemcitabine and capecitabine in patients with advanced biliary cancer: a phase II trial. *J Clin Oncol.* 2005;23:2332–2338.

8. Bajorin DF, et al. Ifosfamide, paclitaxel, and cisplatin for patients with advanced carcinoma of the urothelial tract: final report of a phase II trial evaluating 2 dosing schedules. *Cancer.* 2000;88:1671–1678.

9. Kaufman D, et al. Phase II trial of gemcitabine plus cisplatin in patients with metastatic urothelial cancer. *J Clin Oncol.* 2000;18:1921–1927.

10. Sternberg CN, et al. Methotrexate, vinblastine, doxorubicin, and cisplatin for advanced transitional cell carcinoma of the urothelium: efficacy and patterns of response and relapse. *Cancer.* 1989;64:2448–2458.

11. Harker WG, et al. Cisplatin, methotrexate, and vinblastine (CMV): an effective chemotherapy regimen for metastatic transitional cell carcinoma of the urinary tract: a Northern California Oncology Group study. *J Clin Oncol.* 1985;3:1463–1470.

12. Logothetis CJ, et al. A prospective randomized trial comparing MVAC and CISCA chemotherapy for patients with metastatic urothelial tumors. *J Clin Oncol.* 1990;8:1050–1055.

13. Vaughn D, et al. Phase II study of paclitaxel plus carboplatin in patients with advanced carcinoma of the urothelium and renal dysfunction (E2896). *Cancer.* 2002;95:1022–1027.

14. Campbell M, Baker LH, Opipari M, al-Sarraf M. Phase II trial with cisplatin, doxorubicin, and cyclophosphamide (CAP) in the treatment of urothelial transitional cell carcinoma. *Cancer Treat Rep.* 1981;65:897–899.

15. Kachnic LA, et al. Bladder preservation by combined modality therapy for invasive bladder cancer. *J Clin Oncol.* 1997;15:1022–1029.

16. Moore MJ, et al. Gemcitabine: a promising new agent in the treatment of advanced urothelial cancer. *J Clin Oncol.* 1997;15:3441–3445.

17. Roth BJ, et al. Significant activity of paclitaxel in advanced transitional-cell carcinoma of the urothelium: a phase II trial of the Eastern Cooperative Oncology Group. *J Clin Oncol.* 1994;12:2264–2270.

18. Vaughn D, et al. Phase II trial of weekly paclitaxel in patients with previously treated advanced urothelial cancer. *J Clin Oncol.* 2002;20:937–940.

19. Chu E, DeVita VT. *Physicians Cancer Chemotherapy Drug Manual 2007.* Sudbury, MA: Jones and Bartlett Publishers; 2007.

20. Wilkes G, Barton-Burke M. *Oncology Nursing Drug Handbook 2005.* Sudbury, MA: Jones and Bartlett Publishers; 2005, pp. 94–99, 137–140, 222–226, 310–313.

21. Zometa full prescribing information. Novartis Pharmaceuticals Corporation; 2002.

22. Saad F, et al. Long-term efficacy of zoledronic acid for the prevention of skeletal complications in patients with metastatic hormone-refractory prostate cancer. *J Natl Cancer Inst.* 2004;96:879–882.

23. Rosen LS, et al. Zoledronic acid versus pamidronate in the treatment of skeletal metastases in patients with breast cancer or osteolytic lesions of multiple myeloma: a phase III, double-blind, comparative trial. *Cancer J.* 2001;7:377–387.

24. Kohno N, et al. Zoledronic acid significantly reduces skeletal complications compared with placebo in Japanese women with bone metastases from breast cancer: a randomized, placebo-controlled trial. *J Clin Oncol.* 2005;23:1–8.

25. Rosen LS, et al. Zoledronic acid versus placebo in the treatment of skeletal metastases in patients with lung cancer and other solid tumors: a phase III, double-blind, randomized trial—the Zoledronic Acid Lung Cancer and Other Solid Tumors Study Group. *J Clin Oncol.* 2003;21:3150–3157.

26. Pamidronate full prescribing information. Novartis Pharmaceuticals Corporation; 2005.

27. Stupp R, et al. Radiotherapy plus concomitant and adjuvant temozolomide for glioblastoma. *N Engl J Med.* 2005;352:987–995.

28. Levin VA, et al. Superiority of post-radiotherapy adjuvant chemotherapy with CCNU, procarbazine, and vincristine (PCV) over BCNU for

anaplastic gliomas: NCOG 6G61 final report. *Int J Radiat Oncol Biol Phys.* 1990;18:321–324.

29. DeAngelis LM, et al. Malignant gliomas: who benefits from adjuvant chemotherapy. *Ann Neurol.* 1998;44:691–695.

30. Buckner JC, et al. Phase II trial of procarbazine, lomustine, and vincristine as initial therapy for patients with low-grade oligodendroglioma or oligoastrocytoma: efficacy and associations with chromosomal abnormalities. *J Clin Oncol.* 2003;21:251–255.

31. Yung A, et al. Randomized trial of temodal (TEM) vs. procarbazine (PCB) in glioblastoma multiforme (GBM) at first relapse. *Proc Am Soc Clin Oncol.* 1999;18:139a.

32. Yung A, et al. Multicenter phase II trial of temozolomide in patients with anaplastic astrocytoma or anaplastic oligoastrocytoma at first relapse. *J Clin Oncol.* 1999;17:2762–2771.

33. Raymond E, et al. Multicenter phase II study and pharmacokinetic analysis of irinotecan in chemotherapy-naïve patients with glioblastoma. *Ann Oncol.* 2003;14:603–614.

34. Friedman H, et al. Irinotecan therapy in adults with recurrent or progressive malignant glioma. *J Clin Oncol.* 1999;17:1516–1525.

35. Bear H, et al. The effect on tumor response of adding sequential preoperative docetaxel to preoperative doxorubicin and cyclophosphamide: preliminary results from National Surgical Adjuvant Breast and Bowel Project B-27. *J Clin Oncol.* 2003;21:4165–4174.

36. Fisher B, et al. Two months of doxorubicin-cyclophosphamide with and without interval reinduction therapy compared with 6 months of cyclophosphamide, methotrexate, and fluorouracil in positive node breast cancer patients with tamoxifen-nonresponsive tumors: results from the National Surgical Adjuvant Breast and Bowel Project B-15. *J Clin Oncol.* 2000;8:1483–1496.

37. Jones SE, et al. Phase III trial comparing doxorubicin plus cyclophosphamide with docetaxel plus cyclophosphamide as adjuvant therapy for operable breast cancer. *J Clin Oncol.* 2006;24:5381–5387.

38. Jones S, et al. Final analysis: TC (docetaxel/cyclophosphamide, four cycles) has a superior disease-free survival compared to standard AC (doxorubicin/cyclophosphamide) in 1016 women with early breast cancer. *Proc SABCS.* 2005;(abstract 40).

39. Jones SE, et al. Phase III trial comparing doxorubicin plus cyclophosphamide with docetaxel plus cyclophosphamide as adjuvant therapy for operable breast cancer. *J Clin Oncol.* 2006;24:5381–5387.

40. Hudis C, et al. Sequential dose-dense doxorubicin, paclitaxel, and cyclophosphamide for resectable high-risk breast cancer: feasibility and efficacy. *J Clin Oncol.* 1999;17:93–100.

41. Romond E, et al. Doxorubicin and cyclophosphamide followed by paclitaxel with or without trastuzumab as adjuvant therapy for patients with HER2 positive operable breast cancer: combined analysis of NSABP-B31/NCCTG-N9381. Available at: http://www.asco.org/ac/

1.1003,fl12-002511-00fl18-0034-00fl19-005816-00fl21-001,00. Accessed July 2005.

42. Citron M, et al. Randomized trial of dose-dense versus conventionally scheduled and sequential versus concurrent combination chemotherapy as postoperative adjuvant treatment of node-positive primary breast cancer: first report of Intergroup trial C9741/Cancer and Leukemia Group B trial 9741. *J Clin Oncol.* 2003;21:1431–1439.

43. Martin M, et al. Doxorubicin in combination with fluorouracil and cyclophosphamide (i.v. FAC regimen, day 1, 21) versus methotrexate in combination with fluorouracil and cyclophosphamide (i.v. CMF regimen, day 1, 21) as adjuvant chemotherapy for operable breast cancer: a study by the GEICAM group. *Ann Oncol.* 2003;14:833–842.

44. Aisner J, et al. Chemotherapy versus chemoimmunotherapy (CAF v CAFVP v CMF each +/– MER) for metastatic carcinoma of the breast: a CALGB study: Cancer and Leukemia Group B. *J Clin Oncol.* 1987;5:1523–1533.

45. Bonadonna G, et al. Combination chemotherapy as an adjuvant treatment in operable breast cancer. *N Engl J Med.* 1976;294:405–410.

46. Weiss RB, et al. Adjuvant chemotherapy after conservative surgery plus irradiation versus modified radical mastectomy: analysis of drug dosing and toxicity. *Am J Med.* 1987;83:455–463.

47. Bonadonna G, Zambetti M, Valagussa P. Sequential or alternating doxorubicin and CMF regimens in breast cancer with more than three positive nodes: ten-year results. *JAMA.* 1995;273:542–543.

48. Coombes RC, et al. Adjuvant cyclophosphamide, methotrexate, and fluorouracil versus fluorouracil, epirubicin, and cyclophosphamide chemotherapy in premenopausal women with axillary node-positive operable breast cancer: results of a randomized trial. *J Clin Oncol.* 1996;14:35–45.

49. Marschke RF, et al. Randomized clinical trial of CFP versus CMFP in women with metastatic breast cancer. *Cancer.* 1989;63:1931–1937.

50. Fisher B, et al. Tamoxifen and chemotherapy for lymph node-negative, estrogen receptor-positive breast cancer. *J Natl Cancer Inst.* 1997;89:1673–1682.

51. Howell A, et al. Results of the ATAC (Arimidex, Tamoxifen Alone or in Combination) trial after completion of 5-years' adjuvant treatment for breast cancer. *Lancet.* 2005;365:60–62.

52. Goss PE, et al. Randomized trial of letrozole following tamoxifen as extended adjuvant therapy in receptor-positive breast cancer: updated findings from NCIC CTG MA.17. *J Natl Cancer Inst.* 2005;97:1262–1271.

53. Coombes RC, et al. A randomized trial of exemestane after 2 to 3 years of tamoxifen therapy in postmenopausal women with primary breast cancer. *N Engl J Med.* 2004;350:1081–1092.

54. Sledge GE, et al. Phase III trial of doxorubicin, paclitaxel, and the combination of doxorubicin and paclitaxel as front-line chemotherapy for metastatic breast cancer: an Intergroup trial (E1193). *J Clin Oncol.* 2003;21:588–592.

55. Levine MN, et al. Randomized trial of intensive cyclophosphamide, epirubicin, and fluorouracil chemotherapy compared with cyclophos-

phamide, methotrexate, and fluorouracil in premenopausal women with node-positive breast cancer: National Cancer Institute of Canada Clinical Trials Group. *J Clin Oncol.* 1998;16:2651–2658.

56. O'Shaughnessy J, et al. Superior survival with capecitabine plus docetaxel combination therapy in anthracycline-pretreated patients with advanced breast cancer: phase III trial results. *J Clin Oncol.* 2002;20:2123–2812.

57. Biganzoli L, et al. Moving forward with capecitabine: a glimpse of the future. *Oncologist.* 2002;7(Suppl 6):29–35.

58. Dieras V. Review of docetaxel/doxorubicin combination in metastatic breast cancer. *Oncology.* 1997;11:31–33.

59. Brufman G, et al. Doubling epirubicin dose intensity (100 mg/m2 versus 50 mg/m2) in the FEC regimen significantly increases response rates: an international randomized phase III in metastatic breast cancer: the Epirubicin High Dose (HEPI 010) Study Group. *Ann Oncol.* 1997;8:155–162.

60. Acuna LR, et al. Vinorelbine and paclitaxel as first-line chemotherapy in metastatic breast cancer. *J Clin Oncol.* 1999;17:74–81.

61. Spielman M, et al. Phase II trial of vinorelbine/doxorubicin as first-line therapy of advanced breast cancer. *J Clin Oncol.* 1994;12:1764–1770.

62. Slamon DJ, et al. Use of chemotherapy plus a monoclonal antibody against HER2 for metastatic breast cancer that overexpresses HER2. *N Engl J Med.* 2001;344:783–792.

63. Goldenberg MM, et al. Trastuzumab, a recombinant DNA-derived humanized monoclonal antibody, a novel agent for the treatment of metastatic breast cancer. *Clin Ther.* 1999;21:309–318.

64. Francisco E, et al. Phase II study of weekly docetaxel and trastuzumab for patients with HER2 overexpressing metastatic breast cancer. *J Clin Oncol.* 2002;20:1800–1808.

65. O'Shaughnessy J, et al. Gemcitabine plus paclitaxel (GT) versus paclitaxel (T) as first-line treatment for anthracycline pre-treated metastatic breast cancer (MBC): interim results of a global phase III study. *Proc Am Soc Clin Oncol.* 2003;22:7(abstract 25).

66. Perez EA, et al. A phase II study of paclitaxel plus carboplatin as first-line chemotherapy for women with metastatic breast carcinoma. *Cancer.* 2000;88:124–131.

67. Fitch V, et al. N9332: phase II cooperative group trial of docetaxel (D) and carboplatin (CBCDA) as first-line chemotherapy for metastatic breast cancer (MBC). *Proc Am Soc Clin Oncol.* 2003;22:23(abstract 90).

68. Ixempra (isabepilone) for injection full prescribing information. Princeton, NJ: Bristol-Myers Squibb Company; October 2007.

69. Tykerb (lapatinib) tablets full prescribing information. Research Triangle Park, NC: GlaxoSmithKline; March 2007.

70. Garewal HS, et al. Treatment of advanced breast cancer with mitomycin-C combined with vinblastine or vindesine. *J Clin Oncol.* 1983;1:772–775.

71. Jaiyesimi IA, et al. Use of tamoxifen for breast cancer: twenty-eight years later. *J Clin Oncol.* 1995;13:513–529.

72. Hayes DF, et al. Randomized comparison of tamoxifen and two separate doses of toremifene in postmenopausal patients with metastatic breast cancer. *J Clin Oncol.* 1995;13:2556–2566.

73. Lonning PE, et al. Activity of exemestane in metastatic breast cancer after failure of nonsteroidal aromatase inhibitors, a phase I trial. *J Clin Oncol.* 2000;18:2234–2244.

74. Buzdar A, et al. Anastrozole, a potent and selective aromatase inhibitor, versus megestrol acetate in postmenopausal women with advanced breast cancer: results of overview analysis of two phase II trials. Arimidex Study Group. *J Clin Oncol.* 1996;14:2000–2011.

75. Dombernowsky P, et al. Letrozole, a new oral aromatase inhibitor for advanced breast cancer: double-blind randomized trial showing a dose effect and improved efficacy and tolerability compared with megestrol acetate. *J Clin Oncol.* 1998;16:453–461.

76. Howell A. Future use of selective estrogen receptor modulators and aromatase inhibitors. *Clin Cancer Res.* 2001;7(Suppl 12):4402s–4410s.

77. Kimmick GG, Muss HB. Endocrine therapy in breast cancer. *Cancer Treat Res.* 1998;94:231–254.

78. Baselga J, et al. Phase II study of weekly intravenous trastuzumab (Herceptin™) in patients with HER2/neu-overexpressing metastatic breast cancer. *Semin Oncol.* 1999;26(Suppl 12):78–83.

79. Baselga J, et al. Phase II study of efficacy, safety, and pharmacokinetics of trastuzumab monotherapy administered on a 3-weekly schedule. *J Clin Oncol.* 2005;23:2162–2171.

80. Blum JL, et al. Multicenter phase II study of capecitabine in paclitaxel-refractory metastatic breast cancer. *J Clin Oncol.* 1999;17:485–493.

81. Chan S. Docetaxel vs. doxorubicin in metastatic breast cancer resistant to alkylating chemotherapy. *Oncology.* 1997;11(Suppl 8):19–24.

82. Baselga J, Tabernero JM. Weekly docetaxel in breast cancer: applying clinical data to patient therapy. *Oncologist.* 2001;6(Suppl 3):26–29.

83. Holmes FA, et al. Phase II trial of Taxol™, an active drug in the treatment of metastatic breast cancer. *J Natl Cancer Inst.* 1991;83:1797–1805.

84. Perez EA. Paclitaxel in breast cancer. *Oncologist.* 1998;3:373–389.

85. Fumoleau P, Delozier T, Extra JM, Canobbio L, Delgado FM, Hurteloup P. Vinorelbine (Navelbine®) in the treatment of breast cancer: the European experience. *Semin Oncol.* 1995;22(Suppl 5):22–28.

86. Torti FM, et al. Reduced cardiotoxicity of doxorubicin delivered on a weekly schedule: assessment by endomyocardial biopsy. *Ann Intern Med.* 1983;99:745–749.

87. Carmichael J, et al. Phase II activity of gemcitabine in advanced breast cancer. *Semin Oncol.* 1996;23(Suppl 10):77–81.

88. Ranson MR, et al. Treatment of advanced breast cancer with sterically stabilized liposomal doxorubicin: results of a multicenter phase II trial. *J Clin Oncol.* 1997;15:3185–3191.

89. O'Shaughnessy J, et al. ABI-007 (ABRAXANE), a nanoparticle albumin-bound (nab) paclitaxel demonstrates superior efficacy vs. Taxol™ in

MBC: a phase III trial. *Breast Cancer Res Treat.* 2003;82:(Suppl 1)(abstract 43).

90. O'Shaughnessy JA, et al. Weekly nanoparticle albumin paclitaxel (Abraxane) results in long-term disease control in patients with taxane-refractory metastatic breast cancer. *Breast Cancer Res Treat.* 2004;88:(Suppl 1):S65 (abstract 1070).

91. Hainsworth JD, et al. Carcinoma of unknown primary site: treatment with 1-hour paclitaxel, carboplatin, and extended-schedule etoposide. *J Clin Oncol.* 1997;15:2385–2393.

92. Longeval E, Klastersky J. Combination chemotherapy with cisplatin and etoposide in bronchogenic squamous cell carcinoma and adenocarcinoma: a study by the EORTC lung cancer working party. *Cancer.* 1982;50:2751–2756.

93. Hainsworth JD, Johnson DH, Greco FA. Cisplatin-based combination chemotherapy in the treatment of poorly differentiated carcinoma and poorly differentiated adenocarcinoma of unknown primary site: results of a 12-year experience. *J Clin Oncol.* 1992;10:912–922.

94. Greco FA, et al. Gemcitabine, carboplatin, and paclitaxel for patients with carcinoma of unknown primary site: a Minnie Pearl Cancer Research network study. *J Clin Oncol.* 2002;20:1651–1656.

95. Moertel CG, et al. Streptozocin-doxorubicin, streptozocin-fluorouracil, or chlorozotocin in the treatment of advanced islet-cell carcinoma. *N Engl J Med.* 1992;326:519–526.

96. Moertel CG, et al. Treatment of neuroendocrine carcinomas with combined etoposide and cisplatin. *Cancer.* 1991;68:227–232.

97. Saltz L, et al. Octreotide as an antineoplastic agent in the treatment of functional and nonfunctional neuroendocrine tumors. *Cancer.* 1993;72:244.

98. Sandostatin LAR full prescribing information. Novartis Pharmaceuticals Corporation; February 2005.

99. Rubin J, et al. Octreotide acetate long-acting formulation versus open-label subcutaneous octreotide acetate in malignant carcinoid syndrome. *J Clin Oncol.* 1999;17:606–660.

100. Rose PG, et al. Concurrent cisplatin-based radiotherapy and chemotherapy for locally advanced cervical cancer. *N Engl J Med.* 1995;15:1144.

101. Morris M, et al. Pelvic radiation with concurrent chemotherapy compared with pelvic and para-aortic radiation for high-risk cervical cancer. *N Engl J Med.* 1999;340:1137–1143.

102. Fiorica J, et al. Phase II trial of topotecan and cisplatin in persistent or recurrent squamous and nonsquamous carcinoma of the cervix. *Gynecol Oncol.* 2002;85:89–94.

103. Buxton EJ, et al. Combination bleomycin, ifosfamide, and cisplatin chemotherapy in cervical cancer. *J Natl Cancer Inst.* 1989;81:359–361.

104. Murad AM, Triginelli SA, Ribalta JC. Phase II trial of bleomycin, ifosfamide, and carboplatin in metastatic cervical cancer. *J Clin Oncol.* 1994;12:55–59.

105. Whitney CW, et al. Randomized comparison of fluorouracil plus cisplatin versus hydroxyurea as an adjunct to radiation therapy in stage IIB-IVA carcinoma of the cervix with negative para-aortic lymph nodes: a Gynecologic Oncology Group and Southwest Oncology Group study. *J Clin Oncol.* 1999;17:1339–1348.

106. Pignata S, et al. Phase II study of cisplatin and vinorelbine as first-line chemotherapy in patients with carcinoma of the uterine cervix. *J Clin Oncol.* 1999;17:756–760.

107. Chitapanarux I, et al. Phase II clinical study of irinotecan and cisplatin as first-line chemotherapy in metastatic or recurrent cervical cancer. *Gynecol Oncol.* 2003;89:402–407.

108. Vogl SE, et al. Chemotherapy for advanced cervical cancer with bleomycin, vincristine, mitomycin-C, and cisplatinum (BOMP). *Cancer Treat Rep.* 1980;64:1005–1007.

109. Alberts DS, Garcia DJ. Salvage chemotherapy in recurrent or refractory squamous cell cancer of the uterine cervix. *Semin Oncol.* 1994;21(Suppl 7):37–46.

110. Levy T, et al. Advanced squamous cell cancer (SCC) of the cervix: a phase II study of docetaxel (Taxotere™) 100 mg/m2 intravenously (IV) over 1 hour every 21 days: a preliminary report. *Proc Am Soc Clin Oncol.* 1996;15:292a.

111. Thigpen T, et al. The role of paclitaxel in the management of patients with carcinoma of the cervix. *Semin Oncol.* 1997;24(Suppl 2):41–46.

112. Verschraegen CF, et al. Phase II study of irinotecan in prior chemotherapy-treated squamous cell carcinoma of the cervix. *J Clin Oncol.* 1997;15:625–631.

113. Lacava JA, et al. Vinorelbine as neoadjuvant chemotherapy in advanced cervical carcinoma. *J Clin Oncol.* 1997;15:604–609.

114. Muderspach LI, et al. A phase II study of topotecan in patients with squamous cell carcinoma of the cervix: a Gynecologic Oncology Group study. *Gynecol Oncol.* 2001;81:213–215.

115. Sauer R, et al. Preoperative versus postoperative chemoradiotherapy for rectal cancer. *N Engl J Med.* 2004;351:1731–1740.

116. Minsky BD. Combined modality therapy of rectal cancer with oxaliplatin-based regimens. *Clin Colorectal Cancer.* 2004;4(Suppl 1):S29–S36.

117. O'Connell MJ, et al. Controlled trial of fluorouracil and low-dose leucovorin given for 6 months as postoperative adjuvant therapy for colon cancer. *J Clin Oncol.* 1997;15:246–250.

118. Wolmark N, et al. The benefit of leucovorin-modulated fluorouracil as postoperative adjuvant therapy for primary colon cancer: results from National Surgical Adjuvant Breast and Bowel Project Protocol C-03. *J Clin Oncol.* 1993;11:1879–1887.

119. Benson AB, et al. NCCN practice guidelines for colorectal cancer. *Oncology.* 2000;14:203–212.

120. de Gramont A, et al. Oxaliplatin/5-FU/LV in adjuvant colon cancer: results of the international randomized mosaic trial. *Proc Am Soc Clin Oncol.* 2003;22:253(abstract 1015).

121. Cassidy J, et al. Capecitabine (X) vs. bolus 5-FU/leucovorin (LV) as adjuvant therapy for colon cancer (the X-ACT study): positive efficacy results of a phase III trial. *Proc Am Soc Clin Oncol.* 2004;23:(abstract 3509).

122. Saltz LB, et al. Irinotecan plus fluorouracil and leucovorin for metastatic colorectal cancer. *N Engl J Med.* 2000;343:905–914.

123. Hurwitz H, et al. Bevacizumab plus irinotecan, fluorouracil, and leucovorin for metastatic colorectal cancer. *N Engl J Med.* 2004;350:2335–2342.

124. Hwang JJ, et al. Capecitabine-based combination chemotherapy. *Am J Oncol Rev.* 2003;2(Suppl 5):15–25.

125. Douillard JY, et al. Irinotecan combined with fluorouracil compared with fluorouracil alone as first-line treatment for metastatic colorectal cancer: a multicentre randomized trial. *Lancet.* 2000;355:1041–1047.

126. Andre T, et al. CPT-11 (irinotecan) addition to bimonthly, high-dose leucovorin and bolus and continuous-infusion 5-fluorouracil (FOLFIRI) for pretreated metastatic colorectal cancer. GERCOR. *Eur J Cancer.* 1999;35:1343–1347.

127. de Gramont A, et al. Leucovorin and fluorouracil with and without oxaliplatin as first-line treatment in advanced colorectal cancer. *J Clin Oncol.* 2000;18:2938–2947.

128. Tournigand C, et al. FOLFIRI followed by FOLFOX versus FOLFOX followed by FOLFIRI in metastatic colorectal cancer (MCRC): final results of a phase III study. *Proc Am Soc Clin Oncol.* 2001;20:124a(abstract 494).

129. Andre T, et al. FOLFOX7 compared to FOLFOX4. Preliminary results of the randomized Optimox study. *Proc Am Soc Clin Oncol.* 2003;22:253(abstract 1016).

130. Cunningham D, et al. Cetuximab monotherapy and cetuximab plus irinotecan in irinotecan-refractory metastatic colorectal cancer. *N Engl J Med.* 2004;351:337–345.

131. Scheithauer W, et al. Randomized multicenter phase II trial of two different schedules of capecitabine plus oxaliplatin as first-line treatment in advanced colorectal cancer. *J Clin Oncol.* 2003;21:1307–1312.

132. Kerr D. Capecitabine/irinotecan in colorectal cancer: European early-phase data and planned trials. *Oncology.* 2002;16(Suppl 14):12–15.

133. Goldberg RM, et al. A randomized controlled trial of fluorouracil plus leucovorin, irinotecan, and oxaliplatin combinations in patients with previously untreated metastatic colorectal cancer. *J Clin Oncol.* 2004;22:23–30.

134. Poon MA, et al. Biochemical modulation of fluorouracil: evidence of significant improvement of survival and quality of life in patients with advanced colorectal carcinoma. *J Clin Oncol.* 1989;7:1407–1418.

135. Petrelli N, et al. The modulation of fluorouracil with leucovorin in metastatic colorectal carcinoma: a prospective randomized phase III trial: Gastrointestinal Tumor Study Group. *J Clin Oncol.* 1989;7:1419–1426.

136. Kabbinavar F, et al. Results of a randomized phase II controlled trial of bevacizumab in combination with 5-fluorouracil and leucovorin as first-line therapy in subjects with metastatic CRC. *Proc Am Soc Clin Oncol.* 2004;23:(abstract 3516).

137. Jager E, et al. Weekly high-dose leucovorin versus low-dose leucovorin combined with fluorouracil in advanced colorectal cancer: results of a randomized multicenter trial: Study Group for Palliative Treatment of Metastatic Colorectal Cancer Study Protocol 1. *J Clin Oncol.* 1996;14:2274–2279.

138. de Gramont A, et al. Randomized trial comparing monthly low-dose leucovorin and fluorouracil bolus with bimonthly high-dose leucovorin and fluorouracil bolus plus continuous infusion for advanced colorectal cancer: a French Intergroup study. *J Clin Oncol.* 1997;15:808–815.

139. Mitchell EP, et al. High-dose bevacizumab in combination with FOL-FOX4 improves survival in patients with previously treated advanced colorectal cancer: results from the Eastern Cooperative Oncology Group (ECOG) study E3200. Presented at the 2005 American Society of Clinical Oncology Gastrointestinal Cancers Symposium; January 27–29, 2005, Hollywood, FL (abstract 169a).

140. Hochster HS, et al. Bevacizumab (B) with oxaliplatin (O)-based chemotherapy in the first-line therapy of metastatic colorectal cancer (mCRC): preliminary results of the randomized "TREE-2" trial. Presented at the American Society of Clinical Oncology Gastrointestinal Cancers Symposium; January 27–29, 2005, Hollywood, FL (abstract 241).

141. Blanke, CD, Kasimis B, Schein P, Capizzi R, Kurman M. Phase II study of trimetrexate, fluorouracil, and leucovorin for advanced colorectal cancer. *J Clin Oncol.* 1997;15:915–920.

142. Kemeny N, et al. Phase II study of hepatic arterial floxuridine, leucovorin, and dexamethasone for unresectable liver metastases from colorectal carcinoma. *J Clin Oncol.* 1994;12:2288–2295.

143. Hoff P, et al. Comparison of oral capecitabine versus intravenous fluorouracil plus leucovorin as first-line treatment in 605 patients with metastatic colorectal cancer: results of a randomized phase III study. *J Clin Oncol.* 2001;15:2282–2292.

144. Pitot HC, et al. Phase II trial of irinotecan in patients with metastatic colorectal carcinoma. *J Clin Oncol.* 1997;15:2910–2919.

145. Ulrich-Pur H, et al. Multicenter phase II trial of dose-fractionated irinotecan in patients with advanced colorectal cancer failing oxaliplatin-based first-line combination chemotherapy. *Ann Oncol.* 2001;12:1269–1272.

146. Rougier P, et al. Phase II study of irinotecan in the treatment of advanced colorectal cancer in chemotherapy-naïve patients and patients pretreated with fluorouracil-based chemotherapy. *J Clin Oncol.* 1997;15:251–260.

147. Saltz LB, et al. Phase II trial of cetuximab in patients with refractory colorectal cancer that expressed the epidermal growth factor receptor. *J Clin Oncol.* 2004;22:1201–1208.

148. Vectibix (panitumimab) for injection full prescribing information. Thousand Oaks, CA: Amgen, Inc.; September 2006.

149. Leichman CG, et al. Phase II study of fluorouracil and its modulation in advanced colorectal cancer: a Southwestern Oncology Group study. *J Clin Oncol.* 1995;13:1303–1311.

150. Leichman CG. Schedule dependency of 5-fluorouracil. *Oncology.* 1999;13(Suppl 3):26–32.

151. Hoskins PJ, et al. Paclitaxel and carboplatin alone or with radiation in advanced or recurrent endometrial cancer: a phase II study. *J Clin Oncol.* 2001;19:4048–4053.

152. Thigpen JT, et al. A randomized comparison of doxorubicin alone versus doxorubicin plus cyclophosphamide in the management of advanced or recurrent endometrial carcinoma: a Gynecologic Oncology Group study. *J Clin Oncol.* 1994;12:1408–1414.

153. Deppe G, et al. Treatment of recurrent and metastatic endometrial carcinoma with cisplatin and doxorubicin. *Eur J Gynecol Oncol.* 1994;15:263–266.

154. Fiorica JV. Update on the treatment of cervical and uterine carcinoma: focus on topotecan. *Oncologist.* 2002;7(Suppl 5):36–45.

155. Fleming GF, et al. Phase III trial of doxorubicin plus cisplatin with or without paclitaxel plus filgrastim in advanced endometrial carcinoma: a Gynecologic Oncology Group Study. *J Clin Oncol.* 2004;22:2159–2165.

156. Burke TW, et al. Postoperative adjuvant cisplatin, doxorubicin, and cyclophosphamide (PAC) chemotherapy in women with high-risk endometrial carcinoma. *Gynecol Oncol.* 1994;55:47–50.

157. Muss HB. Chemotherapy of metastatic endometrial cancer. *Semin Oncol.* 1994;21:107–113.

158. Thigpen JT, et al. Oral medroxyprogesterone acetate in the treatment of advanced or recurrent endometrial carcinoma: a dose-response study by the Gynecologic Oncology Group. *J Clin Oncol.* 1999;17:1736–1744.

159. Ball H, et al. A phase II trial of paclitaxel with advanced or recurrent adenocarcinoma of the endometrium: a Gynecologic Oncology Group study. *Gynecol Oncol.* 1996;62:278–282.

160. Wadler S, et al. Topotecan is an active agent in the first-line treatment of metastatic or recurrent endometrial carcinoma: Eastern Cooperative Oncology Group study E3E93. *J Clin Oncol.* 2003;21:2110–2114.

161. Ramirez PT, et al. Hormonal therapy for the management of grade1 endometrial adenocarcinoma, a literature review. *Gynecol Oncol.* 2004;95:133–138.

162. Herskovic A, et al. Combined chemotherapy and radiotherapy compared with radiotherapy alone in patients with cancer of the esophagus. *N Engl J Med.* 1992;326:1593–1598.

163. Heath El, et al. Phase II evaluation of preoperative chemoradiation and postoperative adjuvant chemotherapy for squamous cell and adenocarcinoma of the esophagus. *J Clin Oncol.* 2000;18:868–876.

164. Kies MS, et al. Cisplatin and 5-fluorouracil in the primary management of squamous esophageal cancer. *Cancer.* 1987;60:2156–2160.

165. Ilson DH, et al. Phase II trial of weekly irinotecan plus cisplatin in first line advanced esophageal cancer. *J Clin Oncol.* 1999;17:3270–3275.

166. Ilson DH, et al. Phase II trial of paclitaxel, fluorouracil, and cisplatin in patients with advanced carcinoma of the esophagus. *J Clin Oncol.* 1998;16:1826–1834.

167. Lin LL, Edward H, Lozano R, Karp D. *Color-Matrix Cancer Staging and Treatment Handbook,* 3rd ed. Houston, TX: University of Texas MD Anderson; 2004, p. 75.

168. Ajani JA, et al. Paclitaxel in the treatment of carcinoma of the esophagus. *Semin Oncol.* 1995;22(Suppl 6):35–40.

169. MacDonald JS, et al. Chemoradiotherapy after surgery compared with surgery alone for adenocarcinoma of the stomach or gastroesophageal junction. *N Engl J Med.* 2001;345:725–730.

170. Ajani JA, et al. Docetaxel (D), cisplatin, 5-fluorouracil compare to cisplatin (C) and 5-fluorouracil (F) for chemotherapy-naïve patients with metastatic or locally recurrent, unresectable gastric carcinoma (MGC): interim results of a randomized phase III trial (V3325). *Proc Am Soc Clin Oncol.* 2003;22:249(abstract 999).

171. Wilke M, et al. Preoperative chemotherapy in locally advanced and non-resectable gastric cancer: a phase II study with etoposide, doxorubicin, and cisplatin. *J Clin Oncol.* 1989;7:1318–1326.

172. Findlay M, et al. A phase II study in advanced gastro-esophageal cancer using epirubicin and cisplatin in combination with continuous infusion 5-fluorouracil (ECF). *Ann Oncol.* 1994;5:609–616.

173. Wilke M, et al. Preliminary analysis of a randomized phase III trial of FAMTX versus ELF versus cisplatin/FU in advanced gastric cancer: a trial of the EORTC Gastrointestinal Tract Cancer Cooperative Group and the AIO. *Proc Am Soc Clin Oncol.* 1995;14:206a.

174. Shirao K, Shimada Y, Kondo H, et al. Phase I–II study of irinotecan hydrochloride combined with cisplatin in patients with advanced gastric cancer. *J Clin Oncol.* 1997;15:921–927.

175. MacDonald JS, et al. 5-Fluorouracil, doxorubicin, and mitomycin (FAM) combination chemotherapy for advanced gastric cancer. *Ann Intern Med.* 1980;93:533–536.

176. Kelsen D, et al. FAMTX versus etoposide, doxorubicin, and cisplatin: a random assignment trial in gastric cancer. *J Clin Oncol.* 1992;10:541–548.

177. Cullinan SA, et al. Controlled evaluation of three drug combination regimens versus fluorouracil alone for the therapy of advanced gastric cancer: North Central Cancer Treatment Group. *J Clin Oncol.* 1994;12:412–416.

178. Ajani JA, et al. Multinational randomized trial of docetaxel, cisplatin with or without 5-fluorouracil in patients with advanced gastric or GE junction adenocarcinoma. *Proc Am Soc Clin Oncol.* 2000;20:165a (abstract 657).

179. Ajani, JA, Fodor, MD, Tjulandin, SA, et al. Phase II multi-institutional randomized trial of docetaxel plus cisplatin with or without fluorouracil in patients with untreated, advanced gastric, or gastroesophageal adenocarcinoma. *J Clin Oncol.* 2005;23:5660.

180. O'Connell MJ. Current status of chemotherapy for advanced pancreatic and gastric cancer. *J Clin Oncol.* 1985;3:1032–1039.

181. Ajani JA. Docetaxel for gastric and esophageal carcinomas. *Oncology.* 2002;16(Suppl 6):89–96.

182. Demetri GD, et al. Efficacy and safety of imatinib mesylate in advanced gastrointestinal stromal tumors. *N Engl J Med.* 2002;347:472–480.

183. Sutent [package insert]. New York: Pfizer Inc.; 2006. Available at http://www.pfizer.com/pfizer/download/uspi_sutent.pdf. Accessed March 1, 2006.

184. Shin DM, et al. Phase II trial of paclitaxel, ifosfamide, and cisplatin in patients with recurrent head and neck squamous cell carcinoma. *J Clin Oncol.* 1998;16:1325–1330.

185. Posner M, et al. Multicenter phase I–II trial of docetaxel, cisplatin, and fluorouracil induction chemotherapy for patients with locally advanced squamous cell cancer of the head and neck. *J Clin Oncol.* 2001;19:1096–1104.

186. Shin DM, et al. Phase II study of paclitaxel, ifosfamide, and carboplatin in patients with recurrent or metastatic head and neck squamous cell carcinoma of the head and neck (SCCHN). *Cancer.* 1999;91:1316–1323.

187. Fountzilas G, et al. Paclitaxel and carboplatin in recurrent or metastatic head and neck cancer: a phase II study. *Semin Oncol.* 1997;24(Suppl 2):65–67.

188. Hitt R, et al. A phase I/II study of paclitaxel plus cisplatin as firstline therapy for head and neck cancer. *Semin Oncol.* 1995;22(Suppl 15):50–54.

189. Kish JA, et al. Cisplatin and 5-fluorouracil infusion in patients with recurrent and disseminated epidermoid cancer of the head and neck. *Cancer.* 1984;53:1819–1824.

190. Vokes EE, et al. Cisplatin, 5-fluorouracil, and high-dose oral leucovorin for advanced head and neck cancer. *Cancer.* 1989;63(Suppl 6):1048–1053.

191. Veterans Affairs Laryngeal Cancer Study Group. Induction chemotherapy plus radiation compared with surgery plus radiation in patients with advanced laryngeal cancer. *N Engl J Med.* 1991;324:1685–1690.

192. Forastiere AA, et al. Concurrent chemotherapy and radiotherapy for organ preservation in advanced laryngeal cancer. *N Engl J Med.* 2003;349:2091–2098.

193. Al-Sarraf M, et al. Chemoradiotherapy versus radiotherapy in patients with advanced nasopharyngeal cancer: phase III randomized Intergroup study 0099. *J Clin Oncol.* 1998;16:1310–1317.

194. Forastiere AA, et al. Randomized comparison of cisplatin plus fluorouracil and carboplatin plus fluorouracil versus methotrexate in advanced squamous-cell carcinoma of the head and neck: a Southwest Oncology Group study. *J Clin Oncol.* 1992;10:1245–1251.

195. Gebbia V, et al. Vinorelbine plus cisplatin in recurrent or previously untreated unresectable squamous cell carcinoma of the head and neck. *Am J Clin Oncol.* 1995;18:293–296.

196. Dreyfuss A, et al. Taxotere for advanced, inoperable squamous cell carcinoma of the head and neck (SCCHN). *Proc Am Soc Clin Oncol.* 1995;14:875a.

197. Forastiere AA. Current and future trials of Taxol™ (paclitaxel) in head and neck cancer. *Ann Oncol.* 1994;5(Suppl 6):51–54.

198. Hong WK, et al. Chemotherapy in head and neck cancer. *N Engl J Med.* 1983;308:75–79.

199. Degardin M, et al. An EORTC-ECSG phase II study of vinorelbine in patients with recurrent and/or metastatic squamous cell carcinoma of the head and neck. *Ann Oncol.* 1998;9:1103–1107.

200. Chua DT, et al. A phase II study of capecitabine in patients with recurrent and metastatic nasopharyngeal cancer pretreated with platinum-based chemotherapy. *Oral Oncol.* 2003;39:361–366.

201. Venook AP. Treatment of hepatocellular carcinoma: too many options? *J Clin Oncol.* 1994;12:1323–1334.

202. Okada S, et al. A phase 2 study of cisplatin in patients with hepatocellular carcinoma. *Oncology.* 1993;50:22–26.

203. Aguayo A, et al. Nonsurgical treatment of hepatocellular carcinoma. *Semin Oncol.* 2001;28:503–513.

204. Ireland-Gill A, et al. Treatment of acquired immunodeficiency syndrome-related Kaposi's sarcoma using bleomycin-containing combination chemotherapy regimens. *Semin Oncol.* 1992;19(Suppl 5):32–37.

205. Laubenstein LL, et al. Treatment of epidemic Kaposi's sarcoma with etoposide or a combination of doxorubicin, bleomycin, and vinblastine. *J Clin Oncol.* 1984;2:1115–1120.

206. Gill PS, et al. Randomized phase III trial of liposomal daunorubicin versus doxorubicin, bleomycin, and vincristine in AIDS-related Kaposi's sarcoma. *J Clin Oncol.* 1996;14:2353–2364.

207. Northfelt DW, et al. Efficacy of pegylated-liposomal doxorubicin in the treatment of AIDS-related Kaposi's sarcoma after failure of standard chemotherapy. *J Clin Oncol.* 1997;15:653–659.

208. Gill PS, et al. Paclitaxel is safe and effective in the treatment of advanced AIDS-related Kaposi's sarcoma. *J Clin Oncol.* 1999;17:1876–1880.

209. Gill PS, et al. Multicenter trial of low-dose paclitaxel in patients with advanced AIDS-related Kaposi's sarcoma. *Cancer.* 2002;95:147–154.

210. Real FX, Oettgen HF, Krown SE. Kaposi's sarcoma and the acquired immunodeficiency syndrome: treatment with high and low dose of recombinant leucocyte A interferon. *J Clin Oncol.* 1986;4:544–551.

211. Groopman JE, et al. Recombinant alpha-2 interferon therapy for Kaposi's sarcoma associated with the acquired immunodeficiency syndrome. *Ann Intern Med.* 1984;100:671–676.

212. Linker CA, et al. Improved results of treatment of adult acute lymphoblastic leukemia. *Blood.* 1987;69:1242–1248.

213. Linker CA, et al. Treatment of adult acute lymphoblastic leukemia with intensive cyclical chemotherapy: a follow-up report. *Blood.* 1991;78:2814–2822.

214. Larson R, et al. A five-drug regimen remission induction regimen with intensive consolidation for adults with acute lymphoblastic leukemia: Cancer and Leukemia Group B study 8811. *Blood.* 1995;85:2025–2037.

215. Kantarjian H, et al. Results of treatment with hyper-CVAD, a dose intensive regimen in adult acute lymphoblastic leukemia. *J Clin Oncol.* 2000;18:547–561.

216. Faderl S, et al. The role of clofarabine in hematologic and solid malignancies: development of a next generation nucleoside analog. *Cancer.* 2005;103:1985–1995.

217. Gleevec (imatinib mesylate) tablets full prescribing information. East Hanover, NJ: Novartis Pharmaceutical Corporation; Rev. October 2006.

218. Yates JW, et al. Cytosine arabinoside (NSC-63878) and daunorubicin (NSC-83142) in acute nonlymphocytic leukemia. *Cancer Chemother Rep.* 1973;57:485–488.

219. Preisler H, et al. Comparison of three remission induction regimens and two postinduction strategies for the treatment of acute nonlymphocytic leukemia: Cancer and Leukemia Group B study. *Blood.* 1987;69:1441–1449.

220. Preisler H, et al. Adriamycin-cytosine arabinoside therapy for adult acute myelocytic leukemia. *Cancer Treat Rep.* 1977;61:89–92.

221. Wiernik PH, et al. Cytarabine plus idarubicin or daunorubicin as induction and consolidation therapy for previously untreated adult patients with acute myeloid leukemia. *Blood.* 1992;79:313–319.

222. Santana VM, et al. 2-Chlorodeoxyadenosine produces a high rate of complete hematologic remission in relapsed acute myeloid leukemia. *J Clin Oncol.* 1992;10:364–369.

223. Mayer RJ, et al. Intensive postremission chemotherapy in adults with acute myeloid leukemia: Cancer and Leukemia Group B. *N Engl J Med.* 1994;331:896–903.

224. Sievers EL, et al. Selective ablation of acute myeloid leukemia using antibody-targeted chemotherapy: a phase I study of an anti CD33 calicheamycin immunoconjugate. *Blood.* 1999;11:3678–3684.

225. Ho AD, Lipp T, Ehninfer G, Meyer P, Freund M, Hunstein W. Combination therapy with mitox-antrone and etoposide in refractory acute myelogenous leukemia. *Cancer Treat Rep.* 1986;70:1025–1027.

226. Montillo M, et al. Fludarabine, cytarabine, and G-CSF (FLAG) for the treatment of poor risk acute myeloid leukemia. *Am J Hematol.* 1998;58:105–109.

227. Mandelli F, et al. Molecular remission in PML/RAR alpha-positive acute promyelocytic leukemia by combined all-trans retinoic acid and idarubicin (AIDA) therapy. *Blood.* 1997;90:1014–1021.

228. Trisenox© [package insert]. Seattle, WA: Cell Therapeutics, Inc.; 2003. Trisenox© (arsenic trioxide) injection Nursing Advisory Board Meeting Summary, April 2004. Seattle, WA: Cell Therapeutics, Inc.; 2004.

229. Degos L, et al. All-trans retinoic acid as a differentiating agent in the treatment of acute promyelocytic leukemia. *Blood.* 1995;85:2643–2653.

230. Raphael B, et al. Comparison of chlorambucil and prednisone versus cyclophosphamide, vincristine, and prednisone as initial treatment for chronic lymphocytic leukemia: long-term follow-up of an Eastern Co-

operative Oncology Group randomized clinical trial. *J Clin Oncol.* 1991;9:770–776.

231. Keating MJ, et al. Long-term follow-up of patients with chronic lymphocytic leukemia (CLL) receiving fludarabine regimens as initial therapy. *Blood.* 1998;92:1165–1171.

232. O'Brien S, et al. Results of fludarabine and prednisone therapy in 264 patients with chronic lymphocytic leukemia with multivariate analysis-derived prognostic model for response to treatment. *Blood.* 1993;82:1695–1700.

233. Byrd JC, et al. Randomized phase 2 study of fludarabine with concurrent versus sequential treatment with rituximab in symptomatic untreated patients with B-cell chronic lymphocytic leukemia: results from Cancer and Leukemia Group B9712. *Blood.* 2003;101:6–14.

234. Keating MJ, et al. Early results of a chemoimmunotherapy regimen of fludarabine, cyclophosphamide, and rituximab as initial therapy for CLL. *J Clin Oncol.* 2005;22:4079–4088.

235. Osterborg A, et al. Phase II multicenter study of human CD52 antibody in previously treated chronic lymphocytic leukemia. *J Clin Oncol.* 1997;15:1567–1574.

236. Dighiero G, et al. Chlorambucil in indolent chronic lymphocytic leukemia. French Cooperative Group on Chronic Lymphocytic Leukemia. *N Engl J Med.* 1998;338:1506–1514.

237. Saven A, et al. 2-Chlorodeoxyadenosine activity in patients with untreated chronic lymphocytic leukemia. *J Clin Oncol.* 1995;13:570–574.

238. Keating MJ, et al. Fludarabine: a new agent with major activity against chronic lymphocytic leukemia. *Blood.* 1989;74:19–25.

239. Sawitsky A, Rai KR, Glidewell O, Silver RT. Comparison of daily versus intermittent chlorambucil and prednisone therapy in the treatment of patients with chronic lymphocytic leukemia. *Blood.* 1977;50:1049.

240. Treanda (bendamustine HCL) for injection dull prescribing information. Cephalon Inc., Frazer, PA; March 2008.

241. Guilhot F, et al. Interferon α-2b combined with cytarabine versus interferon alone in chronic myelogenous leukemia. *N Engl J Med.* 1997;337:223–229.

242. Druker BJ, et al. Efficacy and safety of a specific inhibitor of the BCR-ABL tyrosine kinase in chronic myelogenous leukemia. *N Engl J Med.* 2001;344:1031–1037.

243. Hehlmann R, et al. Randomized comparison of busulfan and hydroxyurea in chronic myelogenous leukemia: prolongation of survival by hydroxyurea: the German CML Study Group. *Blood.* 1993;82:398–407.

244. Hehlmann R, et al. Randomized comparison of interferon-alpha with busulfan and hydroxyurea in chronic myelogenous leukemia: German CML Study Group. *Blood.* 1994;84:4064–4077.

245. The Italian Cooperative Study Group on Chronic Myelogenous Leukemia. Interferon alfa-2a as compared with conventional chemotherapy for the treatment of chronic myeloid leukemia. *N Engl J Med.* 1994;330:820–825.

246. Talpaz M. Dasatinib in imatinib-resistant Philadelphia chromosome-positive leukemia. *N Engl J Med*. 2006;354:2531–2541.

247. Sprycel [package insert]. Sprycel (dastinib) tablets. Princeton, NJ: Bristol-Myers Squibb Company.

248. Tasigna (nilotinib) capsules full prescribing information. East Hanover, NJ: Novartis Pharmaceutical Corporation; October 2007.

249. Ontak full prescribing information. Ridgefield Park, NJ: Eisai Inc.; February 2007.

250. Saven A, Piro LD. Treatment of hairy cell leukemia. *Blood*. 1992;79: 1110–1120.

251. Cassileth PA, et al. Pentostatin induces durable remission in hairy cell leukemia. *J Clin Oncol*. 1991;9:243–246.

252. Ratain MJ, et al. Treatment of hairy cell leukemia with recombinant alpha-2 interferon. *Blood*. 1985;65:644–648.

253. Strauss GM, et al. Randomized clinical trial of adjuvant chemotherapy with paclitaxel and carboplatin following resection in stage IB non-small cell lung cancer: CALGB 9633. *J Clin Oncol*. 2004;621S(abstract 7019).

254. Winton T, et al. Vinorelbine plus cisplatin versus observation in resected non-small cell lung cancer. *N Engl J Med*. 2005;352:2589–2597.

255. Langer CJ, et al. Paclitaxel and carboplatin in combination in the treatment of advanced non-small cell lung cancer: a phase II toxicity, response, and survival analysis. *J Clin Oncol*. 1995;13:1860–1870.

256. Giaccone G, et al. Randomized study of paclitaxel-cisplatin versus cisplatin-teniposide in patients with advanced non-small cell lung cancer: the European Organization for Research and Treatment of Cancer Lung Cancer Cooperative Group. *J Clin Oncol*. 1998;16:2133–2141.

257. Fossella F, et al. Randomized, multinational, phase III study of docetaxel plus platinum combinations versus vinorelbine plus cisplatin for advanced non-small cell lung cancer: the TAX 326 Study Group. *J Clin Oncol*. 2003;21:3016–3024.

258. Belani CP, et al. Docetaxel and cisplatin in patients with advanced non-small cell lung cancer (NSCLC): a multicenter phase II trial. *Clin Lung Cancer*. 1999;1:144–150.

259. Georgoulias V, et al. Platinum-based and non-platinum-based chemotherapy in advanced non-small cell lung cancer: a randomized multicentre trial. *Lancet*. 2001;357:1478–1484.

260. Abratt RP, Bezwoda WR, Goedhals L, Hacking DJ. Weekly gemcitabine with monthly cisplatin: effective chemotherapy for advanced non-small cell lung cancer. *J Clin Oncol*. 1997;15:744–749.

261. Langer CJ, et al. Gemcitabine and carboplatin in combination: an update of phase I and phase II studies in non-small cell lung cancer. *Semin Oncol*. 1999;26(Suppl 4):12–18.

262. Frasci G, et al. Gemcitabine plus vinorelbine versus vinorelbine alone in elderly patients with advanced non-small cell lung cancer. *J Clin Oncol*. 2000;18:2529–2536.

263. Smith TJ, et al. Economic evaluation of a randomized clinical trial comparing vinorelbine, vinorelbine plus cisplatin, and vindesine plus cisplatin for non-small cell lung cancer. *J Clin Oncol.* 1995;13:2166–2173.

264. Cremonesi M, et al. Vinorelbine and carboplatin in operable non-small lung cancer: a mono-institutional phase II study. *Oncology.* 2003;64(2): 97–101.

265. Longeval E, et al. Combination chemotherapy with cisplatin and etoposide in bronchogenic squamous cell carcinoma and adenocarcinoma: a study by the EORTC lung cancer working party. *Cancer.* 1982;50: 2751–2756.

266. Gandara D, et al. Consolidation docetaxel after concurrent chemoradiotherapy in stage IIIB non-small cell lung cancer: phase II Southwest Oncology Group Study S9504. *J Clin Oncol.* 2003;21:2004–2010.

267. Sandler A, et al. Paclitaxel-carboplatin alone or with bevacizumab for non-small cell lung cancer. *N Engl J Med.* 2006;355(24):2050–2542.

268. Lilenbaum RC, et al. Single-agent versus combination chemotherapy in advanced non-small cell lung cancer: the Cancer and Leukemia Group B (study 9730). *J Clin Oncol.* 2005;23:190–196.

269. Tester WJ, et al. Phase II study of patients with metastatic non-small cell carcinoma of the lung treated with paclitaxel by 3-hour infusion. *Cancer.* 1997;79:724–729.

270. Miller VA, et al. Docetaxel (Taxotere) as a single agent and in combination chemotherapy for the treatment of patients with advanced non-small cell lung cancer. *Semin Oncol.* 2000;27(Suppl 3):3–10.

271. Hainsworth JD, et al. Weekly docetaxel in the treatment of elderly patients with advanced non-small cell lung cancer. *Cancer.* 2000;89:328–333.

272. Hanna N, et al. Randomized phase III trial of pemetrexed versus docetaxel in patients with non-small cell lung cancer previously treated with chemotherapy. *J Clin Oncol.* 2004;22:1589–1597.

273. Manegold C, et al. Single-agent gemcitabine versus cisplatin-etoposide: early results of a randomized phase II study in locally advanced or metastatic non-small cell lung cancer. *Ann Oncol.* 1997;8:525–529.

274. Perez-Soler R, et al. Phase II study of topotecan in patients with advanced non-small cell lung cancer previously untreated with chemotherapy. *J Clin Oncol.* 1996;14:503–513.

275. Furuse K, et al. Randomized study of vinorelbine (VRB) versus vindesine (VDS) in previously untreated stage IIIB or IV non-small cell lung cancer (NSCLC): the Japan Vinorelbine Lung Cancer Cooperative Study Group. *Ann Oncol.* 1996;7:815–820.

276. Herbst RS. Dose-comparative monotherapy trials of ZD1839 in previously treated non-small cell lung cancer patients. *Semin Oncol.* 2003;30(Suppl 1):30–38.

277. Shepherd FA, et al. A randomized placebo-controlled trial of erlotinib in patients with advanced non-small cell lung cancer (NSCLC) following failure of 1st and 2nd line chemotherapy: a National Cancer Institute of Canada Clinical Trials Group (NCIC CTG) trial. *J Clin Oncol.* 2004;22 (Suppl 1):14S(abstract 7022).

278. Ihde DC, et al. Prospective randomized comparison of high-dose and standard-dose etoposide and cisplatin chemotherapy in patients with extensive-stage small cell lung cancer. *J Clin Oncol.* 1994;12:2022–2034.

279. Viren M, et al. Carboplatin and etoposide in extensive small cell lung cancer. *Acta Oncol.* 1994;33:921–924.

280. Noda K, et al. Irinotecan plus cisplatin compared with etoposide plus cisplatin for extensive small cell lung cancer. *N Engl J Med.* 2002;346: 85–91.

281. Hainsworth JD, et al. Paclitaxel, carboplatin, and extended-schedule etoposide in the treatment of small cell lung cancer: comparison of sequential phase II trials using different dose-intensities. *J Clin Oncol.* 1997;15:3464–3470.

282. Roth BJ, et al. Randomized study of cyclophosphamide, doxorubicin, and vincristine versus etoposide and cisplatin versus alternation of these two regimens in extensive small cell lung cancer: a phase III trial of the Southeastern Cancer Study Group. *J Clin Oncol.* 1992;10:282–291.

283. Aisner J, et al. Doxorubicin, cyclophosphamide, etoposide and platinum, doxorubicin, cyclophosphamide and etoposide for small cell carcinoma of the lung. *Semin Oncol.* 1986;(Suppl 3):54–62.

284. Johnson DH. Recent developments in chemotherapy treatment of small cell lung cancer. *Semin Oncol.* 1993;20:315–325.

285. Johnson DH, et al. Prolonged administration of oral etoposide in patients with relapsed or refractory small cell lung cancer: a phase II trial. *J Clin Oncol.* 1990;8:1013–1017.

286. Hainsworth JD, et al. The current role and future prospects of paclitaxel in the treatment of small cell lung cancer. *Semin Oncol.* 1999;26(Suppl 2):60–66.

287. Ardizzoni A, et al. Topotecan, a new active drug in the second-line treatment of small cell lung cancer: a phase II study in patients with refractory and sensitive disease: the European Organization for Research and Treatment of Cancer Early Clinical Studies Group and New Drug Development Office and the Lung Cancer Cooperative Group. *J Clin Oncol.* 1997;15:2090–2096.

288. Bonadonna G, et al. Combination chemotherapy of Hodgkin's disease with adriamycin, bleomycin, vinblastine, and imidazole carboxamide versus MOPP. *Cancer.* 1975;36:252–259.

289. DeVita VT, Jr, et al. Combination chemotherapy in the treatment of advanced Hodgkin's disease. *Ann Intern Med.* 1970;73:881–895.

290. Klimo P, et al. MOPP/ABV hybrid program: combination chemotherapy based on early introduction of seven effective drugs for advanced Hodgkin's disease. *J Clin Oncol.* 1985;3:1174–1182.

291. Canellos GP, et al. Chemotherapy of advanced Hodgkin's disease with MOPP, ABVD, or MOPP alternating with ABVD. *N Engl J Med.* 1992; 327(21):1478–1484.

292. Bartlett NL, et al. Brief chemotherapy, Stanford V, and adjuvant radiotherapy for bulky or advanced-stage Hodgkin's disease: a preliminary report. *J Clin Oncol.* 1995;13:1080–1088.

293. Diehl V, et al. BEACOPP, a new dose-escalated and accelerated regimen is at least as effective as COPP/ABVD in patients with advanced-stage Hodgkin's lymphoma. *J Clin Oncol.* 1998;16:3810–3821.

294. Tesch H, et al. Moderate dose escalation for advanced Hodgkin's disease using the bleomycin, etoposide, adriamycin, cyclophosphamide, vincristine, procarbazine, and prednisone scheme and adjuvant radiotherapy: a study of the German Hodgkin's Lymphoma Study Group. *Blood.* 1998;15:4560–4567.

295. Radford JA, et al. Results of a randomized trial comparing MVPP chemotherapy with a hybrid regimen, ChlVPP/EVA, in the initial treatment of Hodgkin's disease. *J Clin Oncol.* 1995;13:2379–2385.

296. Longo DL. The use of chemotherapy in the treatment of Hodgkin's disease. *Semin Oncol.* 1990;17:716–735.

297. Colwill R, et al. Mini-BEAM as salvage therapy for relapsed or refractory Hodgkin's disease before intensive therapy and autologous bone marrow transplantation. *J Clin Oncol.* 1995;13:396–402.

298. Santoro A, et al. Gemcitabine in the treatment of refractory Hodgkin's disease: results of a multicenter phase II study. *J Clin Oncol.* 2000;18: 2615–2619.

299. Bagley CM, Jr, et al. Advanced lymphosarcoma: intensive cyclical combination chemotherapy with cyclophosphamide, vincristine, and prednisone. *Ann Intern Med.* 1972;76:227–234.

300. Hochster HS, et al. Results of E1496: A phase III trial of CVP with or without maintenance rituximab in advanced indolent lymphoma (NHL) (abstract). *J Clin Oncol.* 2004;22(abstract 6502).

301. Sonneveld P, et al. Comparison of doxorubicin and mitoxantrone in the treatment of elderly patients with advanced diffuse non-Hodgkin's lymphoma using CHOP versus CNOP chemotherapy. *J Clin Oncol.* 1995; 13:2530–2539.

302. McLaughlin P, et al. Fludarabine, mitoxantrone, and dexamethasone: an effective new regimen for indolent lymphoma. *J Clin Oncol.* 1996;14: 1262–1268.

303. Hochster H, et al. Efficacy of cyclophosphamide (CYC) and fludarabine (FAMP) as first-line therapy of low-grade non-Hodgkin's lymphoma (NHL). *Blood.* 1994;84 (Suppl 1):383a.

304. McKelvey EM, et al. Hydroxydaunomycin (Adriamycin) combination chemotherapy in malignant lymphoma. *Cancer.* 1976;38:1484–1493.

305. Vose JM, et al. Phase II study of rituximab in combination with CHOP chemotherapy in patients with previously untreated, aggressive non-Hodgkin's lymphoma. *J Clin Oncol.* 2001;19:389–397.

306. Wilson WH, et al. EPOCH chemotherapy: toxicity and efficacy in relapsed and refractory non-Hodgkin's lymphoma. *J Clin Oncol.* 1993;11: 1573–1582.

307. Wilson WH. Chemotherapy sensitization by rituximab: experimental and clinical evidence. *Semin Oncol.* 2000;27(Suppl 12):30–36.

308. Klimo P, et al. MACOP-B chemotherapy for the treatment of diffuse large cell lymphoma. *Ann Intern Med.* 1985;102:596–602.

309. Shipp MA, et al. Identification of major prognostic subgroups of patients with large-cell lymphoma treated with m-BACOD or M-BACOD. *Ann Intern Med.* 1986;104:757–765.

310. Longo DL, et al. Superiority of ProMACE-CytaBOM over Pro-MACE-MOPP in the treatment of advanced diffuse aggressive lymphoma: results of a prospective randomized trial. *J Clin Oncol.* 1991;9:25–38.

311. Magrath I, et al. An effective therapy for both undifferentiated lymphomas and lymphoblastic lymphomas in children and young adults. *Blood.* 1984;63:1102–1111.

312. Magrath I, et al. Adults and children with small non-cleaved cell lymphoma have a similar excellent outcome when treated with the same chemotherapy regimen. *J Clin Oncol.* 1996;14:925.

313. Berstein JI, et al. Combined modality therapy for adults with small non-cleaved cell lymphoma (Burkitt's and non-Burkitt's types). *J Clin Oncol.* 1986;4:847–858.

314. Goy AH, et al. Report of a phase II study of proteosome inhibitor bortezomib in patients with relapsed or refractory indolent and aggressive B-cell lymphomas. *Proc Am Soc Clin Oncol.* 2003;22:570(abstract 2291).

315. Coiffier B, et al. Rituximab plus CHOP in combination with CHOP chemotherapy in patients with diffuse large B-cell lymphoma: an update of the GELA study. *N Engl J Med.* 2002;346:235–242.

316. Vose JM, et al. CNOP for diffuse aggressive non-Hodgkin's lymphoma: the Nebraska Lymphoma Study Group experience. *Leuk Lymphoma.* 2002;43:799–804.

317. Velasquez WS, et al. ESHAP-an effective chemotherapy regimen in refractory and relapsing lymphoma: a 4-year follow-up study. *J Clin Oncol.* 1994;12:1169–1176.

318. Velasquez WS, et al. Effective salvage therapy for lymphoma with cisplatin in combination with high-dose ara-C and dexamethasone. *Blood.* 1988;71:117–122.

319. Moskowitz C, et al. Ifosfamide, carboplatin, and etoposide: a highly effective cytoreduction and peripheral blood progenitor cell mobilization regimen for transplant-eligible patients with non-Hodgkin's lymphoma. *J Clin Oncol.* 1999;17:3776–3785.

320. Rodriguez MA, et al. A phase II trial of mesna/ifosfamide, mitoxantrone, and etoposide for refractory lymphoma. *Ann Oncol.* 1995;6:609–611.

321. Abrey LE, et al. Treatment for primary CNS lymphoma: the next step. *J Clin Oncol.* 2000;18:3144–3150.

322. McLaughlin P, et al. Rituximab chimeric anti-CD20 monoclonal antibody therapy for relapsed indolent lymphoma: half of patients respond to a four-dose treatment program. *J Clin Oncol.* 1998;16:2825–2833.

323. Witzig TE, et al. Randomized controlled trial of yttrium-90-labeled ibritumomab tiuxetan radioimmunotherapy versus rituximab immunotherapy for patients with relapsed or refractory low-grade follicular, or transformed B-cell non-Hodgkin's lymphoma. *J Clin Oncol.* 2002;20:2453–2463.

324. Falkson CI. A phase II trial in patients with previously treated low-grade lymphoma.*Am J Clin Oncol.* 1996;19:268–270.

325. Betticher DC, von Rohr A, Ratschiller D, et al. Fewer infections but maintained antitumor activity with lower-dose versus standard-dose cladribine in pretreated low-grade non-Hodgkin's lymphoma. *J Clin Oncol.* 1998;16:850–858.

326. Bexxar [package insert]. Research Triangle Park, NC: Glaxo SmithKline; October 2005.

327. Zolinza (vorinostat) capsules full prescribing information. Whitehouse Station, NJ: Merck and Co., Inc.; October, 2006.

328. Kirkwood JM, et al. Interferon alfa-2b adjuvant therapy of high-risk resected cutaneous melanoma: the Eastern Cooperative Oncology Trial EST 1684. *J Clin Oncol.* 1996;14:7–17.

329. Creagen ET, et al. Phase III clinical trial of the combination of cisplatin, dacarbazine, and carmustine with or without tamoxifen in patients with advanced malignant melanoma. *J Clin Oncol.* 1999;17:1884–1890.

330. DelPrete SA, et al. Combination chemotherapy with cisplatin, carmustine, dacarbazine, and tamoxifen in metastatic melanoma. *Cancer Treat Rep.* 1984;68:1403–1405.

331. Legha SS, et al. A prospective evaluation of a triple-drug regimen containing cisplatin, vinblastine, and DTIC (CVD) for metastatic melanoma. *Cancer.* 1989;64:2024–2029.

332. Falkson CI, et al. Phase III trial of dacarbazine vs. dacarbazine with interferon α-2b vs. dacarbazine with tamoxifen vs. dacarbazine with interferon α-2b and tamoxifen in patients with metastatic malignant melanoma. *J Clin Oncol.* 1998;16:1743–1751.

333. Eton O, et al. Sequential biochemotherapy versus chemotherapy for metastatic melanoma: results from a phase III randomized trial. *J Clin Oncol.* 2002;20:2045–2052.

334. Hwu WJ, et al. Temozolomide plus thalidomide in patients with advanced melanoma: results of a dose finding trial. *J Clin Oncol.* 2002; 20:2607–2609.

335. Luce JK, et al. Clinical trials with the antitumor agent 5-(3,3-dimethyl-1-triazeno) imidazole-4-carboxamide (NSC-45388). *Cancer Chemother Rep.* 1970;54:119–124.

336. Pritchard KI, et al. DTIC therapy in metastatic malignant melanoma: a simplified dose schedule. *Cancer Treat Rep.* 1980;64:1123–1126.

337. Kirkwood JM, et al. Advances in the diagnosis and treatment of malignant melanoma. *Semin Oncol.* 1997;24(Suppl 4):1–48.

338. Parkinson DR, et al. Interleukin-2 therapy in patients with metastatic malignant melanoma: a phase II study. *J Clin Oncol.* 1990;8:1650–1656.

339. Middleton MR, et al. Randomized phase II study of temozolomide versus dacarbazine in the treatment of patients with advanced metastatic malignant melanoma. *J Clin Oncol.* 2000;18:158–166.

340. Ardizzoni A, Rosso R, Salvati F, et al. Activity of doxorubicin and cisplatin combination chemotherapy in patients with diffuse malignant pleural mesothelioma. *Cancer.* 1991;67:2984–2987.

341. Shin DM, et al. Prospective study of combination chemotherapy with cyclophosphamide, doxorubicin, and cisplatin for unresectable or metastatic malignant pleural mesothelioma. *Cancer.* 1995;76:2230–2236.

342. Nowak AK, et al. A multicentre phase II study of cisplatin and gemcitabine for malignant mesothelioma. *Br J Cancer.* 2002;87:491–496.

343. Favaretto AG, et al. Gemcitabine combined with carboplatin in patients with malignant pleural mesothelioma: a multicentric phase II study. *Cancer.* 2003;97:2791–2797.

344. Vogelzang NJ, et al. Phase III study of pemetrexed in combination with cisplatin versus cisplatin alone in patients with malignant pleural mesothelioma. *J Clin Oncol.* 2003;21:2636–2644.

345. Southwest Oncology Group Study. Remission maintenance therapy for multiple myeloma. Arch Intern Med. 1975;135:147–152.

346. Barlogie B, Smith L, Alexanian R. Effective treatment of advanced multiple myeloma refractory to alkylating agents. *N Engl J Med.* 1984;310:1353–1356.

347. Rajkumar SV, et al. Combination therapy with thalidomide plus dexamethasone for newly diagnosed myeloma. *J Clin Oncol.* 2002;20:4319–4323.

348. Case DC, Jr, et al. Improved survival times in multiple myeloma treated with melphalan, prednisone, cyclophosphamide, vincristine, and BCNU. *Am J Med.* 77;63:897–903.

349. Oken MM, et al. Comparison of melphalan and prednisone with vincristine, carmustine, melphalan, cyclophosphamide and prednisone in the treatment of multiple myeloma: results of Eastern Cooperative Oncology Group Study E2479. *Cancer.* 1997;79(8):1561–1567.

350. Orlowski RZ, et al. Phase III study of pegylated liposomal doxorubicin plus bortezomib compared with bortezomib alone improves time to progression in relapsed or refractory multiple myeloma: results from DOXIL-MMY-3001. *J Clin Oncol.* 2007;25:5460–5469.

351. Wever DM, et al. Lenalidomide plus dexamethasone for relapsed multiple myeloma in North America. *N Engl J Med.* 2007;357:2133–2142.

352. Alexanian R, Barlogie B, Dixon D. High-dose glucocorticoid treatment of resistant myeloma. *Ann Intern Med.* 1986;105:8–11.

353. Cunningham D, et al. High-dose melphalan for multiple myeloma: long-term follow-up data. *J Clin Oncol.* 1994;12:764–768.

354. Singhal S, et al. Antitumor activity of thalidomide in refractory multiple myeloma. *N Engl J Med.* 1999;341:1565–1571.

355. Richardson P, et al. A phase II study of bortezomib in relapsed, refractory myeloma. *N Engl J Med.* 2003;348:2609–2617.

356. Browman GP, et al. Randomized trial of interferon maintenance in multiple myeloma: a study of the National Cancer Institute of Canada Clinical Trials Group. *J Clin Oncol.* 1995;13:2354–2360.

357. Kaminskas E, et al. Approval summary: azacytidine for treatment of myelodysplastic syndrome subtypes. *Clin Cancer Res.* 2005;11: 3604–3608.

358. List A, et al. Opportunities for Trisenox (arsenic trioxide) in the treatment of myelodysplastic syndromes. *Leukemia.* 2003;17:1499–1507.

359. List A, et al. Lenalidomide in the myelodysplastic syndrome with chromosome 5q deletion. *N Engl J Med.* 2006;355:1456–1465.

360. Dacogen (decitabine for injection) [package insert]. Bloomington, MN: MGI Pharma, Inc.; May 2006.

361. Kantarjian HM, Issa JP. Decitabine dosing schedules. *Semin Hematol.* 2005;42(3 Suppl 2):S17–S22.

362. Swenerton K, et al. Cisplatin-cyclophosphamide versus carboplatin cyclophosphamide in advanced ovarian cancer: a randomized phase III study of the National Cancer Institute of Canada Clinical Trials Group. *J Clin Oncol.* 1992;10:718–726.

363. Alberts D, et al. Improved therapeutic index of carboplatin plus cyclophosphamide versus cisplatin plus cyclophosphamide: final report by the Southwestern Oncology Group of a phase III randomized trial in stages III and IV ovarian cancer. *J Clin Oncol.* 1992;10:706–717.

364. McGuire WP, et al. Cyclophosphamide and cisplatin compared with paclitaxel and cisplatin in patients with stage III and stage IV ovarian cancer. *N Engl J Med.* 1996;334:1–6.

365. Ozols RE. Combination regimens of paclitaxel and the platinum drugs as first-line regimens for ovarian cancer. *Semin Oncol.* 1995;22 (Suppl 15):1–6.

366. Markman M, et al. Combination chemotherapy with carboplatin and docetaxel in the treatment of cancers of the ovary and fallopian tube and primary carcinoma of the peritoneum. *J Clin Oncol.* 2001;19:1901–1905.

367. D'Agostino G, et al. Phase II study of liposomal doxorubicin and gemcitabine in the salvage treatment of ovarian cancer. *Br J Cancer.* 2003;89: 1180–1184.

368. Nagourney RA, et al. Phase II trial of gemcitabine plus cisplatin repeating doublet therapy in previously treated relapsed ovarian cancer patients. *Gynecol Oncol.* 2003;88:35–39.

369. Jacobus Pfisterer, et al. Gemcitabine plus carboplatin compared with carboplatin in patients with platinum-sensitive recurrent ovarian cancer: an Intergroup trial of the AGO-OVAR, the NCIC CTG, and the EORTC GCG. *J Clin Oncol.* 2006;24:4699–4707.

370. Armstrong DK, et al. Intraperitoneal cisplatin and paclitaxel in ovarian cancer. *N Engl J Med.* 2006;354:34–43.

371. Walker JL, et al. Intraperitoneal catheter outcomes in phase III trial of intravenous verses intraperitoneal chemotherapy in optimal stage III ovarian and primary peritoneal cancer: a gynecological oncology group study. *Gynecol Oncol.* 2006;100:27–32.

372. Markman M. Altretamine (hexamethylmelamine) in platinum-resistant and platinum-refractory ovarian cancer: a gynecologic oncology group phase II trial. *Gynecol Oncol.* 1998;69:226–229.

373. Gordon AN, et al. Phase II study of liposomal doxorubicin in platinum- and paclitaxel-refractory epithelial ovarian cancer. *J Clin Oncol.* 2000; 18:3093–3100.

374. McGuire WP, et al. Taxol: a unique antineoplastic agent with significant activity in advanced ovarian epithelial neoplasms. *Ann Intern Med.* 1989; 111:273–279.

375. Kudelka AP, et al. Phase II study of intravenous topotecan as a 5-day in- fusion for refractory epithelial ovarian carcinoma. *J Clin Oncol.* 1996; 14:1552–1557.

376. Lund B, Hansen OP, Theilade K, Hansen M, Neijt NP. Phase II study of gemcitabine (2929-difluorodeoxycytidine) in previously treated ovarian cancer patients. *J Natl Cancer Inst.* 1994;86:1530–1533.

377. Ozols RF. Oral etoposide for the treatment of recurrent ovarian cancer. *Drugs.* 1999;58(Suppl 3):43–49.

378. Dimopoulos MA, et al. Treatment of ovarian germ cell tumors with a 3-day bleomycin, etoposide, and cisplatin regimen: a prospective multi- center study. *Gynecol Oncol.* 2004;95:695–700.

379. Gastrointestinal Tumor Study Group. Comparative therapeutic trial of radiation with or without chemotherapy in pancreatic carcinoma. *Int J Radiat Oncol Biol Phys.* 1979;5:1643–1647.

380. DeCaprio JA, et al. Fluorouracil and high-dose leucovorin in previously untreated patients with advanced adenocarcinoma of the pancreas: re- sults of a phase II trial. *J Clin Oncol.* 1991;9:2128–2133.

381. Hess V, et al. Combining capecitabine and gemcitabine in patients with advanced pancreatic carcinoma: a phase I/II trial. *J Clin Oncol.* 2003; 21:66–68.

382. Fine RL, et al. The GTX regimen: a biochemically synergistic combina- tion for advanced pancreatic cancer (PC). *Proc Am Soc Clin Oncol.* 2003;22:281(abstract 1129).

383. Heinemann V. Randomized phase III of gemcitabine plus cisplatin com- pared with gemcitabine alone in advanced pancreatic cancer. *J Clin Oncol.* 2006;24:3946–3951.

384. Epelbaum K, et al. Gemcitabine and cisplatin with advanced pancreatic cancer. Proc *J Clin Oncol.* 2003;22:1202.

385. Ko AH, et al. Phase II study of fixed-dose rate gemcitabine with cis- platin formetastatic adenocarcinoma of the pancreas. *J Clin Oncol.* 2006;24:327–329.

386. Poplin E, et al. Phase III trial of gemcitabine (30-minute infusion) ver- sus gemcitabine (fixed-dose-rate infusion [FDR]) versus gemcitabine + oxaliplatin (GEMOX) in patients with advanced pancreatic cancer. *Proc Am Soc Clin Oncol.* 2006;24:1805.

387. Louvet C, et al. Gemcitabine combined with oxaliplatin in advanced pancreatic adenocarcinoma: final results of a GERCOR multicenter phase II study. *J Clin Oncol.* 2002;20:1512–1518.

388. Rocha-Lima C, Savarese D, Bruckner H, et al. Irinotecan plus gemcita- bine induces both radiographic and CA19-9 tumor marker responses in

patients with previously untreated advanced pancreatic cancer. *J Clin Oncol.* 2002;20:1182–1191.

389. Leonard RC, et al. Chemotherapy prolongs survival in inoperable pancreatic carcinoma. *Br J Cancer.* 1994;81:882–885.

390. Moore MJ, et al. Erlotinib plus gemcitabine compared to gemcitabine alone in patients with advanced pancreatic cancer: a phase III trial of the NCIC-CTG. *J Clin Oncol.* 2005;23:16S(abstract 1).

391. No authors listed. Phase II studies of drug combinations in advanced pancreatic carcinoma 5-fluorouracil plus doxorubicin plus mitomycin-C and two regimens of streptozotocin plus mitomycin-C plus 5-fluorouracil: the Gastrointestinal Study Goup. *J Clin Oncol.* 1986;4:1794–1798.

392. Burris HA, et al. Improvements in survival and clinical benefit with gemcitabine as first-line therapy for patients with advanced pancreas cancer: a randomized trial. *J Clin Oncol.* 1997;15:2403–2413.

393. Brand R, et al. A phase I trial of weekly gemcitabine administered as a prolonged infusion in patients with pancreatic cancer and other solid tumors. *Invest New Drugs.* 1997;15:331–341.

394. Cartwright TH, et al. Phase II study of oral capecitabine in patients with advanced or metastatic pancreatic cancer. *J Clin Oncol.* 2002;20:160–164.

395. Eisenberger MA, et al. Prognostic factors in stage D2 prostate cancer: important implications for future trials; results of a cooperative Intergroup study (INT.0036): the National Cancer Institute Intergroup Study #0036. *Semin Oncol.* 1994;21:613–619.

396. Jurincic CD, et al. Combined treatment (goserelin plus flutamide) versus monotherapy (goserelin alone) in advanced prostate cancer: a randomized study. *Semin Oncol.* 1991;18(Suppl 6):21–25.

397. Pienta KJ, et al. Phase II evaluation of oral estramustine and oral etoposide in hormone-refractory adenocarcinoma of the prostate. *J Clin Oncol.* 1994;12:2005–2012.

398. Hudes GR, et al. Phase II study of estramustine and vinblastine, two microtubule inhibitors, in hormone-refractory prostate cancer. *J Clin Oncol.* 1992;11:1754–1761.

399. Hudes GR, et al. Paclitaxel plus estramustine in metastatic hormone-refractory prostate cancer. *Semin Oncol.* 1995;22(Suppl 12):41–45.

400. Tannock IF, et al. Chemotherapy with mitoxantrone plus prednisone or prednisone alone for symptomatic hormone-resistant prostate cancer: a Canadian randomized trial with palliative end points. *J Clin Oncol.* 1996;14:1756–1764.

401. Petrylak DP. Phase I trial of docetaxel with estramustine in androgen-independent prostate cancer. *J Clin Oncol.* 1999;17:958–967.

402. Eisenberger MA, et al. A multicenter phase III comparison of docetaxel (D) + prednisone (P) and mitoxantrone (MTZ) + P in patients with hormone-refractory prostate cancer (HRPC). *Proc Am Soc Clin Oncol.* 2004;23:2(abstract 4).

403. Roth BJ, et al. Taxol in advanced, hormone-refractory carcinoma of the prostate: a phase II trial of the Eastern Cooperative Oncology Group. *Cancer.* 1993;72:2260–2457.

404. Ahmed S, et al. Feasibility of weekly 1 hour paclitaxel in hormone-refractory prostate cancer (HRPC): a preliminary report of a phase II trial. *Proc Am Soc Clin Oncol.* 1998;17:325a.

405. Petrylak DP. Docetaxel (Taxotere) in hormone-refractory prostate cancer. *Semin Oncol.* 2000;27(Suppl 3):24–29.

406. Murphy GP, et al. Use of estramustine phosphate in prostate cancer by the National Prostatic Cancer Project and by Roswell Park Memorial Institute. *Urology.* 1984;23:54–63.

407. Dijkman GA, Debruyne FM, Fernandez del Moral P, et al. A randomized trial comparing the safety and efficacy of the Zoladex 10.8-mg depot, administered every 12 weeks, to that of the Zoladex 3.6-mg depot, administered every 4 weeks, in patients with advanced prostate cancer: the Dutch South East Cooperative Urological Group. *Eur Urol.* 1995;27:43–46.

408. The Leuprolide Study Group. Leuprolide versus diethylstilbestrol for metastatic prostate cancer. *N Engl J Med.* 1984;311:1281–1286.

409. Sharifi R, et al. Leuprolide acetate 22.5-mg 12-week depot formulation in the treatment of patients with advanced prostate cancer. *Clin Ther.* 1996;18:647–657.

410. Schellhammer PF, et al. Clinical benefits of bicalutamide compared with flutamide in combined androgen blockade for patients with advanced prostatic carcinoma: final report of a double-blind, randomized, multi-center trial: Casodex Combination Study Group. *Urology.* 1997;50:330–336.

411. McLeod DG, et al. The use of flutamide in hormone-refractory metastatic prostate cancer. *Cancer.* 1993;72:3870–3873.

412. Janknegt RA, et al. Orchiectomy and nilutamide or placebo as treatment of metastatic prostatic cancer in a multinational double-blind randomized trial. *J Urol.* 1993;149:77–82.

413. Johnson DE, et al. Ketoconazole therapy for hormonally refractive metastatic prostate cancer. *Urology.* 1988;31:132–134.

414. Havlin KA, et al. Aminoglutethimide: theoretical considerations and clinical results in advanced prostate cancer. *Cancer Treat Res.* 1988;39:83–96.

415. Atzpodien J, et al. European studies of interleukin-2 in metastatic renal cell carcinoma. *Semin Oncol.* 1993;20(Suppl 9):22.

416. Rini BI, et al. Phase II trial of weekly intravenous gemcitabine with continuous infusion fluorouracil in patients with metastatic renal cell cancer. *J Clin Oncol.* 2000;18:2419–2426.

417. Fyfe G, et al. Results of treatment of 255 patients with metastatic renal cell carcinoma who received high-dose recombinant interleukin-2 therapy. *J Clin Oncol.* 1995;13:688–696.

418. Minasian LM, et al. Interferon alfa-2a in advanced renal cell carcinoma: treatment results and survival in 159 patients with long-term follow-up. *J Clin Oncol.* 1993;11:1368–1375.

419. Motzer RJ, et al. Prognostic factors for survival in previously treated patients with metastatic renal cell carcinoma. *J Clin Oncol.* 2004;223:454–463.

420. Motzer RJ, et al. Activity of SU11248, a multitargeted inhibitor of vascular endothelial growth factor receptor and platelet-derived growth factor receptor, in patients with metastatic renal cell carcinoma. *J Clin Oncol.* 2006; 24:16–24.

421. Torisel (temsirolimus) for injection, full prescribing information. Philadelphia, PA: Wyeth Pharmaceuticals, Inc.; May 2007.

422. Antman K, et al. An Intergroup phase III randomized study of doxorubicin and dacarbazine with or without ifosfamide and mesna in advanced soft tissue and bone sarcomas. *J Clin Oncol.* 1993;11:1276–1285.

423. Elias A, et al. Response to mesna, doxorubicin, ifosfamide, and dacarbazine in 108 patients with metastatic or unresectable sarcoma and no prior chemotherapy. *J Clin Oncol.* 1989;7:1208–1216.

424. Santoro A, et al. Doxorubicin versus CYVADIC versus doxorubicin plus ifosfamide in first-line treatment of advanced soft tissue sarcomas: a randomized study of the European Organization for Research and Treatment of Cancer, Soft Tissue, and Bone Sarcoma Group. *J Clin Oncol.* 1995;13:1537–1545.

425. Grier HE, et al. Addition of ifosfamide and etoposide to standard chemotherapy for Ewing's sarcoma and primitive neuroectodermal tumor of bone. *N Engl J Med.* 2003;348:694–701.

426. Merimsky O, et al. Gemcitabine in soft tissue or bone sarcoma resistant to standard chemotherapy: a phase II study. *Cancer Chemother Pharmacol.* 2000;45:177–181.

427. Einhorn LH, et al. Evaluation of optimal duration of chemotherapy in favorable-prognosis disseminated germ cell tumors: a Southeastern Cancer Study Group Protocol. *J Clin Oncol.* 1989;7:387–391.

428. Williams SD, et al. Treatment of disseminated germ cell tumors with cisplatin, bleomycin, and either vinblastine or etoposide. *N Engl J Med.* 1987;316:1435–1440.

429. Bosl G, et al. A randomized trial of etoposide + cisplatin versus vinblastine + bleomycin + cisplatin + cyclophosphamide + dactinomycin in patients with good-prognosis germ cell tumors. *J Clin Oncol.* 1988;6:1231–1238.

430. Einhorn LH, et al. Cis-diamminedichloroplatinum, vinblastine, and bleomycin combination chemotherapy in disseminated testicular cancer. *Ann Intern Med.* 1977;87:293–298.

431. Vugrin D, et al. VAB-6 combination chemotherapy in disseminated cancer of the testis. *Ann Intern Med.* 1981;95:59–61.

432. Motzer RJ, et al. Salvage chemotherapy for patients with germ cell tumors: the Memorial Sloan-Kettering Cancer Center experience. *Cancer.* 1991;67:1305–1310.

433. Loehrer PJ, et al. Salvage therapy in recurrent germ cell cancer: ifosfamide and cisplatin plus either vinblastine or etoposide. *Ann Intern Med.* 1988;109:540–546.

434. deWit R, Fizazi K. Controversies in the management of clinical stage I testis cancer. *J Clin Oncol.* 2006; 24:5482–5492.

435. Loehrer PJ, et al. Cisplatin plus doxorubicin plus cyclophosphamide in metastatic or recurrent thymoma: final results of an Intergroup trial. *J Clin Oncol.* 1994;12:1164–1168.

436. Giaccone G, et al. Cisplatin and etoposide combination chemotherapy for locally advanced or metastatic thymoma: a phase II study of the European Organization for Research and Treatment of Lung Cancer Cooperative Group. *J Clin Oncol.* 1996;14:814–820.

437. Fornasiero A, et al. Chemotherapy for invasive thymoma. *Cancer.* 1991;68:30–33.

438. Shimaoka K, et al. A randomized trial of doxorubicin versus doxorubicin plus cisplatin in patients with advanced thyroid carcinoma. *Cancer.* 1985;56:2155–2160.